Seeing and Visualizing

Life and Mind: Philosophical Issues in Biology and Psychology
Kim Sterelny and Rob Wilson, editors

Cycles of Contingency: Developmental Systems and Evolution,
Susan Oyama, Paul E. Griffiths, and Russell D. Gray, editors, 2000

Coherence in Thought and Action, Paul Thagard, 2000

The New Phrenology: The Limits of Localizing Cognitive Processes in the Brain, William R. Uttal, 2001

Evolution and Learning: The Baldwin Effect Reconsidered,
Bruce H. Weber and David J. Depew, editors, 2003

Seeing and Visualizing: It's Not What You Think, Zenon Pylyshyn, 2003

Seeing and Visualizing
It's Not What You Think

Zenon Pylyshyn

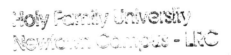
A Bradford Book
The MIT Press
Cambridge, Massachusetts
London, England

This book was set in Sabon by SNP Best-set Typesetter Ltd., Hong Kong, and was printed and bound in the United States of America.

Library of Congress Cataloging-in-Publication Data

Pylyshyn, Zenon W., 1937– .
  Seeing and visualizing : it's not what you think / Zenon Pylyshyn.
    p. cm.—(Life and mind)
  "A Bradford book."
  Includes bibliographical references and index.
  ISBN 0-262-16217-2 (hc. : alk. paper)
  1. Visual perception. 2. Visualization. 3. Mental representation.
  4. Recognition (Psychology). 5. Categorization (Psychology). 6. Cognitive
  science. I. Title. II. Series.

BF241.P95   2003
152.4—dc21   2003046415

10 9 8 7 6 5 4 3 2 1

To my mother
and to the memory of my father

Contents

Preface

This book is about how we see and how we visualize. But it is equally about how we are easily misled by our everyday experience of these faculties. Galileo is said to have proclaimed (Galilei, 1610/1983; quoted in Slezak, 2002), "...if men had been born blind, philosophy would be more perfect, because it would lack many false assumptions that have been taken from the sense of sight." Many deep puzzles arise when we try to understand the nature of visual perception, visual imagery, or visual thinking. As we try to formulate scientific questions about these human capacities we immediately find ourselves being entranced by the *view from within*. This view, which the linguist Kenneth Pike (Pike, 1967) has referred to as the *emic* perspective (as opposed to the external or *etic* perspective), is both essential and perilous. As scientists we cannot ignore the contents of our conscious experience, because this is one of the principal ways of knowing what we see and what our thoughts are about. On the other hand, the contents of our conscious experience are also insidious, because they lead us to believe that we can see directly into our own minds and observe the causes of our cognitive processes.

Such traps are nothing new; psychology is used to being torn by the duality of mental life—its subjective and its objective (causal) side. Since people first began to think about the nature of mental processes, such as seeing, imagining, and reasoning, they have had to contend with the fact that knowing how these achievements appear to us on the inside often does us little good, and indeed often leads us in entirely the wrong direction, when we seek a scientific explanation. Of course we have the option of putting aside the quest for a scientific explanation and setting our goal toward finding a satisfying description in terms that are consonant with how seeing and imagining appear to us. This might be called a phenomenological approach to understanding the workings of the mind, or the everyday folk understanding of vision.

There is nothing wrong with such a pursuit. Much popular psychology revels in it, as do a number of schools of philosophical inquiry (e.g., ordinary language philosophy, phenomenological philosophy). Yet in the long term, few of us would be satisfied with an analysis or a natural history of phenomenological regularities. One reason is that characterizing the systematic properties of how things seem to us does not allow us to connect with the natural sciences, to approach the goal of unifying psychology with biology, chemistry, and physics. It does not help us to answer the *how* and *why* questions: How does vision work? Why do things look the way they do? What happens when we think visually?

The problem with trying to understand vision and visual imagery is that on the one hand these phenomena are intimately familiar to us from the inside so it is difficult to objectify them, even though the processes involved are also too fast and too ephemeral to be observed introspectively. On the other hand, what we do observe is misleading because it is always the *world* as it appears to us that we see, not the real work that is being done by the mind in going from the proximal stimuli, generally optical patterns on the retina, to the familiar experience of seeing (or imagining) the world. The question: How do we see? appears very nearly nonsensical. Why, we see by just looking, and the reason that things look as they do to us is that this is the way that they actually are. It is only by objectifying the phenomena, by "making them strange" that we can turn the question into a puzzle that can be studied scientifically. One good way to turn the mysteries of vision and imagery into a puzzle is to ask what it would take for a computer to see or imagine. But this is not the only way, and indeed this way is often itself laden with preconceptions, as I will try to show throughout this book.

The title of this book is meant to be ambiguous. It means both that seeing and visualizing are different from thinking (and from each other), and that our intuitive views about seeing and visualizing rest largely on a grand illusion. The message of this book is that seeing is different from thinking and that to see is not, as it often seems to us, to create an inner replica of the world we are observing or thinking about or visualizing. But this is a long and not always intuitively compelling story. In fact, its counterintuitive nature is one reason it may be worth telling. When things seem clearly a certain way it is often because we are subject to a general shared illusion. To stand outside this illusion requires a certain act of will and an open-minded and determined look at the evidence. But some things about vision and mental imagery are clear enough now that only deeply ingrained prejudices keep them from being the received view. These facts, which seem to me (if not to others) to be totally persuasive, are the topic of this book. If any of the claims appear radical it is not because they represent a leap into the dark caverns of speculation, but only that some ways of looking at the world are just too comfortable and too hard to dismiss. Consequently, what might be a straightforward story about how we see becomes a long journey into the data and theory, developed mostly over the past thirty years, as well into the conceptual issues that surround them.

The journey begins with the question of why things we see appear to us as they do—a question that has been asked countless times in each generation. In chapter 1, I describe experiments and demonstrations, as well as provide general arguments, to try to persuade you that when you look around, the impression you have that you are creating a large panoramic picture in your head is a total illusion. When you *see*, there is no intermediate *picture* of the world anywhere, your subjective impression notwithstanding; there is just the world and your interpretation of the incoming information (and there are also mechanisms for keeping the two in correspondence, which is the topic of chapters 4 and 5). There is, however, a representation of the visual world; and here the great J. J. Gibson was wrong in trying to develop a theory of direct perception, in which seeing is unmediated by representations and reasoning. But he was right that there is no pictorial object, no stable, spatially distributed, topographically organized representation that we would call a picture, at least not by the time the visual information becomes available to our cognitive mind.

Chapter 2 goes on to make the argument that although the visual system is "smart"—honed by many millennia of evolutionary shaping—it is nonetheless essentially ignorant. The visual system (or at least the part of it I will focus on, the so-called *early-vision* system) does what it was designed to do with neither help nor hindrance from the cognizing mind. How it can do as well as it does in the face of the inherent uncertainty of the incoming visual data is one of the questions that has been explored most successfully in recent decades; it is one of the outstanding achievements of contemporary cognitive science. According to the thesis developed in chapters 2 and 3, there are two primary ways in which the mind (or, as I will say, the cognitive system) affects visual processing. One is that it is able to control where it concentrates its efforts or its limited resources. It does this by determining where to look as well as where to focus attention. The second way is by considering the product of visual processing, together with everything else the whole organism knows and believes, to figure out what is actually in the visual scene. Chapter 3 continues this discussion and goes on to describe some of the recent findings from neuroscience and psychophysics concerning the nature of this largely automatic early vision system.

Chapters 4 and 5 take a second look at the idea introduced in these last two chapters—that focal attention plays an important role in connecting vision and cognition—and suggests that there must be a mechanism, closely related to attention, that also plays a crucial role in connecting visual representations with things in the world. This special connection, which I refer to as visual indexing, allows parts of visual representations to be bound to parts of the visual world so that they can refer to these parts directly, rather than in a way that is mediated by an encoding of the properties that these things have. Visual indexes serve much like what is called demonstrative reference, the sort of reference that we might make in language when we refer to *this* or to *that* without regard to what the *this* and *that* are or what properties they may have. We *pick out* and individuate primitive visual objects as a precursor to focusing attention on them and encoding their properties. Such visual indexes play an important role in attaching mental particulars to things, and they also play a role in allowing mental images to inherit some spatial properties from perceived space. The ideas introduced in chapter 5 fill in some of the missing aspects of the sort of symbolic representations of percepts introduced in chapter 1 and also explain some of the alleged spatial properties of mental images discussed in subsequent chapters.

Finally, the last three chapters build on the ideas introduced in chapters 1 through 5 to make sense of some of the puzzling aspects of mental imagery. The message of these last chapters is that, notwithstanding what it feels like to visualize or to examine a mental image in one's mind's eye, imagining and visualizing are a form of reasoning. And, as with all forms of reasoning, we have little conscious access to the real machinery of the mind, the machinery that encodes our thoughts and that transforms them as we reason, as we draw inferences, as we search our memory, and as we understand the evidence of our senses—including that which arrives in the form of language. Because our intuitions and our introspections are either silent or seriously misleading concerning what our thoughts are like and how they are processed, we need to impose some constraints on our speculations on the subject. In the last three chapters, and especially in chapter 8, I consider these constraints and, drawing on work by Jerry Fodor (1975) as well as our joint work (Fodor and Pylyshyn, 1988), I argue that any form of reasoning, including reasoning by visualizing, must meet the constraints of productivity and systematicity. This leads to the inevitable conclusion that reasoning with mental imagery or reasoning by visualizing or "visual thinking" requires a combinatorial system—a language of thought—that itself is not in any sense "pictorial." Although this conclusion may appear to fly in the face of an enormous amount of evidence collected over the past thirty years showing that thinking using mental images is more like seeing pictures than it is like reasoning with an "inner dialogue," I argue in detail in chapters 6, 7, and 8 that the evidence does not support the assumption that visualizing is special in the way that current theorists have assumed it to be. The data, I will argue, have been widely and seriously misunderstood.

Even if the reader agrees with the general thrust of this discussion, there will no doubt remain many areas of legitimate discomfort. Some of this discomfort concerns the apparent discrepancy between what it feels like to see and to visualize and the nature of vision according to the class of symbolic computational theories that have been developed in cognitive science. This discrepancy is addressed in various places in the book, but in the end it cannot be dismissed, simply because of our deep-seated commitment to what Dan Dennett has called the "Cartesian Theater" view of the mind, a view that is deeply embedded in our psyche. This "explanatory gap" was around long before cognitive science and the computational view of mind (in fact it was the subject of considerable debate between Nicolas Malebranche and Antoine Arnauld in the seventeenth century; see Slezak, 2002). In addition to this deeply held worldview, there are also other aspects of mental imagery where the discomfort owes more to the way we conceive of certain problems than it does to how the contents of our conscious experience strike us. I consider one class of these in chapter 8, where I discuss the close connection that may exist between imagery, imagination, and creativity. I will argue that this connection, although real enough, does not favor one view of the nature of mental imagery over another. It rests, rather, on our ignorance of the nature of creativity and on the puzzle of where new thoughts and ideas come from.

Although the book devotes considerable space to the salubrious task of clarifying many misconceptions that pervade the study of vision and visualization, the principal goal is to provide a new analysis of the nature of visual processing and of mental imagery. The analysis rests on both empirical evidence, some of which comes from the author's laboratory, and on reinterpretations of well-known findings. This book is in many ways a continuation of the investigation of cognition that began with my *Computation and Cognition* (Pylyshyn, 1984a), but it focuses on problems within one of the most highly developed areas in cognitive science, visual perception, and traces the relation between the study of vision, the study of mental imagery, and the study of cognition more generally.

Acknowledgments

Some of the material in chapters 2, 6, and 7 appeared in *Behavioral and Brain Sciences*, 1999, 22 and 2002, 25, where it underwent commentary by other investigators: I am grateful to these writers for their comments, even though there remain many disagreements. I wish to acknowledge the contributions made by my colleagues with whom I discussed many of these ideas, especially Jerry Fodor whose influence should be apparent, Shaun Nichols and Lila Gleitman who made comments on various drafts, and mostly to Peter Slezak, with whom I shared my views about mental imagery and who encouraged me by pointing out that ideas that are so widely believed both in the scientific field and among the public could only be due to shared illusions.

I also wish to acknowledge the influence of students and postdoctoral fellows who contributed in a variety of ways to the ideas that have found their way into this book. I thank my students who worked on the development of the visual index (FINST) theory over the last twenty years: Liam Bannon, Lana Trick, Jacquie Burkell, Chris Sears, Paul McKeever, Roy Eagleson, Brian Acton, Brian Scholl, and Elias Cohen. Ed Stabler, Brian Fisher, Erik Blaser, Christopher Currie, and Vidal Annan were postdoctoral fellows who provided critical input to this work at one time or another. I also acknowledge the participation of members of the Visual Attention Laboratory at the Rutgers Center for Cognitive Science (Diane Kelly, John Dennis, Carly Leonard, Brian Keene, Jonathan Cohen, and research programmers Sharanya Chandrasekar and Amir Amirrezvani) and the undergraduate research interns who worked with me on this research (Ashley Black, Carly Leonard, Emma Gregory, Tatiana Havryliuk, Alex Kushnier, and Parizad Bilimoria). I also thank Carly Leonard for her help with proofreading and indexing. The research was supported over the years by the Natural Science and Engineering Research Council of Canada, the Canadian Institute for Advanced Research (Program in Artificial Intelligence and Robotics), and the National Institutes of Mental Health (Research Grant 1R01 MH60924).

I also acknowledge the permissions I have received from publishers of the various figures I have reproduced in this book (although I have redrawn all the figures except the cartoons and photographs). I thank Judy K. Kliban for permission to reproduce the cartoon from the book *Cat* (figure 1.1), by the late B. Kliban (and also my modification of it in figure 1.20). I thank Sydney Harris for permission to reproduce the cartoon in figure 6.5. All figures taken from published sources are cited in the figure captions. I thank the following publishers for permission to reprint or adapt figures for this book: American Psychological Association for figures 1.13, 3.24, 4.2, 4.3, 4.7, 4.8, 4.9, 4.10, 4.17, 5.10, 5.11, 6.13, 6.14, 7.1; American Association for the Advancement of Science for figures 6.7 and 7.2 from *Science* (and Roger Tootel for supplying the photograph for figure 7.2); Elsevier Publishers for figures 1.10, 1.18, 1.24, 2.5, 3.18, 5.8, 5.13, and 6.6 (from *Vision Research, Acta Psychologica, Cognition,* and *Trends in Cognitive Science*); Pion, London for figure 2.7, parts (c)–(f), and for figures 3.12, 3.13, 3.14, 3.15, 3.23, and 4.16 from the journal *Perception*; Psychology Press for figure 4.12; Lawrence Erlbaum Associates for the center image of figure 6.12 from the *Proceedings of the Cognitive Science Society*; Psychonomics Society for figure 6.8; Thomas Learning, Global Rights Group for figure 2.2; Intellect Books for figures 3.10, 3.20, 3.21, 3.22; Greenwood Publishing Group, Westport, Connecticut for the left image in figure 6.12 from original Ablex publications; McGraw-Hill for figure 3.4; Macmillan Publishers for figures 3.9, 4.14, 4.15, 5.14 reprinted from *Nature*; VSP International Science Publishers for figure 5.6 from *Spatial Vision*; MIT Press for figure 3.11; the American Psychological Society for figure 4.13 from *Psychological Science*; and Columbia University Teachers College for figure 2.7 (a) and (b). I am grateful to Ian Howard for allowing me to adapt figures 1.15 and 1.16 from his unpublished manuscript and to Leo Valdes for permission to reproduce the panels in figure 1.21 from his Web site (http://www.droodles.com) as of October 1997.

Finally I wish to thank my wife, Anne Telford, for her support during the writing of this book.

1

The Puzzle of Seeing

1.1 Why Do Things Look the Way They Do?

Why do things appear to us as they do? We don't even have a clear idea of what kind of story would count as an answer. The whole notion of "appearing" seems problematic. On one hand, it is obvious that things appear to us as they do because, barring illusions, *that's the way they are*! On the other hand, it is also clear that a particular thing's being as it is, is neither necessary nor sufficient for our *seeing* it as we do. We know that things can look quite different to us in different circumstances, and perhaps they do look different to others. So it is not unreasonable for us to ask what is responsible for our seeing things as we do, as opposed to seeing them in some other way.

Despite the dramatic progress that has been made in the study of visual perception in the past half century, the question of why we see things as we do in large measure still eludes us. The question of what and how and why we see are daunting. Surely, the pattern of light arriving at our eyes is responsible for our visual perception. Must this be so—is light both necessary and sufficient for perception? Could we not also "see" if our eye or our brain were electrically stimulated in the right way? And what of the experience of seeing: Is that constitutive of vision; is that what visual perception *is*? Would it make any sense to ask what is the product or even the purpose of visual perception? Could there be full-blooded visual perception in the absence of any awareness of something being seen, without a visual experience? The mystery of the experience of seeing is deep and is at the heart of our understanding (or failure to understand) the nature of consciousness itself. Is it possible to have a scientific understanding of vision without first understanding the mystery of consciousness? The scientific world thinks it is, and it has already made a great deal of progress in acquiring such an understanding. But is this because it has presupposed a view of what it is to see—a set of tacit assumptions about such things as the relation between our experience of seeing and the nature of the information processing performed by the visual system?

I do not intend this book to be about consciousness, or even about our conscious visual experience, because I believe there is little that science can say about this notion at the present time. That's not to say that it is not of the greatest importance and perhaps even central to understanding human nature. It is also not to say that there is nothing worthwhile to be said on the topic of consciousness, since consciousness has become a very active topic of scholarship and a great deal is being said, much of it quite fascinating. Nonetheless, most of what is being said is by way of preliminary scene setting and conceptual clarification. It's about such surprising empirical findings as those showing that certain functions can be carried out without conscious awareness. A lot of the discussion is also about what consciousness is not. It's about such things as why a theory simply misses the point if it says that consciousness *is* such and such a brain property (a certain frequency of brain waves or activity in a certain location in the cortex) or a particular functional property (such as the contents of short-term working memory or the mind's observation of its own functioning). The only part of this discussion that will concern us will be how the content of our experience when we see, visualize, and think misleads us and contaminates many of our scientific theories of vision and of related processes such as visualizing and imagining. For this reason I devote much of the present chapter to a discussion of what vision provides to the mind. The closely related question of how the cognizing mind affects visual perception is raised in chapter 2, and some of that discussion takes us back to the troublesome notion of the nature of visual experience.

1.2   What Is Seeing?

One reason why understanding vision is so difficult is that we who are attempting to understand the process are so deeply embedded in the phenomenology of perception: We know what it *feels* like to see. We look out and see the world, and we cannot escape the impression that what we have in our heads is a detailed, stable, extended, and veridical display that corresponds to the scene before us. Of course, most of us have also seen enough examples of so-called "optical illusions," so we are prepared to admit that what we see is not always what is truly the case. Yet at the same time we have much more difficulty shedding the view that in our heads is a display that our inner first-person self, or our cognitive homunculus, observes. There are other phenomena relating to our experience of seeing a "picture in our head" that are even more problematic. These include the similar experience that we have without any visual input: the experience that accompanies mental imagery or visual thinking. The more we analyze what must be going on and the more we examine the empirical evidence, the more puzzling the process becomes and the less tenable our intuitions. Indeed, we find not only that we must dispense with the "picture in the head," but that we must also revise our ideas concerning the nature of the mechanisms involved in vision and concerning the nature of the internal informational states corresponding to percepts or images. What can never serve as a theory of vision is a theory that says that vision creates a copy of the world inside the head, as the Kliban cartoon in figure 1.1 suggests is the case with a cat. The understanding that this sort of theory will not do is what makes this cartoon funny. Yet it is nontrivial to say what exactly is wrong with a theory that even remotely resembles this sort of story. This I will attempt in the present book, mostly in this chapter and in chapters 6 and 7.

In what follows I will examine some of these counterintuitive aspects of the process of visual perception and mental imagery. For now the following examples will suffice to warn us that our intuitions are a notoriously bad source of ideas as to how the visual system works. The message of these examples is that we should not be surprised to find that our scientific theories will look quite different from how we might imagine them when we try to be faithful to how vision seems to us from the inside—to the phenomenology of visual perception.

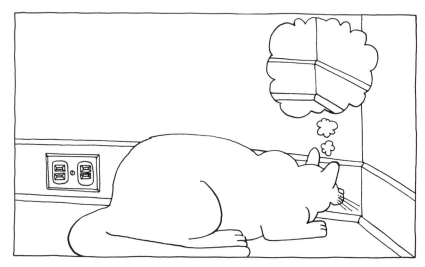

Figure 1.1
A theory of vision such as this is a nonstarter, even for a cat! B. Kliban (American, 1935–1990). From the book *Cat*, by B. Kliban. Used by permission. All rights reserved. Copyright by Judith K. Kliban.

1.3   Does Vision Create a "Picture" in the Head?

1.3.1   The richness of visual appearances and the poverty of visual information

Let's call our conscious experience of how things seem to us when we look at them, the "phenomenal" content of our perception. As we look around, the phenomenal content of our perception is that of a detailed and relatively stable panorama of objects and shapes laid out in three dimensions. Even without turning around, we experience a broad expanse (about 180 degrees of panorama), full of details of the scene: its colors and textures, its shapes and boundaries, and the meaningful things that populate our visual scene—the familiar objects and people that we instantly recognize. Even if there were little or nothing in the scene that we recognized as familiar, say if we had just landed on the surface of Mars, we would still have no trouble seeing shapes and surfaces. We would see a variety of individual objects, set against some background that remained perceptually secondary (i.e., we would experience what Gestalt psychologists call a "figure-ground" separation). We would see each of these objects as having a certain shape and consisting of parts arranged in some spatial relation to one another. We would see some of the objects as further away and some as closer, with the closer objects partially occluding our view of the further objects. We would see that the partly occluded objects continued behind the closer ones; we would *not* see the occluded objects as partial objects or as having the shape of the visible fragment, though it is physically possible that this could in fact be their shape. The phenomenal content of our perception would continue to be that of a world of three-dimensional objects, even though most of every object would be hidden from our view, either by other objects or by the front of the object itself. If we could turn freely to inspect the scene around us, there would be no sharp discontinuity between the part of the scene currently on our retina and the entire 360 degrees of the layout (e.g., we could accurately point to objects behind us, as Attneave and Farrar, 1977, showed).

This phenomenal experience is, as far as we know, universal to our species and probably innate. We don't give it a second thought, because it seems to us that we are seeing what there is to see. But even a cursory examination makes it abundantly clear that much more is going on than we might assume (I am tempted to say that there is more to vision than meets the eye). Consider what the brain has to work with in achieving this familiar experience. The light-sensitive surfaces of the eye (the retinas) are two-dimensional, so the sense of depth must come from other sources of information. We know that at least part of the information comes from the difference between the patterns that the two eyes receive, but why (and how) does this produce the experience of seeing a three-dimensional world? No matter how well we understand the mechanism of stereo perception (and it is one of the most studied problems in visual science), we are very far from breaking through the mystery of this question. The story gets even murkier as we further examine the information that the brain receives from the eyes. The retinas themselves are not uniform. Only a small central region (the fovea), about the size of the area covered by your thumb held at arm's length, has sufficient acuity to recognize printed characters at the normal reading distance. Outside of that region our visual acuity drops off rapidly, and by the time we get to where the edge of a movie screen would normally fall in our field of vision, acuity is so poor that if we thus saw the world generally, we would be considered legally blind. As we move off from the central fovea, the eye also becomes color blind, so almost all color information comes from the tiny area of the fovea (and what color reception there is varies in its degree of responsiveness to the yellow-green dimension depending on how far out from the fovea it is). Moreover, our eye's focal length differs considerably for red and blue colors, so one end of the spectrum is invariably out of focus by about the degree of magnification of off-the-shelf reading glasses. There is also a region of the retina, considerably larger than the fovea and lying about 10 to 13 degrees away, where the retinal nerve fibers come together to form a cable to the brain. This region has no receptors: it is our blind spot. It is easy to show that no information is registered at the location of the blind spot (look at figures 1.2 and 1.3), yet we are unaware of the blind spot: it does not interfere with our

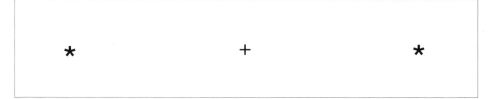

Figure 1.2
If you close your right eye and look at the plus sign with your left eye at a distance of about 10 to 12 inches from the paper (varying the distance as you experiment) you will find that the asterisk on the left disappears from view at some appropriate distance. If you repeat this with your right eye the asterisk on the right will disappear. This is because they fall on the blind spot of each eye. Now repeat the experiment on figure 1.3.

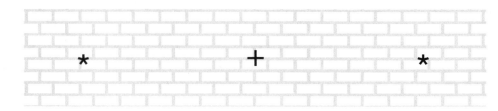

Figure 1.3
If you repeat the experiment from figure 1.2 on this figure, held at the same distance where the asterisk disappeared on the previous figure, you may find that the bricklike pattern, though somewhat indistinct, remains visible without a *gap while the asterisk disappears.* This is a case of what has been called "filling in." But is there some place in your mind/brain where there is an inner display that has filled in the missing pattern?

phenomenal experience of a uniform perceptual world. Even when the spot is located over an elaborate pattern, we do not see a hole in the pattern. In fact, we even see objects move through the blind spot without discontinuity, and we can locate the moving object precisely as being inside the blind spot at the appropriate time (Cai and Cavanagh, 2002). This phenomenon, which many people refer to as "filling in," provides some important clues as to how vision works and how vision, *as an information-processing system*, relates to our phenomenal experience of seeing. We will return to this most perplexing question later.

The properties of the retina (including its blind spot and other distortions of incoming information because it is not flat and the distribution of rods and cones is not uniform) already provide some reason to be concerned about how the brain gets to have such a large expanse of visual experience.[1] But it gets much worse. The eyes are in constant motion, jumping around in rapid saccades several times in each second and generally spending only a fraction of a second gazing in any one direction. The retina, our primary contact with the visual world, is continually being smeared with moving information (moving so rapidly that the nervous system cannot assimilate any detailed information during the rapid saccade, which can take as little as 3 hundredths of a second to sweep its path). And yet the world does not appear to move or flicker, and indeed, we are typically unaware of the saccades. How do we see a rich and stable visual panorama in the face of such dynamic and impoverished information?

The intuitive answer that almost universally leaps to mind is that although the *retina* may get a degraded, nonuniform, rapidly changing,

---

1. In 1604 when Johannes Kepler first described how an image is formed on the retina (Lindberg, 1976) people began to worry about how we manage to see the world right-side-up when the image on the retina is upside-down. These days this no longer bothers most people because they implicitly understand that what counts as *up* for us is determined by how the brain *interprets* the retinal image and how it coordinates properties of the image with our actions on the world. This downplaying of physical image-properties in relation to both our phenomenal experience and our motor behavior toward the perceived world marks the beginning of an appreciation that information processing and phenomenal experience are a long way from the retina and that much goes on in the interval. Yet, as we will see presently, the temptation to mistake the retinal image for the percept continues even today.

peephole view of the world, you, the one who does the seeing, do not receive such impoverished information. What you see is a uniformly detailed, gapless, panoramic, stable view of the world—rather like a three-dimensional picture—built up from the sketchy unstable inputs from the two eyes. This is the first-person view, the world that your "self" (the subject in your claim "I see") gets to examine and enjoy. It is impossible for us to view what happens in our own perception in any other way. I think, my *eyes* may be moving, and they may have poor resolution with a blind spot and all that, but *I, the person observing these events, do not have any of these problems.* What I see is a 3D layout of surfaces and objects that have colors and shapes, and the entire scene stands still and covers a wide panorama (180 or more degrees). Consequently, so the argument goes, there must be something that has these properties of breadth, depth, and stability, and where else could it be but in the head? Enter what Dan Dennett picturesquely calls the "Cartesian Theater," after René Descartes, who, by implication (though not explicitly), proposed such an inner image or screen onto which the eye projects its moving peephole view and paints the larger picture.

But, tempting as it is, the Cartesian Theater creates far more problems than it solves. Dennett (1991) discusses a number of difficulties raised by this "inner eye" idea and shows that it leads to one conceptual impasse after another. The whole idea of an inner screen rests on a well-known fallacy, called the "intentional fallacy" in philosophy and sometimes the "stimulus error" in the structuralist psychology of Wundt and Titchener (in the case of Wundt and Titchener, "stimulus error" meant attributing to one's introspective experience the properties one knows the objective stimulus to possess). The temptation to make the mistake of attributing to a mental representation the properties of what it represents is difficult to avoid. This issue arises in an extreme form in discussions of mental imagery where the temptation appears to be very nearly inescapable (I will return to it in chapters 6 to 8; for an extensive discussion of this point, see Pylyshyn, 2002). What I propose to do in the rest of this chapter is to show that even if it does not create conceptual-philosophical problems, the inner-screen notion is at odds with some well-established facts about human vision. In the course of this discussion I will present a number of experimental results that will serve us later when I will return to the Cartesian Theater in connection with the idea of a mental image, an idea, as it is understood by many contemporary thinkers, that relies heavily on the assumption that there is a Cartesian Theater with a screen and a projector and a homunculus or "mind's eye" sitting in the audience.

While a misinterpretation of our phenomenal experience may be what drives us to the assumption of an inner display in the first place, it is not the only consideration that keeps many psychologists committed to it. In a great many cases the content of phenomenal experience also has observable consequences in objective measures of visual processing. In fact, phenomenal experience plays a central role in the methodology of visual science insofar as theories of vision are typically concerned with explaining the nature of our phenomenal experience. This in itself raises problems that will occupy some of our attention later. For now let us stay with the question of why many scholars of visual perception tacitly assume an inner display in attempting to understand how vision works.

1.3.2   Some reasons for thinking there may be an inner display

The overriding reason for believing in an inner display or image or Cartesian Theater is that the information on the retinas is so totally discrepant from the phenomenal experience of perception. We have already alluded to the peephole scope of retinal information, its rapidly changing contents, and its unnoticed blind spot that gets filled in for phenomenal experience. Then there are frequently noted completion phenomena, where familiar forms appear to get filled in when parts of them are occluded (as in figure 1.4), or where even unfamiliar forms appear to be filled in with illusory contours (illustrated in figure 1.5), or where there is so-called amodal completion (figure 2.5), which will be discussed later. This filling in is a subjective impression in the case of the blind spot, since there is no functional information available for the particular part of the scene corresponding to the scotoma. But in other cases it's not so obvious that *no* information is involved, even though there may be no local information at a particular site. For example, in the case of partially occluded figures, such as in figure 1.5, it is possible that the mind provides the missing information and actually restores the image, if not on the retina, then at some subsequent locus in the brain. In figure 1.4 the missing parts of the words don't just seem to be there, they are functionally present insofar as we are actually able to recognize and read the words.

So-called illusory or virtual contours (such as those seen in the figure on the right of figure 1.5) not only have a phenomenal existence; they

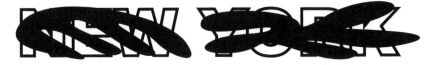

Figure 1.4
Despite the large amount of missing information, the familiar words are easily discerned. Are they "restored" by the visual system on some inner display?

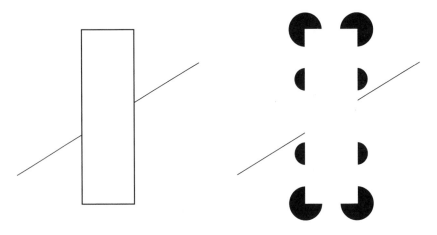

Figure 1.5
The Pogendorff illusion works as well with virtual (illusory) lines as with real ones. The oblique lines in both figures do not looked aligned, even though they are.

act in many ways as though they were actually present in the figures. Take, for example, the Pogendorff illusion, in which an oblique line that crosses a column appears to be broken and not aligned with its geometrical continuation (figure 1.5). When subjects are asked to adjust one part of the diagonal line so it appears to be continuous with the other part, they tend to set the lower line systematically higher than it should be for geometrically correct continuation. This phenomenon happens equally when the column is made up of virtual or illusory lines, as in figure 1.5.

Similarly, one can see that the "completed" figure is the one that is visually prominent by considering the problem of finding a given figure in a jumble (a kind of Where's Waldo game). Consider the simple figure shown here:

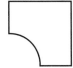

Can you find that target in the jumble in figure 1.6? You may find it easy to identify one such instance, despite the fact that part of it is actually cut off by a circle. But there is another one that is harder to find because the visual system has "completed" it as a square, by adding the part that is hidden by the circular disk.

There are also many examples where visual properties are interrelated or *coupled* (to use Irvin Rock's term). Such visual "couplings" may depend on aspects of the perception that do not exist objectively on the retina. For example, the virtual rectangle created by the array of

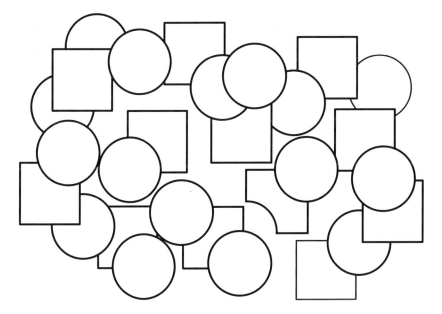

Figure 1.6
The "search set." Find two copies of the target in this set. Have the figures been "completed" in some inner display, making the target that appears to be partly occluded harder to find?

pie-shaped figures in figure 1.5 not only has the phenomenal content of being an opaque surface in front of some disks; it also appears to be brighter than the background by objective psychophysical measures and leads to the Pogendorff illusion shown in the figure. Why would these particular properties (and a large number of other such objective properties) occur *at particular locations* in the display if not because the illusory lines and the surface they define are *actually* present somewhere in the brain and provide the locations where the effect is localized? The "somewhere" in all these examples ends up being the "mental image" or Cartesian display.

The idea that the mind gets to look at a display that has been filled in and built up from separate segments is widespread. Not only is such a display thought to cover a larger spatial extent than the fovea, but it also appears to involve visual information that is no longer present on the retina, though it may have been present in the recent past. In an interesting and thoughtful essay, Julian Hochberg (1968) makes a case that many principles of visual organization seem to hold over arrays larger than those on the retina. He speaks rather cautiously and hesitantly of a visual "immediate memory," though making it clear that such a storage does not retain information in a strictly *visual* or *image* format. One reason why Hochberg speaks of a visual memory at all is that visual forms can be discerned when there are no literal forms on the retina— at least not in the sense of contours defined by luminance gradients— and so it is natural to assume that they must be in some postretinal storage. Here are some examples. In the following, I use the neutral term "discern" instead of "perceive," since I don't want to prejudge whether these count as bona fide cases of visual perception.

Forms can be displayed as contours, dotted lines, or in some cases just the high-information regions, such as vertices alone (figure 1.7).

Forms can be discerned in a field of elements if the subset of elements that lie on a particular (virtual) contour are readily distinguishable—say if they are a different shape or brightness or color from the other elements, or if they are briefly displaced (or wiggled) back and forth. Once again, in this case the form is perceived providing only that the differences are sufficient to constitute what are called "popout" or automatically registered differences (more on this in chapter 5). Figure 1.8 is an example.

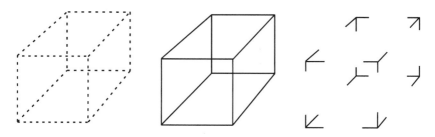

Figure 1.7
Different ways to show a Necker Cube, all of which exhibit equivalent information and lead to similar visual effects.

Forms can also be discerned in random-dot stereograms—an interesting form of visual display invented by Bela Julesz (1971). In these binocularly viewed displays, the perception of a form derives from the retinal disparity of certain regions of the display. Neither eye receives form information, but the distribution of random dots on the two eyes is such that when most of the points on the two retinas are matched, the location of the remaining points in a certain region are discrepant by some retinal distance. This discrepancy (known as "retinal disparity") is what produces the effect of stereo depth in normal binocular vision. When the region of discrepancy is chosen to correspond to a contour region, such as one that defines the line drawing of a Necker cube, a cube is perceived.

Forms can even be discerned if an opaque screen with a narrow slit in it is moved back and forth over a stimulus in a device known as an "anorthoscope." If the motion is fast enough, it appears to "paint" an image that can be discerned, though whether it is actually "perceived" remains an open question. It is reportedly even possible to recognize a form if the stimulus is moved back and forth behind a screen, so that the form is viewed as a stream of views all occurring at a single vertical line on the retina (although the phenomenal impression is not nearly as clear). Perception with these sorts of presentations has been referred to as the "eye-of-the-needle" or the "Zollner-Parks" phenomenon (see figures 1.15 and 1.16 for illustrations of forms presented through an anorthoscope).

The same form can be discerned, more or less clearly and vividly, in all these cases despite the enormous differences in the physical stimuli

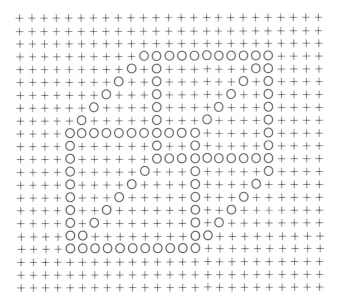

Figure 1.8
The same shape as shown in figure 1.7, but created by local feature differences. Can you *see* the form? Does it look three-dimensional, and does it reverse as you watch it?

and despite the fact that in some of the presentations, such as the random-dot stereograms and the anorthoscopic presentation, *no form at all is present on the retina.* What is important, however, is not just whether the form is recognized, but whether it exhibits the properties associated with what we call early (automatic) vision. As we will see, some of these modes of presentation do, whereas others do not, depending on how quickly they are presented and whether they are distributed over a fixed space. These signature properties of vision include the familiar 2D Gestalt grouping principles (such as grouping by proximity, similarity, common fate, and so on), as well as such 3D principles as apparent motion in 3D and the automatic interpretation of certain contours, shading, and motion cues as depicting a 3D form. The signature properties also include "perceptual coupling" between how parts are interpreted or labeled (see the discussion of labeling constraints in chapter 3). Because of this coupling of interpretations, when the interpretation of one part of a form changes, one can get a spontaneous global change or reversal of a percept, as in the Necker cube (this reversal is

experienced in both figure 1.7 and figure 1.8). When the figure sponta-
neously reverses, the interpretation of individual edges changes, as well
as the relative size of the faces, which depends on which face is perceived
as the front face and which as the rear face. Other properties of early
vision are discussed in chapter 2 (especially pp. 66–68).

Although, as we will see in the next chapter, many of the details of
these claims are problematic in important ways, the basic idea appears
sound enough: various principles of form perception and of visual
organization seem to apply to a unit of display that goes beyond the
current instantaneous content of the retina, and so must necessarily
include visual memory. This provides some reason to think that visual
processes apply to the contents of something like a "visual store," which
is precisely the inner display I have been arguing against. What these
examples do not demonstrate, however, and what I shall argue is not
true, is that the information in the visual store is pictorial in any sense;
i.e., the stored information does not act as though it is a stable and reconstructed extension of the retina.

Other reasons for postulating an inner display are sometimes given as
well. For example, Kosslyn (1994) justifies his postulation of an inner
screen (which he later uses to develop a theory of mental imagery in
which images are projected onto this screen) by arguing that such a
display is independently needed to account for visual stability and for
the ability to recognize objects regardless of their location on the retina
or their retinal size.[2] According to this argument, if you have a central
display, you can expand or contract patterns or move them around (or,
equivalently, move an "attentional window" around) so that they can be
brought into correspondence with a template in a standard location on
the inner screen, even if you can't do so on the retina.

2. In fact, there is evidence that even this apparently bland assumption—that we
can recognize patterns irrespective of their retinal locations—may be false in
some circumstances. Nazir and O'Regan (1990) showed that if the learned
pattern was of a particular size and retinal location it generalized very poorly to
patterns of different sizes and retinal locations. Also Schlingensiepen, et al.
(1986) showed that even simple patterns could not be distinguished without eye
movements so that a static retinal location is a hindrance to pattern perception.
Learning of other perceptual phenomena, such as stereopsis, generalizes very
poorly to new retinal locations (Ramachandran, 1976) and retinal orientation
(Ramachandran and Braddick, 1973).

But as we have seen, there are plenty of reasons to reject the idea of a central display as a way of fusing partial and fleeting images into a coherent large-compass percept. Most vision scientists do not talk about an inner display, and may even be embarrassed when confronted with the fact that their way of talking about certain phenomena appears to tacitly assume such a display. A few, like Kosslyn, actually do explicitly endorse an "inner picture" assumption. Kosslyn (1994) provides a clear case of someone who has built an elaborate theory around the assumption of an inner screen. As he puts it, "If certain properties of the world are internalized, are embodied by properties of our brains, many problems may be solved relatively easily" (1994, p. 85). This assumption will be brought under scrutiny in various places in this book. Later in chapters 6 and 7, I will examine the plausibility of a theory of mental imagery that posits the projection of images onto an inner screen. For the time being, I wish simply to look at the reasons why vision itself does not require such a postulate, and indeed why the theory ought to shun it despite its intuitive plausibility.

1.4   Problems with the Inner-Display Assumption: Part 1, What's in the Display?

1.4.1   How is the master image built up from glances?

We have seen that a form is perceived even when the retinal image is highly impoverished (and perhaps even nonexistent) and even when it is known that the retinal information is not being communicated to the brain (as in the case of the blind-spot or off-foveal parts of the display). We have also seen that off-retinal information combines in some ways with the retinally present information to produce a characteristic percept. All this suggests that information processed by the visual system comes not only from the retina (or the fovea) but also from some form of visual storage. But how does the information get into the storage? For years the common view has been that a large-scope inner image is built up by superimposing information from individual glances at the appropriate coordinates of the master image: as the eye moves over a scene, the information on the retina is transmitted to the perceptual system, which then projects it onto an inner screen in the appropriate location, thus painting the larger scene for the

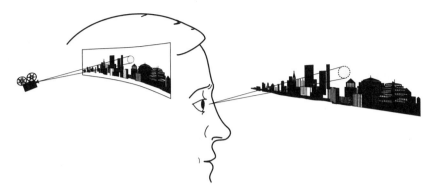

Figure 1.9
The "inner display" explanation of why we appear to see a large panorama, despite the fact that the information the brain receives is limited to a small region at the center of the field of view that is constantly moving across the scene. The idea is that an inner projector moves in registration with the motion of the eye and creates a large and detailed inner image of the scene. This intuitively appealing idea has now been discredited.

"mind's eye" to observe. The general idea behind this view is illustrated in figure 1.9.

This sort of mechanism would clearly explain both the apparent completeness and stability of the percept. This view even had some support from neurophysiological evidence showing that the locus of various visual responses in the brain (the receptive field of visual neurons) shifts when the eye is moved. This theory also received support from the widely accepted "corollary discharge" theory, which claims that when the eye is commanded to move, a copy of the eye-movement command (called the "efference copy") is sent to the "inner projector" and determines where the new information is to be overlaid (an idea that goes back to von Holst and Mittelstaedt, 1971/1950). It has been claimed, for example, that when one tries unsuccessfully to move one's eyes (when, for example, the eye muscles are injured and unable to carry out the command to move), the world appears to move in the opposite direction, since the efference copy of the command tells the projector to place the perceptual signal from the eye where the eye would have been looking had it worked properly. It should be noted here that there is much wrong with this story, not the least of which is that there is serious doubt that the position of an object appears to move to the left when the eye is commanded to move to the right but is unable to. It appears that this widely cited phenomenon may be false—as the amazing experiment by John Stevens and his colleagues (1976) seems to show. Stevens had himself totally paralyzed with curare (except for part of his arm, through which he was able to signal his replies—or call for help!) and performed the experiment in an iron lung. He reported no reverse motion of his percept when he attempted to move his eyes.

More recently, all aspects of this inner-display view have run into serious difficulties, and now the notion of superposition appears to be totally untenable. There are a number of reasons for the demise of this view of how the stable master image is built up.

Recent studies using eye-tracking equipment have provided some rather surprising findings regarding the amount of information taken in at each glance. Carlson-Radvansky (1999), Grimes (1996), Irwin (1991, 1993, 1996), and McConkie and Currie (1996) have shown that very little information is retained from one glance to another when the eyes move, or even when the eyes do not move but the display disappears briefly (Rensink, 2000; Simons and Levin, 1997). If the scene being viewed is changed in even major ways during a saccade, the change goes unnoticed. Observers do not notice changes in the color or location of major parts of a scene (unless they were explicitly attempting to examine those parts), nor do such changes have any consequence on what is perceived. Irwin (1996) showed that very little qualitative information is retained about a simple pattern of dots from one glance to another, and the location of only about 4 or 5 salient points is retained.[3]

A sequence of retinal images does not appear to be superimposed. Experiments have been carried out (O'Regan and Lévy-Schoen, 1983) in which different patterns were presented at known retinal locations before and after a saccade. What observers saw in these cases was not the superposition of the two patterns, as would be expected from, say, the presentation of the figures shown in figure 1.10 when there is a saccade between the two parts of the displays.

3. Recent evidence suggests that accurate information tends to be available from places close to where the eye fell during recent fixations while scanning (Henderson and Hollingworth, 1999). Nonetheless the fact remains that what is retained in immediate memory is generally far from being the sort of detailed pictorial information required by the picture-painting or superposition view.

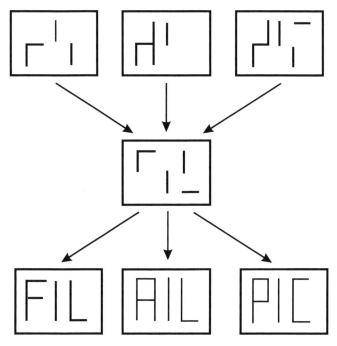

Figure 1.10
In this study described in O'Regan and Lévy-Schoen (1983), an eye movement occurs between presentation of the top figure and presentation of the middle figure. If the two were superimposed, one of the three bottom ones would be seen. There was no evidence of such superposition. (Adapted from O'Regan and Lévy-Schoen, 1983.)

1.4.2   What is the form of nonretinal information?

Despite Hochberg's observation that off-retinal (stored) visual information shows some of the principles of perceptual organization, many important visual properties are not observed when the critical interacting parts are not simultaneously in view, and even those that are observed do not have the phenomenal clarity that they have when they are actually viewed retinally, raising the question of whether they are seen or inferred (see the next section). For example, many of the signature properties of visual perception—such as the spontaneous interpretation of certain line drawings as depicting 3D objects, spontaneous reversals, recognition of the oddity of "impossible objects" such as those in Escher drawings or the so-called Devil's Pitchfork (figure 1.11) do not occur if

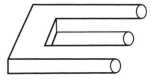

Figure 1.11
In the figure above, it takes just a brief inspection to see that something is amiss—this "devil's pitchfork" cannot be given a consistent 3D interpretation because local information leads to several of the edges having a different interpretation at each end—in other words, the edges receive incompatible labels from local interpretations.

the drawings are made large enough so that the ends are not simultaneously present on the retina. Thus, for example, such well-known figures as the Necker Cube do not appear as reversing 3D shapes and the Devil's Pitchfork does not seem so odd when it is drawn elongated and viewed in such a way that the ends are not simultaneously in the fovea (figure 1.12). Since the phenomenal percept in these cases, as in all perceptual experience involving eye movements, arguably does cover the entire object,[4] the entire object is presumably displayed on the inner screen or the master image.

Other evidence for the claim that off-retinal information (or perhaps I should say "off-foveal information") does not function in the same way as foveal information was obtained by Peterson and Gibson (1991) and Peterson and Hochberg (1983). Using figures such as those in figure 1.13,

4. The question of what is contained in the "phenomenal image" is problematic, to say the least. I am using the term the way many theorists do, although some careful observers, like Hochberg, make a point of emphasizing that the phenomenal experience of what is sensed is quite different from information in memory. Thus, in describing what he saw through the anorthoscope aperture view (such as shown in figure 1.15), Hochberg says:

Let me describe what our . . . aperture view looks like to me: In the aperture itself [is] a clearly *sensory* vertical ribbon of dots . . . ; the ribbon of dots—still quite clear—is part of an entire (largely *unseen*) surface of dots that is moving back and forth *behind* the aperture. . . . There is no real sensory quality to either the shape or its background, where these are occluded by the mask. I'm completely certain that I only *see* those portions of the shape that are behind the aperture at any moment, but I'm equally certain of the extension of the shape behind the mask. Is this "perception," "apprehension," "imagination"? Perhaps we're not dealing with perception at all, in these situations. Maybe merely *knowing* what the pattern is, is sufficient to elicit the different tridimensional ratings, regardless of how this knowledge is gained. (1968, pp. 315–316)

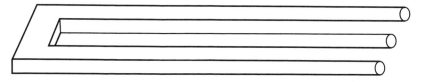

Figure 1.12
In this version, if the picture is held close up so the two ends are not simultaneously on the fovea, it is not nearly so obvious that something is wrong. Integrating the information from the two ends requires an appeal to memory; it is not just a matter of "painting" the larger picture onto the master image.

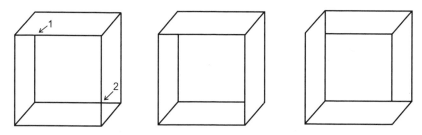

Figure 1.13
The figure on the left is globally unambiguous, yet when attending to the point marked "2" it remains ambiguous between the two orientations shown in the middle and right figures. (Adapted from Peterson and Hochberg, 1993.)

these investigators showed that the figure maintains its ambiguous status and exhibits reversals even though a part of the figure is unambiguous and therefore the entire figure would be unambiguous if the relevant cue that disambiguates the figure were taken into account. In the figure on the left, point 1 disambiguates the figure so that its shape must be that depicted by the middle figure. Yet when attending to point 2, the viewer sees the orientation of the figure alternate between the version shown in the middle and the one shown on the right.

In this example, point 1 should be able to disambiguate the entire figure, since it makes the local portion of the figure univocal. Yet it does not appear to affect how the figure as a whole is perceived; if you focus at point 2, the figure remains ambiguous. In fact, if the distance between the cue and the ambiguous parts is great enough, it has little effect in disambiguating the percept, as can be seen if we elongate the globally unambiguous figure (see figure 1.14).

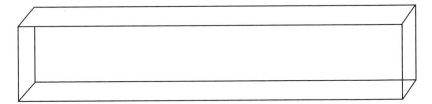

Figure 1.14
This figure, in which the disambiguating cue is farther away from the locally ambiguous parts, is even less likely to be perceived as the unambiguous box such as the middle figure of figure 1.13.

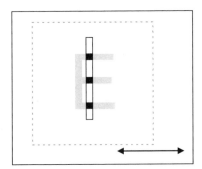 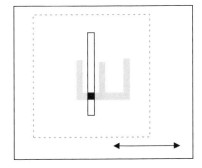

Figure 1.15
In the anorthoscope effect, a slit moves back and forth in front of the pattern. If the speed of the slit is just right, the pattern is perceived. However, the pattern is more easily perceived when there are fewer segments that have to be tracked as they pass in front of the slit (recognizing the E requires keeping track of three segments and checking whether they are joined, whereas recognizing the rotated E only requires tracking one segment and counting the number of crossbars that are passed). (This example is due to Ian Howard and is used with the author's permission.)

The same point can be illustrated by presenting visual patterns in rapid sequence to the eye. As I already remarked, in such cases observers typically feel that they see some larger integrated pattern. I have already mentioned the anorthoscope and the Zollner-Parks phenomenon, studied extensively by Parks (1965) and Rock (1981). In these studies, a pattern, viewed through a moving narrow slit that travels back and forth across the pattern, appears to be seen if the slit moves sufficiently rapidly (see figures 1.15 and 1.16). In fact, it has even been reported as perceived, though not quite as readily or clearly, if the slit is held fixed and the pattern is moved back and forth behind it. Of course, the moving-slit

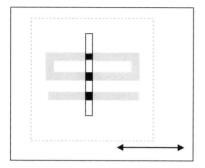 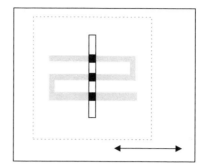

Figure 1.16
Another anorthoscope task. Observers are asked how many distinct line segments there are. These two displays have exactly the same inventory of local features (right angles, vertical and horizontal line segments, etc.). Recognizing which figure has one continuous line segment and which has two separate segments requires keeping track of which currently visible segment was connected to which segment in an earlier part of the viewing sequence. (Example due to Ian Howard.)

version could involve something like a persistent "retinal painting" by the moving-slit display, just as painting a scene on a TV set results in a display larger than the moving dot, though this is unlikely in the fixed-slit, moving-display version of the experiment. Some studies have controlled for the eye movements that would be required to paint the figure across the retina. Also, Rock (1983) showed that "retinal painting" is not in itself a general phenomenon, since simply moving a point of light along a path identical to the one that was traced out in the anorthoscope experiment does not yield a perception of the form. It turns out that the slit itself must be visible in order to get the anorthoscope effect. Not only must the slit be seen in outline; it must also be seen to be occluding the figure as the screen moves over the figure. If the visible portions of the form (the little bits that can be seen through the slits in figure 1.15 and figure 1.16) do not extend to the very edge of the slit, the effect is not observed (as illustrated in figure 3.11, to be discussed later).

Since the anorthoscope effect does not appear to be due to retinal painting, the natural assumption is that the pattern is instead being painted on an inner image, using some unspecified cues as to the motion of the figure behind the slit. But there are many reasons to reject such a view. One is that the ability to see the pattern in the case where the pattern is moving and the slit is fixed depends very much on the memory load imposed by the task of tracking the pattern. For example, in a series of unpublished studies, Ian Howard showed that patterns in which fewer features had to be tracked as they moved across the slit were identified more readily than ones that required more features to be tracked, even when the pattern was actually the same. Thus, for example, in figure 1.15, an E was harder to identify than the same shape lying on its back: the former requires that three segments be tracked as they move behind the slit, while the latter requires only one (together with a count of how many verticals went by). So the image is not just being "painted" on a master image, but must be remembered in a way that is sensitive to how many items there are to recall.

Figure 1.16 shows more clearly what must be remembered as the shape is moved past the slit. In this example, the task is to say whether there are one or two separate curves in the partially seen shape. Clearly, what an observer must do is keep track of the *type* of each line segment as it passes by the slit. This keeping track of line types—and not the operation of the visual system—is precisely the basis, I claim, for all of the demonstrations of "seeing" shapes through the anorthoscope. Such type tracking will be discussed in chapter 3 in terms of the notion of "label propagation." Once again, in the forms shown in figure 1.16 the task is easier when the forms are turned by 90 degrees, since fewer labeled lines must be tracked in that case.

Julian Hochberg (1968) conducted related studies involving serial presentation of patterns. He presented sequences of vertical slices of ambiguous figures, such as the Necker cube, at various speeds. There were two conditions in slicing up the image. In one case, it was sliced up so that slices contained complete vertices. In the other case, slices were made through the tips of the vertices so that the slices contained primarily straight-line segments (thus individual vertices were broken up in the process). The slices were presented at different speeds. Hochberg found that at fast speeds (around half a second to present 6 slices) the figures were perceived equally easily for both types of slices, consistent with other findings of a very-short-term visual buffer. But at slow speeds (more like natural viewing of these figures, in which the entire figure takes 2–3 seconds to examine), only the slices that kept vertices intact provided the information for the perception of tridimensionality.

Similar studies showed that the order in which parts of a figure were displayed through a stationary peephole made a difference in how diffi-

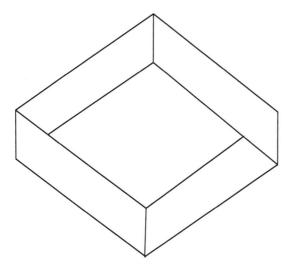

Figure 1.17
Simple "impossible figure" studied by Hochberg (1968) with the sequential presentation shown in figure 1.18.

cult it was to perceive the figure. For example, Hochberg (1968) also studied the perception of anomalous ("impossible") figures when the figure was presented in a piecemeal fashion. He found that anomalous figures (such as figure 1.17) could be detected in sequential presentations if the presentation sequence allowed observers to trace the type of the edges past ambiguous vertices until they reach a vertex where those labels are inconsistent with the requirements of a possible 3D vertex.

An example of a sequence that enables detection of the anomaly is shown in figure 1.18. In this case, however, we do not need to assume that a picture of the global pattern is being built up, because a much simpler explanation is available. It is the idea that observers are keeping track of the type of each line or edge and tracking this edge type from vertex to vertex.[5] The process is more like observers thinking to themselves, "I see this vertex as concave up, so this edge here must be an outside concave edge and must continue to be so when it gets to the next vertex. But if *that*

5. The term "line" is generally used in reference to 2D visual features. When lines are interpreted as parts of 3D objects they are more appropriately referred to as "edges." I will try to maintain this distinction, despite the fact that whether something is a line or an edge is often unclear in many contexts. The same is true of the pair of terms "vertex" and "junction" with the former being a 2D feature.

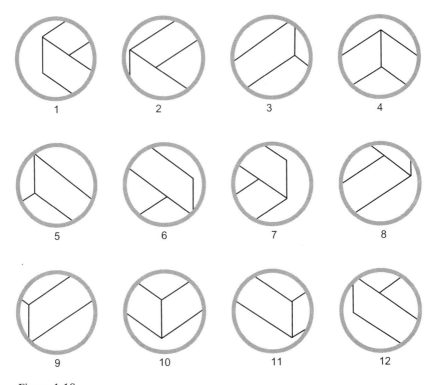

Figure 1.18
Sequence of views similar to that used by Hochberg (1968). Observers were able to detect that the sequence was from a drawing of an impossible figure only if the sequence was presented in the right order. (Adapted from Hochberg, 1968.)

edge is an outside convex edge, then *this* connecting edge must be a concave outside edge as well," and so on. In this way, if the first vertex is seen to reverse, then the rest of the labels change to maintain consistency. Note that such reasoning involves indexical (locative) terms like "this edge" and "that vertex." For such a reasoning sequence to be possible, there must be some way to refer to particular elements in the scene, and that indeed is the focus of a theory of visual indexing, to which we will return in chapter 5. For present purposes I wish merely to point out that the Hochberg experiments, like the anorthoscope examples discussed previously, all point to the importance of the notion of labeling features in a scene and tracking the labels along spatially contiguous elements (such as edges or surfaces) so as to determine whether they are consistent with labels assigned to other parts of the pattern.

The idea of tracking the labels assigned to edges helps to explain why some sequences are easier to see (or perceive as anomalous) than others. In addition, this labeling idea is in fact consistent with a body of research in computational vision that I will describe in some detail in chapter 3. In that context I will relate this labeling technique to an important question that arises concerning how a representation of a 3D world can be reconstructed from its highly incomplete and ambiguous 2D retinal projection. The technique developed in computational vision involves assigning possible sets of labels to the elements in a scene and then pruning the set by taking into account the constraints that must hold among such labels (e.g., the label assigned to an edge at one vertex must be a label possible to assign to that same edge at another vertex).

This provides an alternative way of characterizing the "signature" visual phenomena that led Hochberg to suggest that a "visual buffer" holds information in pictorial form. Such visual phenomena as spontaneous 3D interpretation, spontaneous reversals, and detection of impossible figures can be done by label propagation. This does not require that pictorial information be stored—only that there be a way to keep track of the label assigned to a *currently visible* edge as some vertices connected to that edge come into view and other vertices go out of view. In other words, so long as we can trace a particular edge and track its label continuously over time, we are in a position to interpret the lines as depicting a 3D object or to decide that no such object is possible. Interpretation of line drawings in 3D is a locally supported process, as the example of elongated figures shows (and as Hochberg has argued as well). The interpretation initially comes from cues provided by individual vertices alone. These assign (possibly ambiguous) labels to lines viewed as edges of 3-D objects, which have to be supported or rejected by connected vertices. This does not require any visual storage of off-foveal visual patterns. All it requires is that for each line segment currently in view, there be a record of what label was assigned to it by the vertex that just moved off the retina. This requires tracing, or otherwise identifying, the lines as they appear on successive retinal images. This sort of analysis works perfectly for the anorthoscope examples (the ones in figure 1.16 require an even simpler set of labels: simply keeping track of whether a particular line had ever been connected to any of the other lines in the figure).

1.4.3   How "pictorial" is information in the "visual buffer"?

As I suggested in the previous section, there is good reason for shunning the assumption that information in a "visual buffer" is pictorial. There is also considerable direct evidence that the information we extract from a scene does not have nearly the richness, geometrical completeness, and uniformity of detail that we associate with any kind of picture. In fact, as Bishop Berkeley argued, visual concepts are abstract and highly variable in their details, much as information conveyed by language is (e.g., we can describe what is in a scene in great detail while failing to mention where the things are or only vaguely describing their general shapes, as in "elongated roundish blobs"). If a master inner image were being painted, it is clear that it would have to have some very odd nonpictorial properties, such as labeled regions (what Dennett has described as a "paint-by-numbers" quality). As the examples of extended figures above suggests, once the information gets into the visual system (as opposed to still being on the retina), it no longer seems to function as visual inputs do, in terms of showing such signature properties as automatic three-dimensional interpretation and spontaneous reversals. As we will see in chapter 3, merely getting form information, such as where contours are located, into the visual system does not guarantee that it will serve to drive the usual interpretations, such as three-dimensional shape recovery. Indeed, I will show evidence that contour information provided by clearly perceptible differences in textures and colors does not always enable the visual system to see the form in 3D or in motion. So even if we want to persist in thinking of a master inner image, we will have to greatly modify our idea of what sorts of things can be painted on it—so much so that it will presently become clear that it's not an image at all.

It has been suggested that what we "see" extends beyond the boundaries of both time and space provided by the sensors in the fovea. So we assume that there is a place where the spatially extended information resides and where visual information is held for a period of time while it is integrated with what came before and what is coming in at present. Thus a central function of the "master image" is to provide a short-term visual memory. For this reason, looking at what visual information is stored over brief periods of time (seconds or minutes) may give us some insight as to what the visual system provides to the cognizing mind.[6] If we examine cases where people's visual memory is taxed, we can get an idea of how much detail and what *kinds* of details are registered there. When we do this, we find that the inner image becomes even less plausible as a vehicle for visual representation. Consider the following experimental results (discussed in Pylyshyn, 1978), which suggest that the information provided to the mind by the visual system is *abstract* and is encoded *conceptually*, perhaps in what has sometimes been called the *lingua mentis*, or language of thought.[7]

6. It is generally accepted that the so-called iconic storage retains a complete and detailed image, though only for about a quarter of a second (Sperling, 1960). This is clearly not the storage system that is relevant to the arguments for an inner screen since our phenomenal visual experience, as well as the sorts of empirical phenomena discussed by Hochberg, apply over a much longer period of time and over a wider region than the retina. Some studies (Posner, 1978) have shown that during the first second or so information is transformed from an iconic to a more abstract (categorical) form (for example, it takes longer to judge that "a" and "A" are the same letter when they are presented in rapid succession, compared to when the first letter is presented a few hundred milliseconds earlier, whereas the time it takes to judge that they are typographically the same is less when the two are presented closer in time). Since it is this latter stage of storage that is relevant to our present discussion, this supports what I have been arguing, namely, that information in the visual store is abstract and categorical (e.g., it consists of labels).

7. In a broad defense of the pictorial view (specifically as it pertains to mental imagery), Tye (1991) has criticized these examples on the grounds that (a) they only implicate memory and not the pictorial display itself, and (b) pictures, too, can be noncommittal and abstract. The first of these is irrelevant since one of the ideas I am questioning is precisely the pictorial view of memory representation. Although many proponents of the picture view of mental imagery may have given up on the assumption that long-term memory is pictorial, not everyone has, and certainly at the time of my critique such a view was widespread (see the quotations in Pylyshyn, 1973). As for the notion that images can be noncommittal and have an abstract character, this is simply a play on words. The way pictures get to have noncommittal content is by appealing to conventions by which they may be "read" like linguistic symbols. Sure, you can have a picture of a tilted beaker (such as in figure 1.19) that shows a fluid but is noncommittal about the orientation of the surface: you can paint a blur or a squiggle instead of showing the surface of the fluid, and then you can say that this information is indeterminate. But the blurring is simply an invitation *not to pay attention* to the part of the figure depicting the surface. It's like mumbling when you come to the part of the argument you are not sure about, which, come to think of it, is exactly what is going on in this proposal. In chapters 6 and 7 we will return to the popular shell game in which various ad hoc properties are attributed to the image to hide the fact that the work is being done not by the picture but by the "mind's eye" and the brain behind it.

The first of these examples comes from observing children, who are generally thought to have excellent visual memories. The reason that I present examples taken from observations of children is that we are especially interested in certain kinds of "errors" made in generalizing one visual situation to another (usually a pictorial one), and children tend to be less sophisticated about picturing conventions and so make more errors. We are interested in errors because these tell us what patterns the visual system finds to be most alike, and this in turn tells us something about how the visual patterns are represented in visual memory. First I will present the examples as illustrated in figures 1.19 to 1.24. After describing the results, I will then discuss the moral that might be drawn from them.

In a typical Piagetian task (see Piaget and Inhelder, 1957), a child is shown a tilted glass test tube containing colored water and asked to draw it, or to pick out the drawing that most looks like what she saw. In these experiments the child is most likely to select a drawing in which the water level is either perpendicular or parallel to the sides of the tube, as show in figure 1.19. (Later I will show that adults are not much better at this water-level task!)

If a child is shown a solid block, say a cube, and asked to draw it or to select a drawing that most looks like it from a set of alternatives, the child frequently chooses drawings such as those shown in figure 1.20, rather than the more conventional isometric or perspective projections (such as the Necker Cube show in figure 1.7). This idea was first described by Winston (1974) and led to experiments reported in an M.Sc. thesis by Ed Weinstein (1974).

It is a common observation that a child will frequently reverse a letter of the alphabet and draw its mirror image, as show in figure 1.21. This phenomenon is quite ubiquitous. When presented with any shape and

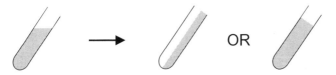

Figure 1.19
Sketch of Piaget's finding (described in Piaget and Inhelder, 1957). A child is shown the figure on the left and mistakenly recalls one of the figures on the right.

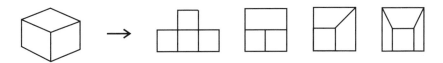

Figure 1.20
Another example of children's recall. A child is shown a real three-dimensional cube and draws one of the drawings shown on the right. (Adapted from Weinstein, 1974.)

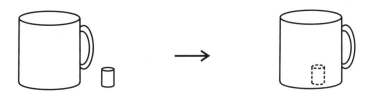

Figure 1.21
Children much more often mistake a figure for its mirror image than for a rotated version of that figure, resulting in the common reversal that has become enshrined in the name of the toy store "Toys Я Us" (Rock, 1973).

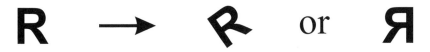

Figure 1.22
Children sometimes make what seem to us like odd errors when they imitate an adult's actions. Here a child is asked to imitate an adult placing a small object beside a cup, but in doing so places the object inside the cup (Clark, 1973). What does this tell us about how the child represents the adult's action?

asked to find the same shape among a set of alternatives, a child tends to mistake the shape and its mirror image more often than the shape and a tilted version of the shape. (Adults tend to make this error as well, though not as frequently.) These and related studies are reported in Rock, 1973.

When asked to imitate an action such as placing a small object close to a container like a cup, children more often place the object *inside* the cup rather than beside it, as illustrated schematically in figure 1.22. Imitating actions is an interesting way of examining how people (or animals) view the action. No act of imitation is ever an exact replica of the action being imitated. Not only are we incapable of perfect imitation of all muscles and movements, an imitation does not need to be a precise physical duplicate to qualify as an accurate imitation. What is required is that the imitation preserve what is essential in the action being imitated, and that in turn tells us something about how the action was perceived or encoded. These studies are part of a series reported in Clark, 1973.

The other examples are drawn from studies with adult subjects, but they illustrate the same general point. Figure 1.23 shows the results of a study on visual memory for chess positions by Chase and Simon (1973). The graph illustrates that when chess masters and novices are shown a midgame chess board for about 5 seconds, the chess master can reproduce it with almost perfect accuracy, while the novice can get only one or two chess positions correct. But when they are shown the same chess pieces arranged in a random pattern, the two groups do equally poorly. The visual-memory superiority of the chess masters is specific to real chess positions.

Figure 1.24 shows an experiment by Steve Palmer (1977) in which subjects are asked to examine two simple line drawings and superimpose them in their mind (presumably on their master images), then to select the drawing most like the superimposed combined image. There is a great

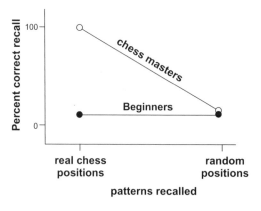

Figure 1.23
This graph shows that chess masters' apparent superior memory of chess positions occurs only when the chess pieces are arranged in a pattern taken from a real chess game. When the same chess pieces are arranged in a random pattern, the chess masters are no better than novices. (This finding is described in Chase and Simon, 1973.)

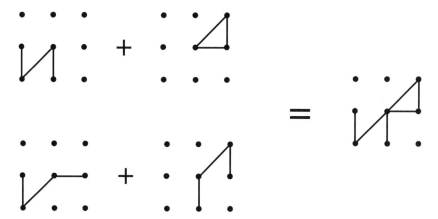

Figure 1.24
When observers are asked to superimpose the figures in the first column with those in the second column and tested as to what the combined figure looks like (in this case it's the one on the right), it matters a great deal whether the figures that are combined constitute a "good subpart" of the combined figure (which they do in the top row and do not in the bottom row*)*. (From Palmer, 1978.)

deal of difference in how well people do, depending on whether or not the two figures fit together as natural subparts to create the complex. It appears that superimposing even simple shapes in the master image is not a matter of mechanically overlaying them: the perceived subpart structure of the resulting figure—whether the two figures form natural groupings when superimposed—matters. Consequently, the two top line drawings in figure 1.24 are easier to combine than the bottom two to produce the same combined image, shown on the right.

This collection of experiments presents some perhaps surprising findings regarding errors in visual recognition commonly made by observers. What do they have in common, and what do they suggest about how the visual system encodes a visual stimulus? If the visual system constructed a master image that persisted and provided the basis for visual memory, then the errors one would expect would be something like the errors that a template-fitting process might produce. Patterns or shapes that differed least in terms of their geometry should be most often mistaken. But that is not what happens in visual memory, and it's not even what we would intuitively expect to happen. After all, when you miss-recall a scene, such as the appearance of the room full of people at your last party, you do not expect that what you will get wrong will be anything like a pictorial distortion—things moved a bit or shapes altered slightly. In fact, in the case of a two-dimensional picture, even a slight difference in vantage point would change the geometry radically without affecting what is represented in the image. People are much more likely to mistake a photograph of a room they had seen with one that was taken from a different point of view, than with one which contained a different person, no matter how large the geometrical difference is in the first case. Even if the image were three-dimensional, like a hologram, it would still be too sensitive to unimportant geometrical deviations in relation to meaningful ones. And it is the meaningful properties, which are often carried by very small pictorial details, that our visual system pays the greatest attention to. As a result, what you might forget in recalling the party scene is that Jones was to the left of Smith, though you might remember that they were close to each other and were talking. Your memory image, however complete and vivid it might seem to you, is also indeterminate and noncommittal in a large number of ways. You can recall that two people were having a good time without any recollection of what they were doing. And you can have what seems to you like a clear *image* of this state of affairs. It is possible to feel that one has a perfectly vivid and complete image of a situation that in fact is highly abstract and sketchy, and that is where one's phenomenal experience leads one astray. I often feel I have a vivid image of someone's face, but when asked whether the person wears glasses, I find that my image is silent on that question: it neither has nor lacks glasses, much as the blind spot neither provides information about the relevant portion of the visual field nor does it contain the information that something is missing. You might note that *sentences* (and other languagelike compositional encoding systems) have this sort of content indeterminacy, whereas pictures do not. You can say things in a language (including any language of thought) that fails to make certain commitments that any picture would have to make (e.g., your sentence can assert that *A* and *B* are beside one another while failing to say which is to the right or left).

In terms of the examples just enumerated, if children's visual experiences are represented not as pictures but as conceptual complexes of some sort (I will not speculate at this point what such a complex might be like, except to point out that it is more like a language of thought than a picture), then the availability of certain concepts could be reflected in the errors they make. There is no way to represent (i.e., describe) the tilted-test-tube display without a concept such as that of allocentric level (or parallel to the surface of the earth). If this concept is not available, then there is no way to capture the special feature that distinguishes between the three displays in figure 1.19. So the child is left with choosing a salient pattern as consistent as possible with what he or she sees, which happens to be a surface that is either parallel or perpendicular to the sides of the tube. Exactly the same can be said of the example in figure 1.20. If shapes are represented conceptually, rather than pictorially, distinguishing a shape from its mirror image requires access to the egocentric concept *left of* or *right of* (try describing a shape in such a way that it can be distinguished from its mirror image without using such terms or their cognates), and these ego-reference concepts are slow to develop compared with concepts like *up* or *down* or *sharp angle* or *perpendicular* or *circular*, and so on. I don't mean that the words "left" or "right," and so on, are not available, but that the underlying concepts that these words conventionally express are not available (although without the concepts, the words could not be learned either).

So long as we appreciate that what the visual system provides is abstract and conceptual, rather than pictorial, we will also not find the other results puzzling. To mimic a movement is not to reproduce it as depicted in an image, it is rather to generate *some* movement (perhaps one that is preferred on some other grounds) that meets the conceptual representation of the movement as it was seen, or as the visual system represented it. Thus if the child represented the action of moving the small object as an action in which the object was placed in some relevant and appropriate proximal relation to a cup, she might choose to place it inside just because she prefers inside-placing (there is certainly evidence that children like to place things inside other things). Similarly, the results of the chess-memory and superposition experiments sketched in figures 1.23 and 1.24 are baffling if one thinks of the visual system as providing a picture that serves as the form of short-term memory. But they are easily understood if one views the memory entry as being conceptual, where the concepts are either learned over the years or are part of the native machinery of visual organization (and for present purposes we need not take a stand on which of these it is). With the right

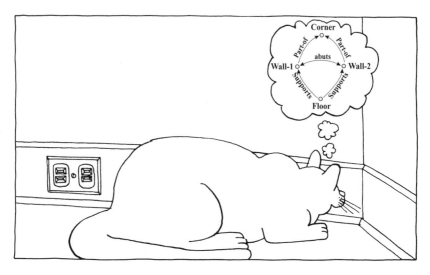

Figure 1.25
Alternative conception of what is in the mind of the cat in the cartoon in figure
1.1. B. Kliban (American, 1935–1990). From the book *Cat*, by B. Kliban. Used
by permission. All rights reserved. © Judith K. Kliban.

concepts, the representation of a scene can be simple and compact and
easily remembered (one may say, with George Miller, that it has been
"chunked"), even if its geometrical or pictorial configuration is not.

These examples, as well as those discussed in section 1.4.2, strongly
suggest that information about a visual scene is not stored in pictorial
form, but rather is stored in a form more like that of a description, which
is characterized by variable grain and abstractness and is based on available concepts. Thus rather than thinking of vision as it was depicted in
the Kliban cartoon in figure 1.1, one should replace the picture in the
thought balloon with a data structure such as that in figure 1.25, in a
format that is typically used in artificial-intelligence applications.

1.5   More Problems with the Inner-Display Assumption: Part 2, Seeing or Figuring Out?

In chapter 2, I will discuss other methodologies for studying visual perception, and in particular for trying to sort out the thorny problem of
which properties of visual apprehension are properties of vision as such,

and which are properties of the cognitive system. I will argue that the empirical data are on the side of a clear separation between these processes, providing we are willing to make the sorts of distinctions and idealizations that are ubiquitous in science. But why do we believe in this separation, and what are we getting ourselves into if we follow this course? As I said earlier, this book is not about the nature of visual experience, as such. Yet we cannot get away without some comment on this question, because visual experience appears to be the main source of data on the operation of the visual system. Even when we appeal to the interaction of visual properties, as I did in some of the examples above, or when we use nonverbal evidence (e.g., pointing, reaching, grasping, event-related potentials, or galvanic skin responses) about perceived objects and thereby get stronger converging evidence, visual experience remains the reference point against which we measure what we mean by *seeing*. The situation is rather similar to that in linguistics, where certain signature properties of grammatical structure, such as intuitions of grammaticality and ambiguity, form the basic data, even though these have to be supplemented by theoretically motivated converging observations and judgments. In the case of vision, we must supplement our use of phenomenal experience as the data of vision, because phenomenal experience is not always available, because we don't want to tie ourselves to the assumption that only consciously experienced percepts constitute genuine vision, and because visual experience is itself a fallible source of evidence. But how can our experience be fallible: are we not the final authority as to how things seem to us? Whether or not we want to claim that we are the final authority on how things seem to us, the question of the *content of our perception* is broader that how things seem to us, because, unlike conscious experience, it is a construct that must serve in information-processing theories and must eventually comport with biological evidence.

1.5.1   A note about terminology

Many of the examples we have considered so far raise questions about when a phenomenon is truly "visual" and when it is conceptually or logically derived or based on figuring out how the world must have been in order to lead to the information we received from the senses. After all, it is possible that the reason we can recognize the words "New York" in our earlier example (figure 1.4) might simply be that we can guess them from the bits of information we can pick up; there may be nothing visual about the process and hence no need to postulate an inner completed display. In the preceding section I claimed that vision and cognition could (and should) be distinguished. But in the everyday use of the terms, the two overlap extensively. Consequently, there are those who object to using a term, such as "vision," in a way that is at variance with its general informal use. We use the term "vision" (or sometimes "early vision") to refer to the part of visual perception that is unique to vision and is not shared by cognition in general. Such a usage has been viewed by some as, at best, terminological imperialism and, at worst, circular, since it assumes that early vision is impenetrable when the very notion is defined in terms of encapsulation from cognition.

In defense of the present usage, however, it should be pointed out that it is perfectly legitimate to adopt a term that refers to that aspect of the brain's function that is distinct and uniquely associated with what goes on in a modality under study (where the exact bound of the "modality" is also an empirical issue; see pp. 126–129). To use the term "vision" to include all the organism's intellectual activity that originates with information at the eye and culminates in beliefs about the world, or even actions, is not very useful, since it runs together a lot of different processes. The same tack was adopted by Chomsky, who uses the term "language" or "language capacity" to refer to that function that is unique to linguistic processing, even though understanding natural-language utterances clearly involves most of our intellectual faculties. It is also the tack I adopted when I use the term "cognition" to refer to processes that operate over representations of knowledge, as distinct from knowledge-independent processes of the "cognitive architecture" (Pylyshyn, 1984a), when I use the term "learning" to refer to certain cognitively mediated changes in cognitive states (Pylyshyn, 1984b, pp. 266–268), and when I use "inference" to refer to any quasi-logical process.[8] Moreover, this use of "vision" is not circular (or at least not

8. The present policy in regard to the use of the term "inference" differs from that of Fodor (1983) and Fodor and Pylyshyn (1981) in that I here do not use it to refer to processes that are systematically restricted as to what type of input they may take and the type of principles that they follow. Thus I consider early vision, which follows the sorts of principles sketched on pp. 66–68 and in

viciously so), since it embodies a strong empirical claim, namely, that there exists a nontrivial part of the overall visual process that is impenetrable. The burden of the next chapter is to argue that a significant part of the intuitive (or prescientific) sense of "visual perception" is in fact impenetrable, and that this part is also complex and covers a great deal of what is special about vision (I will discuss the question of what the visual system, so construed, outputs to other systems in chapter 3).

The reason for this terminological policy is the usual one that applies in any science. A science progresses to the extent that it identifies general empirically valid distinctions, such as between mass and weight, heat and temperature, energy and momentum, and so on. I propose a distinction between vision and cognition in order to try to carve nature at her joints, that is, to locate components of the mind/brain that have some principled boundaries or some principled constraints in their interactions with the rest of the mind. To the extent that we can factor the cognitive system into such components and can specify the nature of the interactions that are permissible among them, we will have taken a step toward understanding how the system works. For the time being, I will take for granted that showing principled macroarchitectural components can be a step toward understanding how a complex system functions (assuming that the description is valid). Given this background we can then ask, Why should we expect there to be a sustainable distinction between cognition and perception? Or more specifically, why do we think that if we draw such a boundary in a principled way, the part that is not "cognition" will include anything more than the sensors? I devote chapters 2 and 3 to arguing the case in favor of the hypothesis that vision and cognition are largely separate functions, i.e., that vision is what I and others have called a module of the mental architecture (see Fodor, 1983). This, I claim, is a major empirical discovery of vision science of the past 30 years.

---

chapter 3, not to merit the ascription "inference." Although it might be possible to characterize the operation of the visual system in terms of "rules," these differ significantly from rules of interence since they only apply to representations arising directly from vision and not to those with a different provenance. Because of their rigidify they are best viewed as the wired-in regularities such as any mechanism must possess. As in the case of the term "vision," something is lost by being too ecumenical in one's linguistic usage: one loses the ability to distinguish between a quasi-logical system of inferences and other sorts of causal regularities.

1.5.2   "Seeing *x*" versus "believing that what you saw is *x*"

There is an important distinction to be made between how you experience a perceptual event and what you believe about your experience, and therefore what you may report about what you saw. People's beliefs are notorious for being filtered through their tacit theories and expectations. Thus it is not clear what to make of such results as those reported by Wittreich (1959). According to Wittreich, a number of married people reported that when two people, one of whom was their spouse, walked across the well-known Ames distorted room, the stranger appeared to change in size (the usual experience), whereas the spouse did not. There are several possible explanations for this surprising phenomenon (if, indeed, it is a reliable phenomenon). One explanation (the one that Wittreich favors) is that the perception of size is affected by familiarity. Another is that a highly familiar person can result in an attentional focus so narrow that it can exclude contextual visual cues, such as those provided by the Ames room and by the accompanying person. Yet another possibility is that because of all the emotional connections one has with a spouse, it is just too hard to accept that the spouse has changed size while walking across the room. As a result, observers may simply refuse to accept that this is how their spouses appeared to them. It is not always possible to describe "how something looks" in terms that are neutral to what you know, although clearly this does happen with illusions, such as the Müller-Lyer illusion (see figure 2.3).

Consider the following related example in which a subject's report of "how things look" may well be confounded with "what I believe I saw" or "how I judge the perceived object to be." In a classical paper, Perky (1910b) reported a study in which observers were told to imagine some particular object (e.g., a piece of fruit) while looking at a blank screen. Unbeknownst to the subjects, the experimenter projected faint images on the screen. Perky found that subjects frequently mistook what they were faintly seeing for what they were imagining (e.g., they reported that the images had certain properties, like orientation or color, that were actually arbitrarily chosen properties of the faintly projected image). One way to view this is as a demonstration that when the visual experience is ambiguous or unclear, subjects' beliefs about their experience are particularly labile to alteration. In this case what the subjects sometimes believed is that they saw nothing but had the experience of imagining something. In other cases, perhaps in this same experiment, the converse obtained: subjects believed they had seen something but in fact they had seen nothing and had only imagined it. Various methodologies, such as signal detection theory, have been developed to try to drive a wedge between the factors leading an observer to decide certain things and factors leading to their detecting things with their senses (for more on the interaction of vision and "mental images," such as in the Perky effect, see section 6.5).

The point is that even if "how something looks" is determined by the visual system, what we believe we are seeing—what we report seeing—is determined by much more. What we report seeing depends not only on vision, but also on a fallible memory and on our beliefs, which in turn depend on a number of factors that psychologists have spent much time studying. For example, it is known that the larger the role played by memory, the more unreliable the report. There is a great deal of evidence that what people believe they saw is highly malleable, hence the concern about the validity of eyewitness testimony (Loftus, 1975). The often dramatic effects of subliminal stimuli, hypnotic suggestion, placebos, and mass hysteria result from the gap (things often do result from a gap!) that exists between seeing, believing, and believing what one has seen. Indeed, because of such malleability of reports of experiences, psychologists long ago came to appreciate that research methods—such as double-blind testing and the use of unobtrusive measures—had to be designed to control for the fact that honest well-meaning people tend to report what they believe they should be reporting (e.g., the "correct" answer or the answer that is wanted—the so-called experimenter-demand effect). It's not a matter of deliberately lying, although the very notion of a deliberate lie came under suspicion long ago with the recognition of unconscious motives (with Freud) and of tacit knowledge, both of which are important foundational axioms in all of the human sciences. What is at issue is not the observer's sincerity, but the plasticity of the belief-determining process. There is no sure methodology for distinguishing between what people experience in a certain perceptual situation and what they (genuinely) *believe* they experienced, although we will discuss a number of methods for refining this distinction later.

1.5.3   Reports of what something "looks like": What do they mean?

There is a further problem with some studies that build on reports of how things look and how these reports can be influenced by beliefs, utilities, expectations, and so on. A problem arises from the fact that a phrase such as "That looks like x" is typically used in a way that merges with something like "My visual experience has convinced me that what I am seeing is x." The terminology of "appearances" is extremely problematic. Wittgenstein provides a typical eye-opening example of how "looks like" runs together appearances and beliefs.

The playwright Tom Stoppard tells the story in his play *Jumpers* by having two philosophers meet. The first philosopher says, "Tell me, why do people always say it was natural for men to assume that the sun goes around the earth rather than that the earth is rotating?" The second philosopher says, "Well, obviously, because it just *looks* as if the sun is going round the earth." To this the first philosopher replies, "Well, what would it have looked like if it had looked as if the earth was rotating?"

Examples closer to our immediate concerns are easily found. For instance, it is commonly reported that how big something "looks" depends on the presence of size cues in the form of familiar objects (so, for example, when you are shown a photograph of an unfamiliar shape, it is common to include something familiar, such as a person or a hand, in the photograph). But this may well be a different sense of "looks like" than what is meant when we say that in the Müller-Lyer illusion one line looks longer than the other. In the case of the "perceived size" of an unfamiliar object, the object may not actually look different, depending on nearby size cues; it may simply be judged to be a different size.

Sometimes claims that some stimulus is "seen" in a particular way have been contested on the grounds that perception and inference have been conflated. For example, a disagreement arose between Theodore Parks and Ralph Haber regarding whether what has been called the eye-of-the-needle or anorthoscope phenomenon demonstrates "post-retinal storage" (Haber, 1968; Haber and Nathanson, 1968; Parks, 1965; Parks, 1968). In the original anorthoscope effect discussed earlier (and illustrated in figure 1.15), I claimed that people could "see" a stimulus pattern that was viewed through a slit in a screen that moved back and forth in front of the stimulus. As I already suggested, this sort of seeing is different from the usual kind in that there is a memory load imposed by the task that shows up in differences in the ability to recover the shape depending on the order in which parts of the figure are presented. Haber and Nathanson (1968) raised the question of whether what is stored in the anorthoscope effect is an image or more abstract information that allows an interpretation to be inferred (rather than seen). The question of when some episode constitutes a case of visual perception (i.e., of "seeing"), as opposed to being merely a case of drawing an inference from fragmentary visual cues, is more than a terminological one—it has implications for theories of visual memory and mental imagery.

An even more extreme case of the overly inclusive way in which the term "see" or "looks like" is used is provided by the case of "Droodles"—a type of humorous visual puzzles first developed by Roger Price, such as the ones in figure 1.26. These have sometimes been cited (e.g., Hanson, 1958) to illustrate that what you see depends on what you know. (Look at each figures and then ask yourself, What does it look like? Then do it again after reading the captions in note 9.)

Like Gestalt closure figures (or fragmented figures, discussed in chapter 2 and illustrated in figures 2.6 and 2.7), these appear to come together suddenly to make a humorous closure. But unlike the fragmented figures, these interpretations clearly depend on collateral information. The question is, Do these cases illustrate the operation of the visual system, or are they more like puns or jokes in which the punch line causes one to cognitively reinterpret or reframe what came before (or what was seen)?

Ordinary language uses terms like "appears" or "seems" in ways that do not distinguish plausible functions of the visual system from inferences based partly on visual cues and partly on other (nonvisual) information. For example, we speak of someone "looking sick" or of a painting "looking like a Rembrandt." Whatever is involved in this sort of "looking like," it is unlikely to be the basis for building a scientific theory of vision, since it clearly involves more than vision in the sense in which this term is used in science (I will return to this issue in the next chapter).

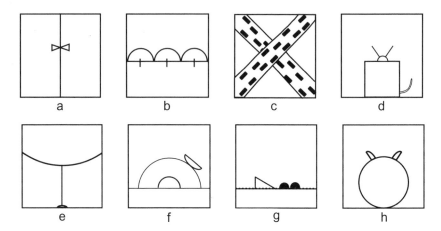

Figure 1.26
Examples of visual puns invented by Roger Price, known as "droodles." What do you see in each of these panels? Reproduced with permission from Mr. Leo Valdes, who maintains the droodles home page at http://www.droodles.com.[9]

1.5.4   Vision and conscious appearance: Can they be separated?

Although the intuitive sense of "how things look" provides the starting point in a study of visual phenomena, this is not the only way to determine what the visual system does or what it produces. For example, vision leads not only to the phenomenal experience of *seeing* (I will have more to say about this experience on pp. 350–357), it also leads to our being able to act appropriately towards objects (e.g., point to them, grasp them, and so on). When certain properties are perceived, we can also make certain judgments about the objects that have those properties; for

9. Droodles (a), (b), and (c) are originals by Roger Price. The others are contributions (ca. 1997) to the Droodles home page maintained by Leo Valdes (http://www.droodles.com), reproduced with permission of Mr. Valdes. The original captions are:

(a)   Man wearing a bow tie entered an elevator and the door closed on his tie.

(b)   Rear view of the starting line for a rat race.

(c)   Giraffes in love.

(d)   Cat watching TV.

(e)   Flea holding up an elephant.

(f)   Igloo with a satellite dish.

(g)   Shark returning from a holiday at Disneyland.

(h)   Rabbit blowing a large bubble.

example, we can discriminate them or recognize them to be different. When surfaces with different properties, such as different colors, are placed side by side, we can judge that there is a visible boundary between them (in the extreme, when we cannot discriminate any boundary between surfaces that have different spectral properties, we say that those properties are "metamers," meaning that they are visually indiscernible). In addition, under certain circumstances we can also show that perception of properties leads to certain physiological responses (such as the galvanic skin response, which is the basis of lie-detector tests) or neurological responses (such as patterns of EEGs called event-related potentials), and so on. Another way to try to distinguish between purely visual phenomena and phenomena involving beliefs is to appeal to the interaction between two visual phenomena, one of which is independently known to occur in early vision. This is what was done in the interaction between "perceived virtual contours" and the Pogendorff illusion (figure 1.5) and when I appealed to certain "signature properties" of vision, such as automatic figure-ground separation, interpretation in 3D, reversals, and apparent motion. I also hinted at other methods, such as the use of signal-detection theory, event-related potentials, the galvanic skin response.

To understand whether certain phenomena are purely visual, we can also the appeal to clinical cases of brain damage that show deficits in reports of visual perception and in the ability to recognize objects, but without concomitant deficits in related cognitive skills. For example, there are remarkable cases of what is called "blindsight" (studied extensively by Weiskrantz, 1997), in which some patients with cortical damage have as a result large blind regions in their visual fields (often as large as half the visual field). When objects are held up before them in these "blind" regions, the patients say that they seen nothing there. Yet when they are forced to guess or to reach for the objects (just to humor the experimenter), they perform significantly above chance in both types of tasks. Such reports of not seeing accompanied by performance indicating that visual information is being processed also occur with split-brain patients (patients who had their corpus collosum surgically cut in order to alleviate epileptic seizures, or who were born without the connecting fibers). In these patients there is almost no communication between the two hemispheres of the brain, so that the left half, which has the language skills, cannot communicate with the right half, which gets input from the left half of each retina. Such people exhibit amazing symptoms (Gazzaniga, 2000). For example, they report that they do not see objects presented to the left half of their visual field. Yet their left hand (which is connected to the half of the cortex that is receiving visual information about the objects) is able to reach for the objects quite normally. In fact, they can often recognize the objects by their feel or the sound they make when moved. Once the left hand brings the object into view of the right hemisphere, these people can report seeing them. Other related visual disorders also suggest that equating seeing with being able to report a conscious visual experience may unnecessarily limit the scope of the evidence for vision.

The point is that there is no limit to the type of evidence than can in principle be marshaled to help us understand visual perception. As I already remarked, even though perceptual experience may define the clear cases, the strategy in visual science, as in all human sciences, is then to let various convergent measures and the developing body of theory determine where the boundary between perception and cognition will fall. Thus there is no reason in principle why we should not include in the category of perception cases of unconscious perception. Indeed, perhaps one might even have good reason to call certain mental states cases of unconscious perceptual *experiences*. None of these issues can be prejudged in the absence of at least a partial theory of what it is to have a conscious experience; once again, common sense is no help in these matters. The everyday notion of seeing is too fluid and all encompassing to be of scientific use. Science needs to make certain distinctions and to identify what Simon (1969) refers to as "partially decomposable" systems. But then such distinctions invariably belie the everyday prescientific ideas.

1.6   Where Do We Go from Here?

This chapter has provided a sketch of some of the reasons why many people have assumed that vision provides us with an inner version of the world more complete, detailed, and extended, and more responsive to our beliefs, desires, and expectations, than is the retinal information we are forced to deal with in the first instance. In the course of this discussion I have hinted that in formulating a scientific theory of vision, we will more than likely have to shed much of our intuitively comfortable view. In particular, we will have to jettison the phenomenal image or display and come to grips with the information-processing task that vision carries out. But we will also have to come to terms with other equally uncomfortable conceptual issues. For example, in the discussion so far I spoke freely about the *visual system* and the *visual process*. But what if there is no specifically visual process, but only an undifferentiated cognitive process. For example, many people view vision as being quite close in spirit to the process of science itself, where people use all the intellectual apparatus at their disposal to come up with theories, which they then attempt to confirm or disconfirm, leading to newer (and hopefully better) theories, and so on in an endless cycle. If this picture is correct, then it is highly unlikely that there will ever be a theory of visual perception, any more than there is a theory of science. Indeed, the nature of the scientific process, or the problem of induction, remains one of the most difficult puzzles in philosophy. But we are here embarked on a more optimistic venture: I will defend the thesis that there is such a thing as a *visual system*, apart from the entire system of reasoning and cognizing that humans and other organisms possess. I will examine the claim that vision is, as Fodor (1983) puts it, a *module*, informationally encapsulated from the rest of cognition and operating with a set of autonomously specifiable principles. More particularly, I will argue that an important part of what we normally would call visual perception is *cognitively impenetrable*. Earlier I suggested that it is problematic to distinguish between vision and visual memory because space and time can be traded off in the visual process (as happens routinely when we scan our eyes around). What I now want to claim, in contrast, is that there *is* a distinction between "seeing" and "thinking."

2

The Independence of Vision and Cognition

2.1 Is Vision Distinct from Reasoning?

2.1.1 What determines what we see? Do we see what we expect to see?

If the first major seduction of our phenomenal experience is the belief that vision constructs an inner world or inner display, then the next one is that "seeing is believing," or that there is little or no distinction between the visual system and the general reasoning system, other than that the former gets some of its initial information from the eyes. It is widely, if not universally, accepted that what we see is heavily conditioned by our beliefs and expectations. The view that perception and cognition are continuous is particularly believable because it comports well with everyday experience as well as with the zeitgeist—the spirit of the times—which celebrates the plasticity of the mind. The beginning of the second half of the twentieth century was characterized by a belief in biologically unlimited human potential. An advertisement on the American Public Television System declares, "If it can be imagined, it can be done: This is America!" In the debate between nature and nurture, nature had its day in the 1950s with the dominance of philosophical empiricism. That brought with it not only the view that the mind is a blank *tabula rasa*, upon which experience writes the entire adult intellectual capacity, but also the view that the newborn perceptual system provides the infant only with what William James called "a blooming buzzing confusion." One part of this ideology was a perceptual relativity: the view that how we perceive the world is conditioned by our beliefs, our culture, our moods, and so on. The average person takes it for granted that how we see the world is radically influenced by our mental state—by our beliefs;

our expectations; and our needs, hopes, and fears; and above all, by our language and culture. And there are plenty of reasons to take this view. One of the more dramatic illustrations of this is magic, where the magician manipulates what we see by setting up certain false expectations. We are also told that when people are thirsty in a desert, they often see oases. And who has not had the experienced of being afraid and then being "spooked" by harmless shadows that he mistakes for signs of something awful. The popularity among the literate public of what is known as the Sapir-Whorf hypothesis of linguistic relativity (which gave us the apocryphal story that Eskimos have 17 different words for snow because their perceptual discrimination of types of snow is more refined, i.e., because they have 17 different ways of *seeing* snow) also supports this general view, as does the widespread belief in the cultural effect on our *ways of seeing* (e.g., the books by Carlos Castaneda). The remarkable placebo effect of drugs and of authoritative suggestions by people wearing white coats also bears witness to the startling malleability of perception, not to mention the effects of suggestions given under hypnosis.

In this chapter I will examine some of the reasons why this view has been generally held, not just by the public, but also by psychologists, and I will also examine some evidence against this view of vision. To anticipate the conclusion, I will argue that visual perception, in the everyday sense of the term, does indeed merge seamlessly with reasoning and other aspects of cognition. But the everyday sense of the term is too broad to be of scientific value precisely because it fails to make distinctions that "cut nature at her joints." I will argue that within the broad category of what we call "vision" is a highly complex information processing system, which some have called "early vision," that functions independently of what we believe. This system individuates, or picks out, objects in a scene and computes the spatial layout of visible surfaces and the 3D shape of the objects in the scene.[1] It thus covers a lot of what one means by "visual

1. Notice that it is critical for our thesis that the notion of early vision includes, among other things, such functions as the individuation of objects (which will be the topic of ch. 5), as well as the computation of what are referred to as "surface layouts"—the shape of the visible surfaces in our field of view. If it were not for the fact that early vision includes such complex features of the visible world, the independence theses would be trivial; everyone believes that

perception." What it does not do is *identify* the things we are looking at, in the sense of relating them to things we have seen before, to the contents of our memory. And it does not make judgments about how things really are. In other words, this aspect of vision is not the sole determiner of our perceptual beliefs—our beliefs about what we are seeing. In this sense, then, seeing is not the same as believing; far from it.[2] Believing depends on all your wits and intelligence and knowledge of how the world works, whereas early vision does not. Early vision depends on how the visual system was wired up by evolution as well as on biological, chemical, and physical principles, and on the incoming patterns of light, but on little else. In would not be a great exaggeration to say that early vision—the part of visual processing that is prior to access to general knowledge—computes just about everything that might be called a "visual appearance" of the world *except* the identities and names of the objects. This view, which I have referred to as the "independence thesis" or the "modularity-of-vision thesis," flies in the face of a great deal of received wisdom, both in and out of visual science, and requires some elaboration. In particular, it requires drawing some conceptual distinctions and explaining a great deal of apparently contradictory evidence. By the time we are through with this topic, we will have distinguished between seeing and believing, between "seeing" and "seeing as," and between the processes carried out by the visual system and the previsual

---

something is detected by the visual system without regard for beliefs and expectations—otherwise we would only see what we wished to see. The more conventional view (e.g., that was held by empiricists and perhaps by "New Look" theorists discussed on pp. 52–56) is that the only thing that is isolated from cognition is the operation of the sensors. We will return to the question of the nature of the output of early vision in the next chapter.

2. Having made the distinction between the ordinary sense of vision and what I call "early vision," I will often fall into the habit of referring to the latter as "vision" and of this process as resulting in "seeing." I do this because the narrow technical sense of "vision" is precisely that part of visual perception that is unique to, and therefore constitutive of, visual perception. The broader sense is simply a confounding of several distinct processes. The policy of using the general term when referring to the part of a process that forms the unique core of that process is precisely what Chomsky (1976) does when he uses the term "language" to refer to that part of our entire linguistic ability that is unique to language, even though understanding and generating linguistic signs involves all of our cognitive faculties.

process of deciding where to focus attention or the postvisual process of deciding what the visual system reveals about the scene.

But first, let us look more closely at the basis for the belief in the relativity and plasticity of vision. The reasons for believing that vision and cognition are very closely linked go deeper than just our everyday experience. The view is backed by an enormous amount of experimental evidence from psychology and social sciences more broadly (including cross-cultural observations). It is also supported by work in artificial intelligence that attempts to build computer systems that can recognize objects and scenes. Below I present some of the experimental evidence that persuaded many scientists that vision is continuous with cognition. I do this to illustrate the reasons for the received wisdom, and also to set the stage for some critical distinctions and for some methodological considerations related to the interpretation generally given to the evidence.

2.2   The Case for the Continuity of Vision and Cognition

2.2.1   The "new look" in the psychology of perception
In 1947 Jerome Bruner published an extremely influential paper called "Value and need as organizing factors in perception" (cited in Bruner, 1957). This paper presented evidence for what was then a fairly radical view: that values and needs determine how we perceive the world, down to the lowest levels of the visual system. As Bruner himself relates in a later review paper (Bruner, 1957), the "Value and need" essay caught on beyond expectations, inspiring about 300 experiments in the following decade, all of which showed that perception was infected through and through by perceivers' beliefs about the world and about the particular scene before them: hungry people were more likely to see food and to read food-related words, poor children systematically overestimate the size of coins relative to richer children, and anomalous or unexpected stimuli tend to be assimilated to their regular or expected counterparts.

Bruner's influential theory formed the basis of what became known as the "new look in perception," a movement that flourished in the 1960s and 1970s and continues to be influential even today in many areas of social science. According to this view, we perceive in conceptual categories. There is no such thing as a "raw" appearance or an "innocent eye": we see something *as* a chair or a table or a face or a particular person, and so on. As Bruner put it, "all perceptual experience is necessarily the end product of a categorization process," and therefore "perception is a process of categorization in which organisms move inferentially from cues to category identity and . . . in many cases, as Helmholtz long ago suggested, the process is a silent one." Perception, according to Bruner, is characterized by two essential properties: it is categorical, and it is inferential. Thus perception might be thought of as a form of problem solving in which part of the input happens to come in through the senses and part through needs, expectations, and beliefs, and in which the output is the category of the object being perceived. Because of this there is no essential distinction between the processes of perception and thought.[3]

This view opposed the earlier position that had been adopted by psychologists from as wide a perspective as structuralists (like Titchener, 1915), gestaltists (like Wallach, 1976), and even the early work of James J. Gibson (1966). Adherents of all these schools had accepted some sort of distinction between a pure stimulus event and a stimulus event that had interacted with past experience or, as it was sometimes put, between the "visual field" and the "visual world" or between perception and conception (or, as the latter was sometimes called, *apperception*—the process of assimilating perception to one's cognitive world). It would not be a misstatement to say that these thinkers accepted that there is a difference between appearances and beliefs, even though they would not have put it in those terms.

The new look fit well with the zeitgeist, which saw the organism as highly malleable by its environment, both in the short term and in the longer term (in the latter case this malleability was called "learning"). It was also a reaction against sense-data views of perception, views that had attained some currency with the structuralist and introspectionist schools of perception. Sense-data theories assumed that percepts were

3. Bruner (1957) characterized his claim as a "bold assumption" and was careful to avoid claiming that perception and thought were "utterly indistinguishable." In particular he explicitly recognized that perception "appear[s] to be notably less docile or reversible" than "conceptual inference." This lack of "docility" will play a central role in the present argument for the distinction between perception and cognition.

constructed out of more basic elements of experience called "sensations." Sensations were different in kind from percepts; they were not perceptual categories but the raw material of the senses. This version of perceptual atomism lost much of its popularity with the fall of the introspective method, as well as with the general disenchantment with perceptual atomism and the rise of Gestalt psychology. It seemed that basic perceptual atoms, especially ones that could be consciously sensed, were not to be had; perception was, as the gestalt psychologists would say, always greater than the sum of its more elementary parts. In this spirit, the field was ripe for a holistic all-encompassing theory of perception that integrated it into the general arena of induction and reasoning.

There were literally thousands of experiments performed from the 1950s through the present time showing that the perception of almost any pattern, from the perception of sentences in noise to the recognition of familiar stimuli at short exposures, could be influenced by observers' knowledge and expectations. Bruner cites evidence as far-ranging as findings from basic psychophysics to psycholinguistics and high level perception—including social perception. For example, Bruner cited evidence that magnitude estimation is sensitive to the response categories with which observers are provided, as well as to the anchor points and adaptation levels induced by the set of stimuli, and from this he concluded that cognitive context affects such simple psychophysical tasks as magnitude judgments. In the case of more complex patterns there is even more evidence for the effects of what Bruner calls "readiness" on perception. The recognition threshold for words decreases as the words become more familiar (Soloman and Postman, 1952). The exposure time required to report a string of letters shown in the flash-exposure instrument known as the tachistoscope, which was becoming extremely popular in psychology laboratories at that time, varies with the predictability of the string (Miller, Bruner, and Postman, 1954): random strings (such as YRULPZOC) require a longer exposure for recognition than strings whose sequential statistics approximate those of English text (such as VERNALIT, which is a nonword string constructed by sampling 4-letter strings from a corpus of English text); the greater the order of approximation to the statistical properties of English text, the shorter the exposure required for recognition. The level of background noise at which listeners can still recognize a word is higher if that word is part of a sentence (where it can be predicted more easily) or even if it occurs in a list of words whose order statistically approximates English (Miller, 1962). More generally, words in sentences can be recognized more easily and in more adverse conditions that can words alone or in random lists.

Similar results were found in the case of nonlinguistic stimuli. For example, the exposure duration required to correctly recognize an anomalous playing card (e.g., a black ace of hearts) is higher than the time required to recognize a normal card (Bruner and Postman, 1949). Also, as in letter and word recognition, the perceptual thresholds reflect the likelihood of occurrence of the stimuli in a particular context and even their significance to the observer (the latter being illustrated by studies of so-called "perceptual defense," in which pictures previously associated with shock show elevated recognition thresholds). The reconstruction of partially occluded figures was also taken as showing that vision makes use of knowledge to restore familiar shapes, as in the "New York" example in figure 1.4.

The results of these experiments were explained in terms of the accessibility of perceptual categories and the hypothesize-and-test nature of perception (where the "hypotheses" can come from any source, including immediate context, memory, and general knowledge). There were also experiments that investigated the hypothesize-and-test view more directly. One way this was done was by manipulating the "availability" of perceptual hypotheses. For example, Bruner and Minturn (1955) manipulated what they called the "readiness" of the hypothesis that stimuli were numbers as opposed to being letters (by varying the context in which the experiment was run), and found that ambiguous number-letter patterns (e.g., a "B" with gaps so that it could equally be a "13") were reported more often as shapes congruous with the preset hypothesis. Also if a subject settles on a false perceptual hypothesis in impoverished conditions (e.g., with an unfocused picture), then the perception of the same stimulus is impaired, so it takes longer or requires a better display before a figure is correctly recognized when it is first presented unfocused. When subjects make incorrect guesses as the focus is gradually improved, they eventually perform worse in comparison with when they do not make a false hypotheses (Bruner and Potter, 1964; Wyatt and Pola, 1979).

Because of these and other types of experiments showing contextual effects in perception, the belief that perception is thoroughly contaminated by such cognitive factors as expectations, judgments, beliefs, and so on, became the received wisdom in much of psychology, with virtually all contemporary elementary texts in human information processing and vision taking that point of view for granted (Lindsay and Norman, 1977; Sekuler and Blake, 1994). The continuity view also became widespread within philosophy of science. Thomas Kuhn (1972) gathered a cult following with his view of scientific revolutions, in which theory change was seen as guided more by social considerations than by new data. The explanation was that theoretical notions in different theories are essentially incommensurable, and so evidence itself is contaminated by the theoretical systems within which scientists worked. Philosophers of science like Feyerabend (1962) and Hanson (1958) argued that there was no such thing as objective observation, since every observation was what they called "theory laden." These scholars frequently cited the new-look experiments showing cognitive influences on perception to support their views. Mid-nineteenth-century philosophy of science welcomed the new all-encompassing holistic view of perception that integrated it into the general framework of induction and reasoning.

2.2.2 The perspective of neuroscience

During the heyday of the new look (in the 1960s and the 1970s), speculative neuropsychology, such as the influential work of the Canadian psychologist Donald Hebb, was in general sympathy with the interactionist view (see Hebb, 1949). However, the important discovery of single-cell receptive fields and the hierarchy of simple, complex, and hypercomplex cells (Hubel and Wiesel, 1962) gave rise to the opposing idea that perception involves a hierarchical process in which larger and more complex aggregates are constructed from more elementary features. In fact, the hierarchical organization of the early-vision pathways sometimes encouraged an extreme hierarchical view of visual processing in which the recognition of familiar objects by master cells was assumed to follow from a succession of categorizations by cells lower in the hierarchy. This idea seems to have been implicit in some neuroscience theorizing, even when it was not explicitly endorsed. Of course, such an assumption is not warranted by the mere existence of cells that responded to more and more abstract properties, since any number of processes, including inference, could in fact intervene between the sensors and the high-level pattern-neurons.

There were some early attempts to show that some top-down or centripetal influences (i.e., from higher brain regions to sensors) also occurred in the nervous system. For example, Hernandez-Péon, Scherrer, and Jouvet (1956) showed that the auditory response in a cat's cochlear nucleus (the first neural way station from the ear) was attenuated when the cat was paying attention to some interesting visual stimulus. More recently, the notion of *focal attention* has begun to play a more important role in behavioral-neuroscience theorizing, and some evidence has been obtained showing that the activity of early parts of the visual system can indeed be influenced by selective attention (e.g., Haenny and Schiller, 1988; Moran and Desimone, 1985; Mountcastle et al., 1987; Sillito et al., 1994; van Essen and Anderson, 1990). There is even recent evidence that attention can have long-term effects as well as transitory ones (Desimone, 1996). Some writers (e.g., Churchland, 1988) have argued that the presence of outgoing (centripetal) nerve fibers running from higher cortical centers to the visual cortex constitutes prima facie evidence that vision must be susceptible to cognitive influences. However, the role of the centripetal fibers remains unknown except where it has been shown that they are concerned with the allocation of attention. I will argue later that allocation of focal attention is indeed a principal means by which top-down effects can occur in vision, but that these do not constitute cognitive penetration.

What the evidence shows is that attention can selectively sensitize or gate certain regions of the visual field as well as certain stimulus properties. Even if such effects ultimately originate from "higher" centers, they constitute one form of influence that I claim is prior to the operation of early vision—in particular, they constitute an attentional selection of relevant properties. By and large, the neuroscience community (at least since the influential work of neurocomputationalist David Marr) is now interested in how the visual system decomposes into separate modules and is comfortable with the idea that vision itself is far less dependent on cognition than assumed by the more behavioral psychologists of the same era. I will look at some of the evidence considered relevant to this newer perspective in section 2.3 below.

2.2.3   The perspective of robot vision

Another line of support for the idea that vision implicates reasoning and memory comes from the field of artificial intelligence, or computer vision, where the goal has been to design systems that can "see" or exhibit visual capacities of some specified type. The approach of trying to design systems (i.e., robots) that can see well enough to identify objects or to navigate through an unknown environment using visual information has the virtue of at least posing a clear problem to be solved. In computer vision the goal is to design a system that is *sufficient* to the task of exhibiting properties we associate with visual perception. The sufficiency condition on a theory is an extremely useful constraint, since it forces one to consider possible mechanisms that could accomplish certain parts of the task. Thus it behooves the vision researcher to consider the problems that computer-vision designers have run into, as well as some of the proposed solutions that have been explored. And indeed, modern vision researchers have paid close attention to work on computer vision and vice versa. Consequently, it is not too surprising that the history of computer vision closely parallels the history of ideas concerning human vision.

Apart from some reasonably successful early "model-based" vision systems capable of recognizing simple polyhedral (block-shaped) objects when the scene was restricted to only such objects (Roberts, 1965), most early approaches to computer vision were of the data-driven or so-called "bottom-up" variety. They took elementary optical features as their starting point and attempted to build more complex aggregates, leading eventually to the categorization of the pattern. Many of these hierarchical models were statistical pattern-recognition systems inspired by ideas from biology, including Rosenblatt's Perceptron (Rosenblatt, 1959), Uttley's Conditional Probability Computer (Uttley, 1959), and Selfridge's Pandemonium (Selfridge, 1959).

In the 1960s and 1970s a great deal of the research effort in computer vision went into the development of various "edge-finding" schemes in order to extract reliable features to use as a starting point for object recognition and scene analysis (Clowes, 1971). Despite this effort, the edge finders were not nearly as successful as they needed to be if they were to serve as the primary inputs to subsequent analysis and identification stages. The problem is that if a uniform intensity-gradient threshold is used as a criterion for the existence of edges in the image, it invariably results in one of two undesirable situations. If the threshold is set low, it leads to the extraction of a large number of features that corresponded to shadows, lighting and reflectance variations, noise, or other luminance differences unrelated to the existence of real edges in the scene. On the other hand, if the threshold is set higher, then many real scene edges clearly perceptible by human vision are missed. This dilemma led to attempts to guide the edge finders into more promising image locations or to vary the edge threshold according to whether an edge was more likely at those locations than at other places in the image.

The idea of guiding local edge-finding operators using knowledge of the scene domain may have marked the beginning of attempts to design what are known as knowledge-based vision systems. At MIT the slogan "heterarchy, not hierarchy" (Winston, 1974) was coined to highlight the view that there had to be context-dependent influences from domain knowledge, in addition to local image features such as intensity discontinuities. Guided line-finders were designed, e.g., by Kelly (1971) and Shirai (1975) based on this approach. The idea that knowledge is needed at every level to recognize objects was strongly endorsed by Freuder (1986) in his proposal for a system that would use a great deal of specialized knowledge about certain objects (e.g., a hammer) in order to recognize these objects in a scene. Riseman and Hanson also took a strong position on this issue, claiming, "It appears that human vision is fundamentally organized to exploit the use of contextual knowledge and expectations in the organization of visual primitives. . . . Thus the inclusion of knowledge-driven processes at some level in the image interpretation task, where there is still a great degree of ambiguity in the organization of the visual primitives, appears inevitable" (1987, p. 286). Indeed, a rather heated debate ensued between supporters of the bottom-up view (Clowes, 1971), which utilized line-finders in the initial stage of processing, and those who believed that vision systems would have to be heavily knowledge-based all the way down (Michie, 1986).

The knowledge-based approach is generally conceded to be essential for developing high-performance computer-vision systems using current technology. Indeed, virtually all currently successful automatic-vision systems for robotics or for such applications as analyzing medical images or automated manufacturing are model-based (e.g., Grimson, 1990); that is, their analysis of images is guided by some stored model of possible objects that could occur in the input scene. Although some model-based systems neither use general knowledge nor draw inferences, they fall in the knowledge-based category because they quite explicitly use knowledge about particular objects in deciding whether a scene contains instances of those objects.[4] In addition, it is widely held that the larger the domain over which the vision system must operate, the less likely that a single type of stored information will allow reliable recognition. This is because, in the general case, the incoming data are too voluminous, noisy, incomplete, and intrinsically ambiguous to allow univocal analysis. Consequently, so the argument goes, a computer-vision system must make use of many different domain "experts," or sources of knowledge at various levels of organization and concerning different aspects of the input domain, from knowledge of optics to knowledge of the most likely properties to be found in the particular domain being visually examined.

The knowledge-based approach has also been exploited in a variety of speech-recognition systems. For example, the early speech-recognition systems developed at BBN Technologies (Woods, 1978) (known as SPEECHLIS or HWIM, for "Hear What I Mean") is strongly knowledge-based. Woods has argued for the generality of this approach and has suggested that it is equally appropriate in the case of vision. HEARSAY (described by Reddy, 1975) and Harpy (described by Newell, 1980a), two speech-recognition systems developed at Carnegie-Mellon University, also use multiple sources of knowledge and introduced a general scheme for bringing knowledge to bear in the recognition process. These speech-recognition systems use a so-called blackboard architecture, in which a common working memory is shared by a number of "expert" processes, each of which contributes a certain kind

4. An alternative, which is sometimes also referred to as a "model-based" approach, that uses some form of "general purpose" model of objects (Lowe, 1987; Zucker, Rosenfeld, and David, 1975)—or even of parts of such object (Biederman, 1987)—does not fall into this category because the models are not selected on the basis of expectations about the particular situation being observed (where the latter depends on what the observer knows and believes). This type of constrained perception falls into the category of "natural constraint" approaches that will be discussed in chapter 3.

of knowledge to the perceptual analysis. Each knowledge source contributes "hypotheses" as to the correct identification of the speech signal, based on its area of expertise. Thus, for example, the acoustic expert, the phonetic expert, the syntactic expert, the semantic expert (which knows about the subject matter of the speech), and the pragmatic expert (which knows about discourse conventions) each propose the most likely interpretation of a certain fragment of the input signal. The final analysis is a matter of negotiation among these experts. What is important here is the assumption that the architecture (the relatively fixed structural properties of the system) permits any relevant source of knowledge to contribute to the recognition process at every stage. This general scheme has also been used as the basis for vision systems, such as those developed by Freuder (1986) and Riseman and Hanson (1987). Figure 2.1, which shows the structure of such a system (showing both speech and vision experts), illustrates how each expert can give and receive input at any stage in the analysis, thus making for a completely open system.

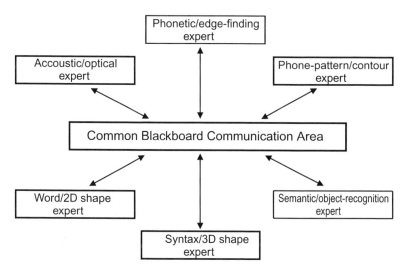

Figure 2.1
Sketch of the "blackboard architecture" used by the HEARSAY speech understanding system, as well as by some computer vision systems. In this architecture each "expert" process can communicate with every other process, so the information flow is unconstrained, in contrast to a modular style of architecture advocated in this chapter.

The idea of complete freedom of communication among different "experts" (through the common "blackboard") received wide recognition in many areas of psychology and artificial intelligence. In fact, it was for a time the received wisdom for how such pattern recognizers as systems for reading text might be organized. A popular idea, closely related to the blackboard architecture, was based fairly directly on Selfridge's Pandemonium idea, in which various experts competed for the attention of an executive decision maker, as illustrated in figure 2.2 in a popular text on human information processing (Lindsay and Norman, 1977).

While it is true that computational systems that make use of knowledge do better than ones that do not, I will argue later that one needs to distinguish between systems that access and use knowledge, such as those just mentioned, and systems that have constraints on interpretation built into them that reflect certain properties of the world. The latter embody an important form of "visual intelligence" that is perfectly compatible with the independence thesis and will be discussed in chapter 3.

2.2.4   Seeing and knowing: Where do we stand?

The experimental and informal psychological evidence in favor of the idea that vision involves the entire cognitive system appears to be so ubiquitous that you might wonder how anyone could possibly believe that vision is separate and distinct from cognition. The answer, I claim, lies not in denying the evidence that shows the importance of knowledge for visual apprehension (although in some cases we will need to reconsider the evidence itself), but in making certain distinctions. It is clear that what we believe about the world we are looking at does depend on what we know and expect. In that sense we can easily be deceived, as in magic tricks. But as I noted earlier, seeing is not the same as believing, the old adage notwithstanding. To understand visual perception, it is essential to distinguish certain stages in the process—in particular a stage, which I call *early vision* (after David Marr and other vision scientists), that is prohibited from accessing relevant knowledge of the world or of the particular scene—and other stages that are permitted, or in some cases are even required by the nature of the task (e.g., recognizing a familiar face), to access such knowledge. The knowledge-dependent (or cognitively penetrable) stages include a *preperceptual*

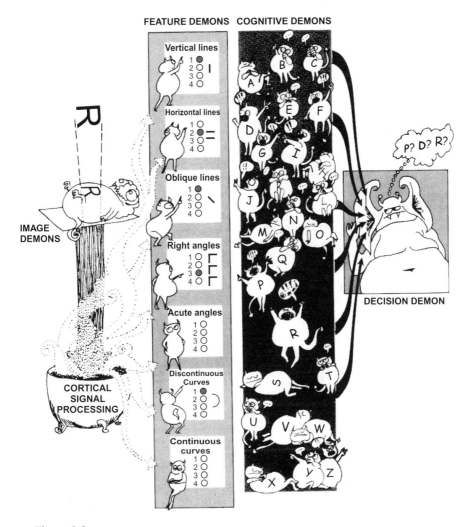

Figure 2.2
A caricature of the "Pandemonium" style of processing, proposed by Selfridge (1959), in which "demons" specializing in various aspects of the recognition problem compete for recognition by a master "decision demon." In this example this idea is applied to the problem of recognizing printed text. (From Lindsay and Norman, 1977.)

stage, wherein vision is directed at relevant places or objects in a scene, and a *postperceptual stage*, in which memory is accessed and judgments are made about what is in the scene. The idea of drawing a sharp distinction between visual perception and cognition, or between stages of visual perception, has been anathema to much of psychology and contemporary scholarship in general, although Fodor (1983) has done much to revive its popularity. In what follows, I will suggest some reasons why such a distinction is empirically justified.

2.3 Some Reasons for Questioning the Continuity Thesis

Before getting into the details of some methodological and experimental findings supporting the thesis that a major part of the visual process is cognitively impenetrable, I provide a brief summary of why I believe this to be the case despite the sorts of evidence already sketched. Here are four general reasons why it makes sense to consider the possibility that there is a principled demarcation between early vision and cognition.

2.3.1 Evidence of the cognitive impenetrability of illusions
As Bruner himself noted (see note 3): perception appears to be rather resistant to rational influence. It is a remarkable fact about the perceptual illusions that knowing about them does not make them disappear: Even after you have had a good look at the Ames room—perhaps even built it yourself—it still looks as though the person on one side is much bigger than the one the other side (Ittelson and Ames, 1968). Knowing that you measured two lines to be exactly equal does not make them look equal when arrowheads are added to them to form the Müller-Lyer illusion, or when a background of converging perspective lines are added to form the Ponzo illusion, as shown in figure 2.3.

For another example in which the visual system's internal mechanisms override your knowledge, consider the tables in figure 2.4. Which of the top faces of tables A or C is identical in size and shape (except for being rotated) to face B? If you check using a ruler or by cutting the figures out of paper, you will find that the face labeled A is identical to the face labeled B, while C is quite different. Notice that such illusions are not just stubborn, in the way some people appear unwilling to change their

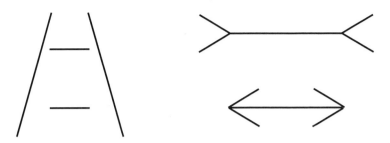

Figure 2.3
Illustrations of the Ponzo illusion (on the left) and the Müller-Lyer illusion (on the right). In both cases the horizontal lines above one another are the same length.

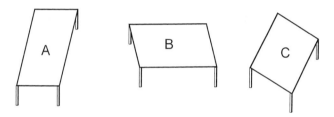

Figure 2.4
Which of these figures has the same top face as B, except for rotation (A or C)? The problem is made difficult in this case because you cannot suppress the automatic interpretation of certain figures as three-dimensional objects, even if you try.

minds in the face of contrary evidence: it is simply impossible to make something look to you the way you know it really is. What is noteworthy is not that there are perceptual illusions; it is that in these cases there is a very clear separation between what you see and what you know is actually there—what you believe. What you believe depends on how knowledgeable you are, what other sources of information you have, what your utilities are (what's important to you at the moment), how motivated you are to figure out how you might have been misled, and so on. Yet how things look to you appears to be impervious to any such factors, even when what you know is both relevant to what you are looking at and at variance with how you see it. Later in section 2.5, I will examine (and reject) claims that certain kinds of illusions (e.g.,

reversals of ambiguous figures and perceptual closure of difficult percepts) are susceptible to cognitive influences.

2.3.2 Independence of principles of visual organization and principles of inference

Many regularities in visual perception—some of them highly complex
and subtle—are automatic, depend only on the visual input, and often
follow principles quite different from the principles of rational reasoning. These principles of perception differ from the principles of inference
in two ways.

First, unlike the principles of inference, perceptual principles are
responsive only to visually presented information. One way to think of
the difference between visual representations and thoughts is to think of
the representations that occur within the visual system as being in a
proprietary vocabulary, distinct from the vocabulary that occurs in
representations of thoughts and beliefs. This vocabulary encodes such
perceived properties as which regions of a scene go together as a single
object, which contours go with which surfaces, which surfaces partially
occlude other surfaces, and so on. Perceptual principles specify how
certain encoded properties (or "scene labels") go with other encoded
properties. In computer vision, a major part of early vision is concerned
with what is called *scene labeling* or *label-propagation* (Chakravarty,
1979; Rosenfeld, Hummel, and Zucker, 1976), wherein principles
of label consistency are applied to represented features in a scene to
compute the correct labeling (we will see examples of this sort of labeling in the next chapter, pp. 99–106). Principles of visual interpretation
explain why it is that how you perceive one aspect of a visual scene determines how you perceive another aspect of the scene. When a percept of
an ambiguous figure (like a Necker Cube) reverses, a variety of properties (such as the perceived relative size and luminance of the faces) appear
to automatically change together to maintain a coherent percept, even if
it means a percept of an impossible 3-D object, as in Escher drawings.
Such intravisual regularities have been referred to as "perceptual couplings" (Epstein, 1982; Rock, 1997). Gogel (1997/1973) attempted to
capture some of these regularities in what he called *perceptual equations.*
Such equations provide no role for what the perceiver knows or expects,
because the perception of visual form is *not* sensitive to the beliefs that

perceivers have about what the scene being examined *should* look like, given what they know about the circumstances of that scene. The question of why certain principles (or equations) should be embodied in our visual systems is one that can only be answered by examining the function that vision has served in allowing organisms to survive in our kind of world. The particular equations or couplings may be understood in relation to the organism's needs and the nature of world it typically inhabits (see chapter 3 for a discussion of perceptual coupling; a more extensive discussion of the notion of *natural constraints* is provided on p. 94).

Second, the principles of visual organization are quite different from those of logical inference and often do not appear to conform to what might be thought of as tenets of "rationality." Particularly revealing examples of the difference between the organizing principles of vision and the principles of inference are to be found in the phenomenon of "amodal completion." This phenomenon, first studied by Michotte, refers to the fact that partially occluded figures are not perceived as the fragments of figures that are actually in view, but as whole figures that are partially hidden from view behind the occluder (a distinction that is phenomenally quite striking). It is as though the visual system "completes" the missing part of the figure, yet the completed portion, though it is constructed by the mind, has real perceptual consequences (see figure 1.6). The form taken by an amodal completion (the shape that is "completed" or amodally perceived to be behind the occluder) follows complex principles of its own—principles that are generally not rational principles, such as semantic coherence or even something like maximum likelihood. As Kanizsa (1985) and Kanizsa and Gerbino (1982) have persuasively argued, these principles do not appear to reflect a tendency for the simplest description of the world, and they are insensitive to knowledge and expectations, even to the effects of learning (Kanizsa, 1969). For example, figure 2.5 shows a case of amodal completion in which the visual system constructs a complex and asymmetrical completed shape rather than the simple octagon, despite the presence of the adjacent examples. In this and very many other such examples (many are discussed by Kanizsa in the papers cited) the figure chosen is not the *simplest* one, but rather one that conforms to some special principle that applies to local regions of the image. It is precisely because of this that

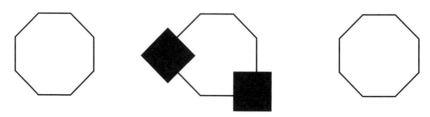

Figure 2.5
Illustration of "amodal completion." What is the shape of the figure partly hidden by the squares in the middle panel? The completion preferred by the visual system is not the simplest figure despite the flanking examples of simple figures. (After Kanizsa, 1985.)

there are visual illusions; the visual system *cannot* ignore its wired-in geometrical principles in favor of what the perceiver knows to be true.[5]

2.3.3 Neuroscience evidence for top-down attenuation and gating of visual signals

On pp. 56–57, I mentioned the existence of top-down neural pathways in vision. I also pointed out that the primary function of these pathways appears to be to allow attention to selectively sensitize or gate certain objects or regions of the visual field, as well as certain physical properties of the stimuli. Even if such effects ultimately originate from "higher" centers, they constitute a form of influence that I claimed was prior to the operation of early vision—that is, they constitute an early attentional selection of relevant properties.

Where both neurophysiological and psychophysical data show top-down effects, they do so most clearly in cases where the modulating signal originates *within* the visual system itself (roughly identified with

5. Of course, if the principles by which vision constructs a representation of the world were totally capricious we would find ourselves walking into walls and generally not faring well in our commerce with the world. So the principles must be ones that more often than not yield a true description of the world in typical situations, even if they do it not by rational inferential means, but by virtue of local geometrical principles. We will return to this point (in ch. 3), referred to as the tendency of the visual system to embody *natural constraints*, since this is an important general principle that explains why vision, which is insensitive to knowledge and processes of rational inference, nevertheless manages to solve visual problems mostly the way they need to be solved for the purposes of survival.

the visual cortex, as mapped out, say, by Felleman and Van Essen, 1991). There are two major forms of modulation, however, that appear to originate from outside the visual system. The first is one to which I have already alluded—modulation associated with focal attention, which can originate either from events in the world that automatically attract attention (exogenous control) or from voluntary cognitive sources (endogenous control). The second form of extravisual effect is the modulation of certain cortical cells by signals originating in both visual and motor systems. A large proportion of the cells in the posterior parietal cortex, and in what Ungerleider and Mishkin (1982) identified as the dorsal stream of the visual or visuomotor pathway, are activated jointly by specific visual patterns together with specific undertaken (or anticipated) behaviors that are related to these visual patterns (see the extensive discussion in Milner and Goodale, 1995, as well as the review in Lynch, 1980). There is now a great deal of evidence suggesting that the dorsal system is specialized for what Milner and Goodale (1995) call "vision for action." What has not been reported, to my knowledge, is comparable evidence to suggest that cells in any part of the visual system (and particularly the ventral stream that appears to be specialized for recognition) can be modulated similarly by higher-level cognitive influences. While there are cells that respond to such highly complex patterns as a face, and some of these may even be viewpoint-independent (i.e., object-centered) (Perrett, Mistlin, and Chitty, 1987), there is no evidence that such cells are modulated by nonvisual information about the identity of the face (e.g., whether it was the face expected in a certain situation). More general activation of the visual system by voluntary cognitive activity has been demonstrated by PET and fMRI studies (Kosslyn, 1994), but no clearly content-specific modulations of patterns of activity have been shown (i.e., there is no evidence for patterns of activity particular to certain *interpretations* of visual inputs), as it has in the case of motor-system modulation (I will take up this topic again in chapter 7).

At issue is not the visual complexity of the class to which the cell responds, nor whether the cell is modulated in a top-down manner, but whether or not the cell responds to how a visual pattern is *interpreted*, where the latter depends on what the organism knows or expects. If vision were cognitively penetrable, one might expect there to be cells that respond to certain interpretation-specific perceptions. In that case whether or not some cell responds to a certain visual pattern would appear to be governed by the cognitive system in a way that reflects how the pattern is conceptualized or understood.[6] Studies of macaque monkeys by Perrett and his colleagues suggest that cells in the temporal cortex respond only to the *visual* character of the stimulus and not to its cognitively determined (or conceptual) interpretation. For example, Perrett et al. (1990) describe cells that fire to the visual event of an experimenter "leaving the room"—and not to comparable experimenter movements that are not directed towards the door. Such cells clearly encode a complex class of events (perhaps involving the relational property "towards the door"), which the authors refer to as a "goal centered" encoding. However, they found no cells whose firing was modulated by what they call the "significance" of the event. The cells appear to fire equally no matter what the event means to the monkey. As Perrett et al. put it, "The particular significance of long-term disappearance of an experimenter . . . varies with the circumstances. Usually leaving is of no consequence, but sometimes leaving may provoke disappointment and isolation calls, other times it provokes threats. It would . . . appear that [for the firing of certain cells] it is the visual event of leaving the laboratory that is important, rather than any emotional or behavioral response. In general, cells in the temporal cortex appear to code visual objects and events independent of emotional consequences and the resulting behavior" (1990, p. 195). In terms of the present thesis, I would say that although what such cells encode may be complex, it is not sensitive to the cognitive context.

6. Changes in attenuation or sensitivity can result in different percepts. Whether or not this constitutes cognitive penetration depends on two things: (a) what kinds of perceptual changes can be underwritten by changing activation levels and (b) whether the particular changes can be attributed to appropriate differences in the contents of beliefs and expectations. As for (a), it is dubious that the sort of influence that allows people to see a word whose meaning is predicted from the context, to see monsters when they are afraid, or to see food when they are hungry (as claimed by the New Look school), can be supported by differences in attenuation or sensitivity (see the discussion of this issue in ch. 4). But (b) is even more germane because it matters whether the influence comes from within the visual system or from outside. We know that how you interpret a certain portion of an image depends on how you interpret other parts of the image. Such intravisual effects do not constitute cognitive penetration. Unfortunately, the neuroanatomical data do not cast light on that question.

2.3.4   Evidence of dissociation of visual and cognitive functions in the brain

One intriguing source of evidence that vision can be separated from cognition comes from the study of pathologies of brain function that demonstrate dissociations among various aspects of vision and cognition. Even when, as frequently happens, no clear lesion can be identified, the pattern of deficits can provide evidence of certain dissociations and co-occurrences of skill components. They thus constitute at least initial evidence for the taxonomy of cognitive skills. The discovery that particular skill components can be dissociated from other skill components (particularly if there is evidence of a double-dissociation in which each component occurs without the other), provides a prima facie reason to believe that these skills might constitute independent systems.

Consider the example of visual agnosia, a rather rare family of visual dysfunctions in which a patient is often unable to recognize formerly familiar objects or patterns. In these cases (many of which are reviewed in Farah, 1990) there is typically no impairment in sensory, intellectual, or naming abilities. A remarkable case of classical visual agnosia is described in a book by Glyn Humphreys and Jane Riddoch (1987). After suffering a stroke that resulted in bilateral damage to his occipital lope, the patient was unable to recognize familiar objects, including faces of people well-known to him (e.g., his wife), and found it difficult to discriminate among simple shapes, despite the fact that he did not exhibit any intellectual deficit. As is typical in visual agnosias, this patient showed no purely sensory deficits, showed normal eye-movement patterns, and appeared to have close-to-normal stereoscopic depth and motion perception. Despite the severity of his visual impairment, the patient could perform many other visual and object-recognition tasks. For example, even though he could not recognize an object in its entirety, he could recognize its features and could describe and even draw the object quite well—either when it was in view or from memory. Because he recognized the component features, he often could figure out what the object was by a process of deliberate problem solving, much as the continuity theory claims occurs in normal perception, except that for this patient it was a painstakingly slow process. From the fact that he could describe and copy objects from memory and could recognize objects quite well by touch, it appears that there was no deficit in his memory for shape. These deficits seem to point to a dissociation between the ability to recognize an object (from different sources of information) and the ability to compute from visual inputs an integrated pattern that can serve as the basis for recognition. As Humphreys and Riddoch put it, this patient's pattern of deficits "supports the view that 'perceptual' and 'recognition' processes are separable, because his stored knowledge required for recognition is intact," and inasmuch as recognition involves a process of somehow matching perceptual information against stored memories, this case also "supports the view that the perceptual representation used in this matching process can be 'driven' solely by stimulus information, so that it is unaffected by contextual knowledge" (1987, p. 104).

It appears that in this patient the earliest stages in perception—those involving computing contours and simple shape features—are spared. So is the ability to look up shape information in memory in order to recognize objects. What, then, is damaged? It appears that an intermediate stage of "integration" of visual features fails to function as it should. The pattern of dissociation shows that an intact capacity to extract features, together with the capacity to recognize objects from shape information, is insufficient for visual recognition so long as the unique visual capacity for integration is absent. But "integration," according to the new-look (or Helmholtzian) view of perception, comes down to no more than making inferences from basic shape features—a capacity that appears to be spared.

2.3.5 Evidence that cognitive penetration occurs in pre- and postperceptual stages

Finally, there are methodological questions that can be raised in connection with the interpretation of empirical evidence favoring the continuity thesis. There are certain methodological arguments favoring the view that the observed effects of expectations, beliefs, and so on, while real enough, operate primarily on a stage of processing after what I have called early vision (some of these are summarized in the next section, but they are treated at greater length in Pylyshyn, 1999). Thus the effect of knowledge can often be traced to a locus subsequent to the operation of vision proper—a stage where decisions are made as to the category of the stimulus or its function or its relation to past perceptual experiences.

There is also evidence that in other cases where beliefs and past experience appear to influence what we see, such as in perceptual learning and in the effect of "hints" on the perception of certain ambiguous stimuli, the cognitive effect may be traced to a preperceptual stage in which the perceiver learns to allocate attention to different features or places in a stimulus. Both these cases are briefly reviewed in the next section.

2.4   Distinguishing Perceptual and Decision Stages: Some Methodological Issues

Some of the arguments among researchers concerning whether early vision is cognitively penetrable or encapsulated rest on certain considerations of experimental methodology. The question of whether vision is encapsulated might be approached by trying to divide visual processing into stages, for example, a stage that might correspond to what I have called early vision and a stage that is concerned with making decisions about what the stimulus was and what response to make to it. Such distinctions raise questions of experimental method: given that context affects how observers respond to a stimulus, how does one tell whether this is because the context affects how they see it, what they recognize it to be (i.e., what they see it as), how they classify it in relation to things they have seen before, or what they decide to do in a particular experimental context (i.e., what response they decide to make)? The attempt to distinguish such stages has a venerable history in the study of perception, going back to the earliest days of experimental psychology. The question received a major impetus in the 1950s with the development of such theoretical instruments as signal-detection theory (SDT) and the use of certain patterns of electrical potentials on the scalp (called event-related potentials, or ERPs) and other techniques for dividing the information process into stages and for determining which stage is responsible for certain observed phenomena.

Quite early in the study of sensory processes it was known that some aspects of perceptual activity involve decisions, whereas others do not. Bruner (1957) himself even cites research using the newly developed technique of signal-detection theory (Tanner and Swets, 1954) in support of the conclusion that psychophysical functions involve decisions. What Bruner glossed over, however, is that the work on signal-detection analysis not only shows that decisions are involved in such psychophysical tasks as threshold measurements; it also shows that such tasks typically involve at least two stages, one of which, sometimes called "stimulus detection," is immune from cognitive influences, while the other, sometimes called "response selection," is not. In principle, the theory provides a way to separate these two stages and to assign independent performance measures to them: To a first approximation, detection is characterized by a sensitivity measure, usually denoted as d', while response selection is characterized by a response bias or response criterion measure, denoted as β. Only the second of these measures was thought to capture the decision aspect of certain psychophysical tasks, and therefore, according to this view, it is the only part of the process that ought to be sensitive to knowledge and utilities.

The idea of factoring visual information processing into roughly a stimulus-processing stage and a response-selection stage inspired a large number of experiments directed at "stage analysis" using a variety of methodologies in addition to signal-detection theory, including the "additive-factors method" (Sternberg, 1969), such techniques as the "attention operating characteristic" (Sperling and Melchner, 1978), event-related potentials (ERPs), and other methods devised for specific situations. Numerous experiments have shown that certain kinds of cognitive malleability observed in experiments on perception is due primarily to the second of these stages—the stage at which a response decision is made (Samuel, 1981). But not all the results support this conclusion; a few studies have also shown that stages prior to response selection are also changed by changes in expectations (i.e., by the cognitive context). When I began a review of techniques for analyzing information processing into stages (which led to the analysis presented in Pylyshyn, 1999), I had hoped that these techniques would allow us to separate those effects attributable to the perceptual stage from those attributable to subsequent decision stages. This goal was only partly achieved, however, because it turned out that the stages distinguished by these techniques are too coarse for this purpose and do not correspond exactly to the distinction relevant to the independence thesis. What the techniques are able to show is that certain influences, sometimes taken to demonstrate the cognitive penetration of vision, have their locus in the selection of a response and in the preparation of an actual overt response.

When the effect is found to lie outside the response-selection stage, however, the methods are unable to distinguish whether this occurs in what I have been calling early vision or in some other part of the information-processing stream. There is clearly much more going on in perception than detecting a stimulus followed by the preparation of a response. For example, apart from various shape and surface computations, there is the *recognition* of the stimulus pattern as one that has been seen before. Since this sort of recognition (seeing the stimulus *as* something familiar) inherently involves accessing memory, it falls outside what I call early vision, and yet it is not a case of preparing an actual response. Thus the use of such methods as those of signal detection theory and ERPs provides an asymmetrical test of the cognitive penetrability of vision. Showing that the effect of changing beliefs or expectations operates entirely at the response-selection stage (i.e., that it affects β but not d') shows that in this case the belief change does not influence early vision. On the other hand, showing that the effect operates at the so-called stimulus-detection stage (or operates by influencing the sensitivity measure d' and not β) does *not* show that early vision is cognitively penetrable, because the detection stage includes more than just early vision.

The problem with all the techniques of stage analysis that have so far been proposed is this: Whether the technique is simple or sophisticated, it usually ends up distinguishing a stage of response preparation from everything else concerned with processing visual information. But that distinction is too coarse for our purposes if our concern is whether an intervention affects the visual process or the postperceptual recognition-inference-decision-response process. To determine whether early vision is cognitively penetrable, one needs to make further distinctions within what stage-theorists call the stimulus-detection or stimulus-evaluation stage. In particular, one needs to factor out functions such as categorization and identification, which require accessing general memory, from functions of early vision, such as individuating objects and computing spatial relations among them, which, by hypothesis, do not. That is why we find, not surprisingly, that some apparently visual tasks are sensitive to what the observer knows, since the identification of a stimulus clearly requires both inferences and access to memory and knowledge. (A more detailed technical discussion of this claim is provided in

Pylyshyn, 1999, and the reader who is interested in the underlying assumptions is invited to consult that paper.)

2.5   Some Examples in Which Knowledge Is Claimed to Affect Perception

2.5.1   "Intelligent" interpretations of inherently ambiguous information

A number of writers (Gregory, 1970; Rock, 1983) have noted that the visual system delivers unique interpretations of visual (optical) information that is inherently ambiguous, and that when it does so, it invariably produces an interpretation that is "intelligent" in that it appears to take into account certain cues in a way that suggests that, to use an anthropomorphic phrase, "it knows how things in the world work." These examples are indeed among the most interesting cases to consider from the perspective of the independence thesis, both because they constitute impressive demonstrations of smart vision and also because they provided major challenges to theories of computer vision as well as led to some of its most impressive successes. The successes followed the seminal work of David Marr (1982) and are based on the discovery of certain constraints inherent in the visual system (so-called "natural constraints"). Because of the importance and far-reaching implications of this idea, I will postpone this discussion until the next chapter, where I consider the nature of the "architecture," or relatively fixed structural properties of the visual system.

2.5.2   Experience and hints in perceiving ambiguous figures and stereograms

So far I have suggested that many cases of apparent penetration of visual perception by cognition are either cases of top-down effects occurring within the visual system (discussed on pp. 68–70) or cases in which knowledge and utilities are brought to bear at the preperceptual stage (by determining where to focus attention) or at the postperceptual stage (by determining which possible interpretation provided by early vision to favor). But there are some alleged cases of penetration that, at least on the face of it, do not seem to fall into either of these categories. One is the apparent effect of hints, instructions, and other knowledge contexts on the ability to resolve certain ambiguities or to achieve a stable percept in certain difficult-to-perceive stimuli. A number of such cases have been reported, though these have generally been based on informal observations rather than on controlled experiments. Examples include so-called fragmented figures (such as figure 2.6 or figure 2.7), ambiguous figures, and stereograms, including the famous Magic Eye™ posters that show 3D images based on what are known as autostereograms. I will now suggest that these apparent counterexamples, though they may sometimes be phenomenally persuasive (and indeed have persuaded many vision researchers), are not sustained by careful experimental scrutiny.

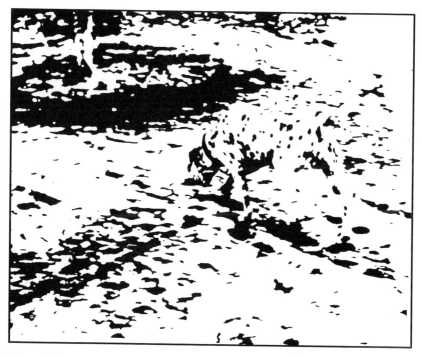

Figure 2.6
A famous picture of a Dalmatian dog, by Ronald C. James, which usually appears suddenly as a clear percept (from Carraher and Thurston, 1996). (Salvador Dalí, who was very interested in the question of the minimum information necessary for perception, incorporated this image into his 1969–1970 autobiographical painting *The Hallucinogenic Toreador*.)

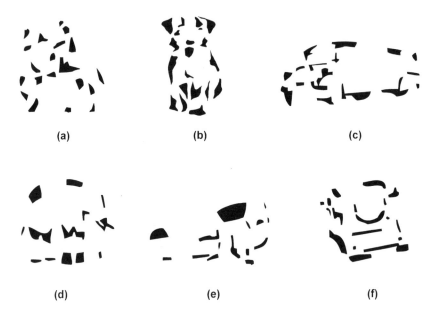

(a)   (b)   (c)

(d)   (e)   (f)

Figure 2.7
Examples of fragmented or "closure" figures used by Reynolds (1985). Figures
(a) and (b) are based on Street (1931). When closure is achieved these are seen
as "horse and rider," "dog," "bus (or truck)," "elephant," "airplane," and
"typewriter," respectively.

It is widely believed that providing hints can improve a person's ability
to recognize a fragmented figure, such as that shown in figure 2.6, and
other so-called closure figures, such as those devised by Street (1931),
some of which are shown in figure 2.7. Yet that claim has rarely been
tested experimentally. There is some evidence that priming with completed pictures does improve recognition performance, although Gollin
(1960) showed that training with fragmented pictures using an ascend-
ing method of limits produced more learning than extensive training with
completed pictures. In a related finding, Snodgrass and Feenan (1990)
showed that perceptual closure can best be primed by showing partially
completed fragmented figures. Priming with complete figures was much
poorer than priming with partially completed figures. These cases,
however, only show the effect of visually presented information on perceptual closure, and even then they show that partial information is
better than complete information in priming identification. Since com-

plete pictures carry full information about the identity of the objects, it seems that it is not knowing the identity of the objects that is most effective in priming, but some other perceptual factor. Perhaps the attempt to obtain closure in the partially completed figures initiates a search for visual cues, which then helps to focus attention. The partially completed figures used by Snodgrass and Feenan allow the viewer to see both the identity of the complete figure and also the nature and location of some of the fragments that form part of the completed figure, so it provides better cues as to where to focus attention in the fragmented figure.

The effectiveness of verbal hints was investigated directly by Reynolds (1985). Reynolds used figures taken from Street's Gestalt Completion Test (Street, 1931), a few of which are shown in figure 2.7, and found that providing the instruction that a meaningful object exists in the figure greatly improved recognition time and accuracy (in fact, when subjects were not told that the figure could be perceptually integrated to reveal a meaningful object, only 9% saw such an object). On the other hand, telling subjects the class of object increased the likelihood of eventual recognition but did not decrease the time it took to do so (which in this study took around 4 seconds—much longer than any picture-recognition time, but much shorter than other reported times to recognize other fragmented figures, where times in the order of minutes are typically observed).[7] The importance of expecting a meaningful figure is quite general and parallels the finding that knowing that a figure is reversible or ambiguous is important for arriving at alternative percepts (perhaps even necessary, as suggested by Girgus, Rock, and Egatz, 1977, and Rock and Anson, 1979). But this is not an example in which knowledge acquired through hints affects the content of what is seen—which is what

7. Keith Humphrey, at the University of Western Ontario, has arranged class demonstrations in which he shows fragmented figures in class to a group of students, some of whom have been given written hints in advance. Judging by the latency of hand-raises, the hints tend to speed up the recognition. Given the informal nature of this demonstration, the results should be received with caution; a controlled version of the experiment seems merited. But an interesting observation that Humphrey reports is that the time taken for closure is very long—in the order of minutes, rather that the fractions of a second required for normal perception of such simple forms. Clearly something other than visual recognition is involved in such cases—most likely some sort of problem solving based on searching for critical cues.

cognitive penetration requires. If anything, the fact that the principle effect on perception comes from knowing that a meaningful figure could be seen (in the case of fragmented figures) or from knowing that a figure was ambiguous adds more credence to the earlier suggestion that such information initiates a search for cues as to where to focus attention, as opposed to a perceptual process. This would also explain why closure of fragmented figures takes so long to attain, compared to the very short time to perceive a picture (which appears to be on the order of a tenth of a second; see, for example, Potter, 1975).

Notice that the fragmented-figure examples constitute a rather special case of visual perception, insofar as they present the subject with a problem-solving or search task. Subjects are asked to provide a report under conditions where they would ordinarily not see anything meaningful. Knowing that the figure contains a familiar object results in a search for cues. As fragments of familiar objects are found, the visual system can be directed to the relevant parts of the display, leading to a percept. That a search is involved is also suggested by the long response latencies (see note 7) compared with the very rapid speed of normal vision (on the order of tenths of a second when response time is eliminated).

What may be going on in the time it takes to reach perceptual closure on these figures may be simply the search for a locus at which to apply the independent visual process. This search, rather than the perceptual process itself, may thus be the process that is sensitive to collateral information. This is an important form of intervention, from my perspective, since it represents what is really a preperceptual stage during which the visual system is indeed directed by voluntary cognitive processes—though not in terms of the content of the percept but in terms of the location at which the independent visual process is to be applied. In chapter 4, I will argue that an important way in which cognition can affect the outcome of visual perception is by directing the independent visual system to focus attention at particular (and perhaps multiple) places in the scene.

A similar story concerning the locus of cognitive intervention applies in the case of other ambiguous displays. When one percept is attained and observers know that there is another one, they can engage in a search for other organizations by directing their attention to other parts of the display (hence the importance of the knowledge that the figure is ambiguous). It has sometimes been claimed that we can will ourselves to see one or another of the ambiguous percepts. For example, Churchland claims to be able to make ambiguous figures "flip back and forth at will between the two or more alternatives, by changing one's assumptions about the nature of the object or about the conditions of viewing" (1988, p. 172). This is not what has been reported in experiments with naive subjects, where the only factor that has been found to be relevant is the knowledge that the stimulus is ambiguous. Moreover, as I have already suggested, there is a simple mechanism available for some degree of control of such phenomena as figure reversal—the mechanism of spatially focused attention. Kawabata (1986) and Peterson and Gibson (1991) have shown that the locus of attention is important in determining how one perceives ambiguous or reversing figures such as the Necker cube. Some parts of a figure tend to have a bias toward one interpretation, while other parts have a bias toward another interpretation; consequently, changing the locus of attention may change the interpretation (e.g., there appears to be a bias toward seeing the attended parts of a figure as being closer to the viewer). If there is a bias in the interpretation of a part of the figure, this will tend to influence the interpretation of the remainder of the figure. But there is no evidence that voluntarily "changing one's assumptions about the object" has any direct effect on how one perceives the figure.

There are other cases where it has been suggested that hints and prior knowledge affect perception. For example, the fusion of stereo images—such as figure 3.18 and even more so with stereo images made of random dots, a form of presentation invented by Julesz (1971) called "random dot stereograms"—is often quite difficult and was widely thought to be improved by giving people information about what they should see (the same is true of the popular autostereograms).[8] There is evidence, however, that merely telling a subject what the object is or what it looks like does not make a significant difference. In fact, Frisby and Clatworthy (1975) found that neither telling subjects what they "ought to see" nor showing them a 3-D model of the object provided any

---

8. A commercial version of these autostereograms are the Magic Eye 3D posters. As of this writing, examples of these may be seen at http://www.magiceye.com. Other stereo demonstrations can be found at http://www.vision3d.com/sghidden.html.

significant benefit in fusing random-dot stereograms. What does help, especially in the case of large-disparity stereograms, is the presence of prominent monocular contours, even when they do not themselves provide cues as to the identity of the object. Saye and Frisby (1975) argued that these cues help facilitate the required vergence eye movements and that in fact the difficulty in fusing random-dot stereograms in general is due to the absence of features needed for guiding the vergence movements of the eyes required to fuse the display. One might surmise that it may also be the case that directing focal attention to certain features (thereby making them perceptually prominent) can help facilitate eye movements in the same way. In that case, learning to fuse stereograms, like learning to see different views of ambiguous figures, may be mediated by learning where to focus attention.

2.5.3   Learning to "see" differently: A case of controlling focal attention?

There is general agreement that focal attention can be directed, either extrinsically (by virtue of certain properties of the stimulus) or intrinsically (by central processes, operating voluntarily). Whichever form of attention allocation occurs, both the conditions triggering automatic allocation and the conditions that determine voluntary allocation may be modified over time. There is evidence that just as eye movements can be modulated by experience (e.g., Shapiro and Raymond, 1989), so can the allocation of attention. This being the case, one might reasonably wonder whether some or all of the effects studied under the category of "perceptual learning" might not be attributable to the indirect effect of learning to allocate attention.

Clearly, we can decide to focus our attention on certain parts of a scene rather than others. Earlier I claimed that this allocation of attention was one of the two principle ways for cognition to intervene in influencing visual perception, the other being the postvisual determination of the identity of familiar scene contents. I suggested that such attention allocation was responsible for speeding up perceptual closure after exposure to a previous instance of the closure figure. Similarly, the effect of certain types of experience on our ability to fuse random-dot stereograms and autostereograms was attributed to learning to focus attention on features that guide appropriate eye vergence. For example, the main thing that makes a difference in the ease of fusing a stereogram is having seen the stereogram before. Frisby and Clatworthy (1975) found that repeated presentation had a beneficial effect that lasted for at least 3 weeks. In fact, the learning in this case, as in the case of improvements of texture segregation with practice (Karni and Sagi, 1995), is extremely sensitive to the retinal location and orientation of the visual displays—so much so that experience generalizes poorly to the same figures presented in a different retinal location (Ramachandran, 1976) or a different orientation (Ramachandran and Braddick, 1973). An important determiner of stereo fusion (and even more important in the case of popular autostereogram posters) is attaining the proper vergence of the eyes. Such a skill depends on finding the appropriate visual features to drive the vergence mechanism. It also involves a motor skill that one can learn; indeed, many vision scientists have learned to free-fuse stereo images without the benefit of stereo goggles. This suggests that the improvement with exposure to a particular stereo image may simply be learning where to focus attention and how to control eye vergence.

The improvement in a perceptual skill following learning which features are critical to the skill is a quite general phenomenon. In chapter 1 this claim was illustrated with the case of chess masters, whose memory for chess positions was found to be highly dependent on whether or not the chess positions could be interpreted in terms of a real chess match. This was taken as evidence that chess masters differ from beginners because (1) masters have a code for a large number of positions and (2) masters know where to look for significant chess-relevant patterns. It is frequently the case that expertise in a visual skill depends on finding and encoding certain special features that are diagnostic for the particular distinctions defining the expertise in question. I will present some quite general cases of this principle below.

Cultural and linguistic effects on perception   It was widely believed that how people see the world is conditioned by their culture and even by the language they speak. This thesis, called linguistic relativity, was articulated by the anthropologist Benjamin Lee Whorf and the linguist Edward Sapir and is sometimes referred to as the Sapir-Whorf hypothesis. The thesis was widely accepted during the time when the new look in perception held sway. It was congenial to the *tabula rasa* view of human nature that pervaded both philosophical and psychological behaviorism, as well as view of the "perfectibility of human nature" that grew out of the Enlightenment. It is the view that human nature is largely the product of our experiences. Although linguistic relativity in the strong Worfian form has been discredited in the past several decades, a modified and somewhat weaker version of this hypothesis has once again seen some support (e.g., Gumperz and Levinson, 1996). Most of the recent work only supports the claim that language provides resources over and above the nonlinguistic concepts needed to encode the visual world (and even so, many believe that the new relativism also rests on shaky foundations; see Li and Gleitman, 2002; Pinker, 1994). Notice that the new linguistic relativism is not the same as the new-look view, which claims that what we see and how we see depends on our beliefs. Even if the newer evidence and arguments are sustained, the claims that they make only concern long-term effects of language on visual interpretation and encoding, not the sort of effects that support the idea that vision and cognition merge continuously into one another.

The case of "expert" perceivers   Another apparent case of penetration of vision by knowledge occurs in the case of "expert" perceivers of various kinds—people who are able notice patterns that the rest of us fail to see (bird watchers, art authenticators, radiologists, aerial-photo interpreters, sports analysts, chess masters, and so on). Not much is known about such perceptual expertise, since such skills are typically highly deft, rapid, and unconscious. When asked how they do it, experts typically say that they can "see" certain properties by "just looking." But what research is available shows that often what the expert has learned is not a "way of seeing" as such, but rather some combination of task-relevant mnemonic skills (knowing what kinds of patterns to look for) and knowledge of where to look or where to direct his attention.

The first type of skill is reminiscent of the conclusion reached by Haber (1966) that a "preparatory set" operates primarily through mnemonic encoding strategies. It is most clearly illustrated in the work of Chase and Simon (1973), who showed that what appears to be chess masters' rapid visual processing and better visual memory for chess boards only manifests itself when the board consists of familiar chess positions and not at all when it is a random pattern of the same pieces (beginners, of course, do equally poorly on both; see figure 1.23). Chase and Simon interpret this as showing that rather than having learned to see the board differently, chess masters have developed a very large repertoire (they call it a "vocabulary") of patterns that they can use to classify or encode genuine chess positions, though not random positions. Thus what is special about experts' vision in this case is the system of classification they have learned that allows them to recognize and encode a large number of relevant patterns. But, as I argued earlier, such a classification process is postperceptual insofar as it involves decisions that require accessing long-term memory.

The second type of skill, the skill to direct attention in a task-relevant manner, is documented in what is perhaps the largest body of research on expert perception—the study of performance in sports. It is obvious that fast perception, as well as quick reaction, is required for high levels of sports skill. Despite this truism, very little evidence of faster visual information processing has been found among athletes (e.g., Abernethy, Neil, and Koning, 1994; Starkes et al., 1994). In most cases the difference between sports novices and experts is confined to the specific domains in which the experts excel—and there it is usually attributable to the ability to anticipate relevant events. Such anticipation is based, for example, on observing initial segments of the motion of a ball or puck or the opponent's gestures (Abernethy, 1991; Proteau, 1992). Except for a finding of generally better attention-orienting abilities (Castiello and Umiltà, 1992; Greenfield et al., 1994; Nougier, Ripoll, and Stein, 1989) visual expertise in sports, like the expertise found in the Chase and Simon studies of chess skill, appears to be based on nonvisual abilities related to the learned skills of identifying, predicting, and therefore attending to the most relevant places. Indeed, a report published in the May 5, 1969, issue of *Sports Illustrated* gave the reaction time of the great heavyweight boxer Muhammed Ali in responding to a light as 190 ms, which is within the normal range (reported in Keele, 1973, p. 76). Presumably Ali's lightening-fast performance in the ring was due in part to his being able to anticipate his opponent's moves—that and the fact that he could move his arm 16.5 inches in only 40 ms after his initial reaction time! Being a fast reactor in a visual-motor skill does not always mean processing visual information better or more quickly.

An expert's perceptual skill frequently differs from a beginner's in that the expert has learned where the critical distinguishing information is located within the stimulus pattern. In that case the expert can direct focal attention to the critical locations, allowing the independent visual process to do the rest. A remarkable case of such expertise, investigated by Backus (1978) and Biederman and Shiffrar (1987), involves expert "chicken sexers." Determining the sex of day-old chicks is both economically important and also apparently very difficult. In fact, it is so difficult that it takes years of training (consisting of repeated trials) to become one of the rare experts. By carefully studying the experts, Biederman and Shiffrar found that what distinguished good sexers from poor ones is, roughly, where they look and what distinctive features they look for. Although the experts were not aware of it, what they had learned was the set of contrasting features and, even more important, where exactly the distinguishing information was located. Biederman and Shiffrar found that telling novices where the relevant information was located allowed them quickly to became experts themselves. What the telling teaches, and what the experts had tacitly learned, is how to bring the independent visual system to bear at the right spatial location and what types of patterns to encode into memory—both of which are functions lying outside the visual system itself.

Note that this is exactly how hints work, as I suggested, in cases of fragmented or ambiguous figures and cases of binocular fusion. In all these cases the mechanism of spatially focused attention plays a central role. I believe that this role is in fact quite ubiquitous and can help us understand a large number of phenomena involving cognitive influences on visual perception (see below and section 6.5 for more on this claim).

Attention and perceptual learning   There is a large literature on what is known as "perceptual learning," much of it associated with the work of Eleanor Gibson and her students (e.g., Gibson, 1991). The findings show that, in some general sense, how people apprehend the visual world can be altered through experience. For example, how people categorize objects and properties—and even whether they can discriminate features—can be altered through prior experience with the objects. In this same tradition, recent studies (Goldstone, 1994, 1995) showed that the discriminability of stimulus properties is altered by preexposure to different categorization tasks. Schyns, Goldstone, and Thibaut (1998) have argued that categorization does not rely on a fixed vocabulary of features, but that featurelike properties are "created under the influence of higher-level cognitive processes ... when new categories need to be learned."

This work is interesting and relevant to the general question of how experience can influence categorization and discrimination. Without doubt, a fixed repertoire of features at the level of cognitive codes (though clearly not at the level of basic sensory receptors) is inadequate for categorization (for more on this, see Fodor, 1998). However, none of these results is in conflict with the independence or impenetrability thesis as I have been developing it here for the following reasons:

First, although some perceptual-learning researchers have claimed that basic early-vision processes may be altered, this is far from clear from the results themselves. In all reported cases, what is actually being measured is observers' differential use of certain features compared with their use of other available features. But this could be the result of one of the two processes lying outside of early vision that were discussed earlier. These are (a) selective attention being applied to one physically specifiable dimension over another (e.g., one location over another, color over luminance, height over width, and so on) or (b) one perceptual feature being weighted more or less than another and/or combined in different (nonlinear) ways in the postperceptual categorization process (which could, in effect, result in the creation of different feature clusters).

Second, even if the claim that there is low-level learning in early vision can be sustained (i.e., even if the effect is due neither to learning to allocate focal attention nor to postperceptual decision processes) the claims are not directly relevant to the discontinuity thesis. The shaping of basic sensory processes by experience is not the same as cognitive penetration. The latter entails that the content of percepts (not just the discriminability of features) is rationally connected to beliefs, expectations, values, and so on, regardless of how the latter are arrived at or altered. That is the type of influence that the new look was concerned with, and that is the kind of influence that concerns us here. It is this kind of influence that is at the core of the discontinuity thesis and the issue of architectural constraints. The tuning of the sensitivity of sensory systems (not only organs but also cortical centers) by evolution or by prolonged experience is not the same as cognitive penetration—the determination of what we see in any particular instance by our immediate expectations, beliefs, needs, or inferences.

Finally, with regard to the genesis of visual expertise, it should be noted that there is no a priori reason why a postperceptual decision process might not, with time and repetition, become automatized and cognitively impenetrable, and therefore indistinguishable from the encapsulated visual system. Such automatization creates what I have elsewhere referred to as "compiled transducers" (Pylyshyn, 1984a). Compiling complex new transducers is a process by which formerly postperceptual processing may become part of early vision by becoming automatized and encapsulated, and may even have its own local storage (see Pylyshyn, 1984a, chap. 9, for more on this point). If the resulting process is cognitively impenetrable, and therefore systematically loses access to general memory, then, according to the view being advocated here, it becomes part of the visual system. Consequently, it is consistent with the present framework that new complex processes could become part of the early-vision system over time: cognitive impenetrability and diachronic change are not incompatible. How processes can become "compiled" into the visual system remains unknown, although according to the Allan Newell's levels-taxonomy (Newell, 1990), the process of altering the encapsulated visual system should take one or two orders of magnitude longer to accomplish than the duration of basic cognitive operations themselves (i.e., on the order of minutes as opposed to fractions of a second) and would very likely require repeated experience, as is the case with many perceptual-learning phenomena.

2.5.4   Focal attention as an interface between vision and cognition

One of the features of perceptual learning already noted is that learning may lead to attention being focused on the most relevant objects, regions, or properties of the visual field. Spatial and object-based (see chapter 4) focusing of attention is perhaps the most important mechanism by which the visual system rapidly adjusts to an informationally dense and dynamic world. It thus represents the main interface between cognition and vision—an idea that has been noted in the past (e.g., Julesz, 1990; Pylyshyn, 1989). Visual attention is a fundamental mechanism in both vision and visualization (or mental imagery), and a careful analysis of the various forms and functions of focal attention goes a long way toward explaining many phenomena of perceptual learning, perceptual organization, mental imagery, and even the source of certain phenomenal experiences of the spatial extension and spatial stability of both visual percepts (discussed in chapter 1 and chapter 5) and mental images (discussed in section 6.5). Chapters 4 and 5 will be devoted to a discussion of these issues. For present purposes I wish merely to note that there are two logically possible loci where a mechanism like selective attention could operate. First, it might operate on the input to the visual system, by enhancing and/or attenuating certain properties of the input. For example, it might enhance certain spatial locations or certain regions that constitute individual visual objects. Second, it might operate by enhancing and/or attenuating the availability of certain perceptual categories, as proposed by Bruner. This is what Bruner meant by "perceptual readiness"—the *ready availability* of categories of perception. From my perspective, the latter locus of attention occurs *after* the early-visual process and may even include selective encoding into memory or selective retrieval from memory. If selective attention operates on input prior to early vision, then it must operate on properties that are primitive and preperceptual, such as spatial location or perhaps spatial frequency; otherwise, appeal to selective attention would be circular. In that case perceptual learning might consist of learning where to look or something equally basic (as suggested in section 2.5.3). On the other hand, if attention is viewed as being at least in part a postperceptual process, operating on the outputs of the visual system, then there is room for much more complex forms of "perceptual learning," including learning to recognize paintings as genuine Rembrandts, learning to identify tumors in medical x rays, and so on. But in that case the learning is not strictly within the visual system, but rather involves postperceptual decision processes based on knowledge and experience, however tacit and unconscious these may be. In the everyday use of the term "attention," these two loci are not distinguished. Attention is viewed as any process that selects some aspect of perception from other aspects. As a consequence, the attempt to judge whether attention occurs early or late in vision has had mixed results: evidence for both "early selection" and "late selection" theories has been found. But it remains possible, and indeed seems reasonable, that attention operates at both loci. My position is that attention operates at both loci but *not* in between, i.e., not *within* the early-vision system itself.

2.6   Conclusions: Early Vision as a Cognitively Impenetrable System

In this chapter I have considered the question of whether early visual perception is continuous with cognition or whether it is best viewed as a separate process, with its own principles and possibly its own internal memory, isolated from the rest of the mind except for certain well-defined and highly circumscribed modes of interaction. In the course of this analysis I have touched on many reasons why it appears on the surface that vision is part of general cognition and thus thoroughly influenced by our beliefs, desires, and utilities. Opposed to this interactionist view we found a great deal of psychophysical evidence attesting to the autonomy and inflexibility of visual perception and its tendency to resolve ambiguities in a manner that defies what the observer knows and what is a rational inference. As Irvin Rock, one of the champions of the view that vision is "intelligent," nevertheless noted, "Perception must rigidly adhere to the appropriate internalized rules, so that it often seems unintelligent and inflexible in its imperviousness to other kinds of knowledge" (1983, p. 340).

Most of this chapter concentrated on showing that many apparent examples of cognitive effects in vision arise either from a postperceptual decision process or from a preperceptual attention-allocation process. To this end I examined some alleged cases of "hints" affecting perception, of perceptual learning, and of perceptual expertise. I argued that in the cases that have been studied carefully, as opposed to reported informally, hints and instructions rarely have an effect, but when they do, it is invariably by influencing the allocation of focal attention, by the attenuation of certain classes of physically specifiable signals, and in certain circumstances by the development of such special skills as the control of eye movements and eye vergence. We arrived at a similar conclusion in the case of perceptual learning and visual expertise, where the evidence pointed to the improvement being due to learning where to direct attention—in some cases aided by better domain-specific knowledge that helps anticipate where the essential information will occur (especially true in the case of dynamic visual skills, such as in sports). Another relevant aspect of the skill that is learned is contained in the inventory of pattern types that the observer assimilates (and perhaps stores in a special visual memory) and that helps in choosing the appropriate mnemonic encoding for a particular domain.

I also noted a number of clinical findings concerning the dissociation of cognition and perception that tend to substantiate the view that vision and cognition are independent systems (some more evidence will be presented in the next chapter). Very little has been said about the general issue of the nature of the output from the visual system. I will take up this question in the next chapter, where it will be concluded that the output consists of shape representations involving at least surface layouts, occluding edges (where these are parsed into objects), and other details sufficiently rich to allow looking up parts of the stimulus in a shape-indexed memory for identification. I will also considered the possibility that more than one form of output is generated, directed at various distinct postperceptual systems. In particular, I will examine the evidence that motor-control functions may be served by different visual outputs than recognition functions, and that both are cognitively impenetrable.

In examining the evidence that vision is affected by knowledge and expectations, I also devoted some space to methodological issues concerned with distinguishing various stages of perception. Although the preponderance of evidence locates cognitive influences in a postperceptual stage, we found that the sort of stage-analysis methods in general use within experimental psychology provide a decomposition that is too coarse to establish whether the locus of cognitive effects is inside or outside early vision proper. In particular, both signal-detection measures and event-related potentials fail to provide a way to examine a stage that corresponds to what I have been calling early vision. So, as in so many examples in science, there is no simple and direct method—no methodological panacea—for answering the question of whether a particular observed effect has its locus in vision or in pre- or postvisual processes.

The idea that early vision is both complex and impervious to such cognitive influences as expectations, beliefs, and desires will play an important role in our subsequent discussion about how vision interacts with the world and with what we know—with our cognitive representations. What I call "early vision" I might as well call "vision," since it is the part of the extensive overall process of acquiring knowledge through the visual modality that is *special* or proprietary to visual processing. Henceforth, in speaking about the connection between vision and the world or vision and visualization (mental imagery), "vision" will refer to the system that was identified in this chapter—the early-vision system. The rest of what goes on when we visually perceive, being part of reasoning, recall, judgment and so on, will not be counted as part of the visual system proper. If the entire visual-cognition process were to count as "vision," then one would be forced to conclude that there is no such thing as vision proper, only cognizing. In that case there would be nothing particular to say about whether (and how) we reason using the visual system, or how what we see connects with the perceived world— at least no more to say about those connections than about the connection between how we reason about fashion and how we reason about physics, or how we reason about any topic or subject matter. But as we have seen, vision is not just another subject matter to be thought about by the reasoning system. It is a system that has well-defined properties and principles of its own, so it is of considerable interest to ask how (if at all) *these* principles interact with the principle by which we reason, recall, make judgments, and understand language. Such questions could not be studied with any precision if it had turned out that there was no such thing as *the visual system* as a separate and autonomous set of processes. Luckily for us, and for a science of visual perception, this appears to be far from the case. Rather, there appears to be a rich set of mechanisms and processes that we may say are *proprietary* to vision. The question of just *how* rich and complex these mechanisms and processes are is the burden of much that follows. In particular, if this technical sense of "vision" is to be of much interest, it must include a lot more than merely converting a retinal image into a mental image; it must include the process that allows us to see as much as we do see without benefit of what we know about the scene we are observing. We begin to explore this question in the next chapter.

3

The Architecture of the Early-Vision System: Components and Functions

3.1 Some Intrinsic Architectural Factors Determining What We See

In the last chapter I suggested that many contextual and other apparently "intelligent" effects in vision come about *after* the visual system has completed its task—in other words, that they have a postperceptual locus. But not all top-down effects in vision are cases that can be explained in terms of postperceptual processes. Top-down effects are extremely common in vision, and I will consider a number of examples in this section. In particular, I will consider examples that appear on the surface to be remarkably like cases of inference. In these cases the visual system appears to "choose" one interpretation over other possible ones, and the choice appears to be notably "rational." The important question is whether these cases constitute cognitive penetration. I argue that they do not, for reasons that cast light on the subtlety, efficiency, and autonomy of visual processing.

In what follows I consider two related types of apparent "intelligence" on the part of the visual system. The first has seen some important recent progress, beginning with the seminal work of David Marr (1982). It concerns how the visual system recovers the 3D structure of scenes from proximal 2D data that are logically insufficient or intrinsically ambiguous. The second type of case, which has a longer tradition, consists in demonstrations of what Rock (1983) has called "problem solving," wherein vision provides what appear to be "intelligent" interpretations of certain systematically ambiguous displays (but see Kanizsa, 1985, for a different view concerning the use of what he calls a "ratiomorphic" vocabulary). I will suggest that it is likely that these two forms of apparent intelligence have a similar etiology.

3.1.1 Natural constraints in vision

Historically, an important class of argument for the involvement of reasoning in vision comes from the fact that the mapping from a three-dimensional world to our two-dimensional retinas is many-to-one and therefore noninvertible. Noninvertibility is a mathematical property commonly found in nature. For example, if you know the area of a rectangle you cannot derive the lengths of the sides, because there is an unlimited number of pairs of lengths that give the same product when multiplied (i.e., there are an unlimited number of different-shaped rectangles with the same area). In general, there is an infinite number of 3D stimuli corresponding to any 2D image. Thus, for example, figure 3.1 shows a two-dimensional version of this infinite ambiguity. The line L_1 on the retina can be the projection of any (or all) of the edges E_1, E_2, E_3, ... in the world (as long as all these lines lie on a common plane with the projected line).

This problem is quite general, and the mathematical noninvertibility persists so long as no restrictions are imposed to prevent it. And yet we do not perceive a range of possible alternative worlds when we look out at a scene. We invariably see a single unique layout. Somehow the visual system manages to select one of the myriad logical possibilities. This is not because of some magical property of our visual systems: the interpretation our visual systems provide really is underdetermined by the information available to our eyes. Because the information available to the visual system underdetermines the true state of affairs in the world,

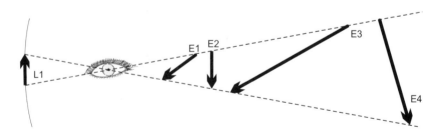

Figure 3.1
An unlimited number of oblique edges in the environment (E1, E2, E3, E4 ...) project to the same 2D line (L1) on the retina. Consequently it is a mathematical truth that if you know the exact retinal project of an edge you cannot compute the distal layout with certainty. For this reason, the 3D-to-2D projection is said to be noninvertible.

the unique interpretation we get always *could*, in principle, be the wrong one. When we discover a wrong interpretation, we are surprised because we have learned to assume that vision is veridical. And indeed, the visual system does provide a unique interpretation that is normally consistent with the interpretation one would get from other sorts of evidence (e.g., from the evidence of touch or from walking around and observing the scene from many angles). When you do get an obviously wrong interpretation, it is usually because you assimilate an unusual situation to a normal one, as in illusions such as those created by the Ames room, which is constructed to mimic an ordinary rectilinear room when viewed from a particular vantage point, but which is, in fact, highly distorted. But the converse can also occur. Richard Gregory (1970) constructed a real three-dimensional object which, when viewed from a particular vantage point, is perceived as an impossible one. Figure 3.2 shows the percept of an "impossible triangle," which is, of course, not impossible at all. The figure on the right shows how to construct it, but from a specific viewpoint the viewer sees something that can't exist!

In almost all cases our visual system provides a unique percept (usually in 3D) for each 2D image, even though it is possible that other options might have been computed and rejected in the process. The uniqueness of the percept (except for the case of reversing figures, like the Necker cube) means that there is something else that must be entering into the process of inverting the mapping. Helmholtz, as well as most vision

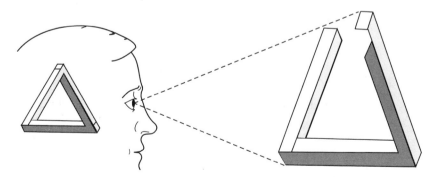

Figure 3.2
A real 3D object (on the right), which, when viewed from a particular viewpoint, is seen as the impossible object illustrated in the viewer's mind.

researchers in the 1950s through the 1970s, assumed that this was *inference from knowledge of the world* because the inversion was almost always correct (e.g., we see the veridical 3D layout even from 2D pictures). The one major exception to this view was that developed by J. J. Gibson, who argued that inference is not needed, since vision consists in the "direct" pickup of relevant information from the optic array by a process more akin to "resonance" than to inference. Gibson's research program (which he called "direct realism") was an interesting and ambitious one, but it failed primarily because it left no room for representations of any kind. (I will not discuss this approach here, since Fodor and I devoted considerable attention to it in Fodor and Pylyshyn, 1981.)

Beginning with the work of Marr (1982), however, a great deal of theoretical analysis has shown that there is another option for how the visual system can uniquely invert the 3D-to-2D mapping. All that is needed is that the computations carried out in early processing embody (without explicitly representing and drawing inferences from) certain very general constraints on the interpretations that it is allowed to make. These constraints do not guarantee the correct interpretation of all stimuli (the noninvertibility of the mapping ensures that this is not possible in general because there *really are* other 3D configurations that could have caused the same 2D image). All that is needed is that the natural constraints lead to the correct interpretation under specified conditions that frequently obtain in our kind of physical world. If we can find such generalized constraints, and if their deployment in visual processing is at least compatible with what is known about the nervous system, then we would be in a position to explain how the visual system solves this inversion problem without "unconscious inference."

Researchers have proposed and studied a substantial inventory of such constraints, which have been called "natural constraints" because they are typically stated as if they were assumptions about the natural physical world (see, for example, Brown, 1984; Marr, 1982; Richards, 1988; Ullman and Richards, 1990). One of the earliest is the "rigidity" constraint (Ullman, 1979), which has been used to explain the kinetic depth effect. In the kinetic depth effect, a set of randomly arranged moving points is perceived as lying on the surface of a rigid (though invisible) 3D object. The requirement for this percept is primarily that the points move in a way that is compatible with this interpretation. In this case there is a natural constraint that derives from the assumption that most points in the perceived world lie on the surface of a rigid object. This assumption leads mathematically to the "structure from motion" principle, which states that if a set of points moves in a way that is consistent with the interpretation that they lie on the surface of a rigid body, then they will be so perceived. The conditions under which this principle can lead to a unique percept are spelled out, in part, in a uniqueness theorem (Ullman, 1979). This theorem states that three or more distinct 2D projections of four noncoplanar points that maintain fixed 3D interpoint distances uniquely determine the 3D spatial structure of those points. Hence if the display consists of a sequence of such views, the principle ensures a unique percept, which, moreover, will be veridical if the scene does indeed consist of points on a rigid object. Since in our world all but a very small proportion of feature points in a scene do lie on the surface of rigid objects, this principle ensures that the perception of moving sets of feature points is more often veridical than not.[1] It also explains why we see structure from certain kinds of moving dot displays, as in the "kinetic depth effect" (Wallach and O'Connell, 1953).

Another set of constraints that apply to a world consisting only of blocks of polyhedral objects (the so-called "blocks world" that was often used as a test bed for investigating ideas in computer vision) concerns the requirement of consistency on labels of edges. If an edge is assumed to be concave at one end, where if forms part of a vertex, then it must also be concave at its other end, where it forms part of another vertex. But if such a labeling of the second vertex is physically impossible in the blocks world, then that label must be discarded as inconsistent. Such a simple label-consistency constraint arises in part from the physical nature of edges and vertices and turns out to be a strong constraint that makes it possible to give a unique labeling to most images of scenes containing blocks. The way this sort of constraint propagates until it uniquely determines the 3D labeling of a scene is typical of how natural constraints operate in vision. In this way a constraint that arises from physical properties of (our sort of) world, together with certain assumptions (e.g., that

1. The "rigidity" constraint is not the only constraint operative in motion perception, however. To explain the correct perception of "biological motion" (Johansson, 1950) or the simultaneous motion and deformation of several objects, additional constraints must be brought to bear.

the scene consists entirely of rigid blocks), makes it possible to recover the 3D structure of a blocks world despite the fact that such a recovery is logically not unique (i.e., there is an unbounded number of real-world 3D edges that could lead to any of the 2D images projected onto our retinas).

But the nature of the physical world is only part of the reason that the vertex-labeling system works. The other part is that we may be justified in making certain assumptions about the nonaccidental nature of the image projected on our retinas. In a world like ours, certain things are overwhelmingly more likely to occur than others. A good example is the assumption that three coterminal lines in an image arise from three edges of objects that come together at one point in 3D space. Not only does such an assumption not follow from the laws of physics or geometry, it is easily thwarted by simply constructing a collection of wire segments, or even edges of different blocks, as shown in figure 3.3. But such a coincidence of edges in 3D would be *accidental* in a special technical sense, namely, that if you changed your point of view even slightly, the edges would no longer project as lines that come together at a common point.

The rarity and vulnerability of such special alignments to even small movements warrants the assumption that if a pattern such as a Y, involving the coincidence of three lines, does occur in an image, it is most likely due to the fact that three edges do actually meet at a common point in

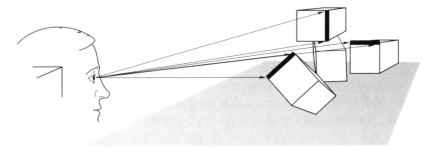

Figure 3.3
It is easy to set up a situation in which certain patterns occur "accidentally" in their two-dimensional projection on the retina. The visual system appears to shun such interpretations, preferring the "nonaccidental" construal (such as the one illustrated in the viewer's mind), even though the accidental ones are logically possible.

the 3D scene. Such properties are called "nonaccidental" and form the basis for a number of principles, which, while not inevitably true, are ones that it would be reasonable to build into a visual system. Nonaccidental properties are particularly important in human and animal vision because we generally move about and can easily discover whether or not such image properties as cotermination of edges are maintained with small changes in viewpoint. These image properties allow one to interpret a 3D scene by following certain simple principles of "natural constraints."

An example of the use of natural constraints in feature labeling   To illustrate how such natural constraints can be used to restrict the permissible 2D-to-3D mapping, consider the simplified world of blocks. Perception of such a "microworld" was one of the first applications where natural constraints were used in computer vision (see Mackworth, 1973, for a clear description of the historical development of techniques in this area). In this approach, parsing a scene consisting of blocks proceeds by the assignment of "labels" to individual edges in the 2D image. These labels allow us to group the parts (or features) as belonging to the same object, and to specify which object is in front and which object is behind, and so on. The goal is to be able to provide a qualitative description of a scene that is rich enough to make it possible to recognize the objects in the scene and to characterize their shapes and relative locations.

Consider a scene such as the one in figure 3.4, consisting of rectilinear blocks of various sizes arranged in a haphazard manner. Let us assume that the lines in the image corresponding to the edges of blocks are clearly identified. What is the minimum information that we need to have a useful analysis of the scene? Clearly, we need to segregate (or "individuate") each of the blocks and specify which edges, vertices, and surfaces belong with which block. We also need to characterize the spatial layout of the blocks: which blocks are in front of which, which are on top of which, and so on. A qualitative solution to part of this problem would be achieved if we could label each line in the 2D scene in some coherent and meaningful way. For example, we should be able to say that a certain line in the 2D scene corresponds to the top edge of a particular block, another line corresponds to the edge of a certain block

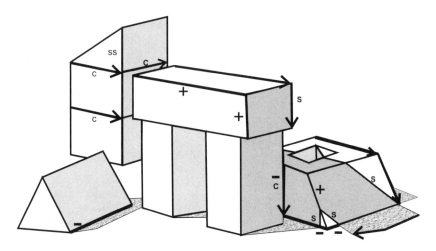

Figure 3.4
A typical blocks scene that can be analyzed using the Waltz labeling system. The
analysis would reveal which lines go together to form faces and blocks, which
lines separate shadow from light, which faces are in front of (and occlude) other
faces, which are the outside (bottom or back) faces, and so on, thus providing
a qualitative description of the scene. The labels on some of the edges are discussed in the text. (Adapted from Waltz, 1975.)

that occludes another block, and so on. In building a system that generates such a description, much thinking and experimenting must go into
the selection of an appropriate set of labels so that in the end these two
conditions are met: (1) it is possible to assign a unique set of labels to a
scene that is perceptually unique (at least to human observers), and (2)
the labeling so assigned provides a meaningful analysis of the scene that
can be used for such subsequent purposes as scene recognition. A set of
labels meeting these conditions was developed by David Waltz in his
Ph.D. dissertation (see an abridged version in Waltz, 1975). He found a
basic set of 11 line labels that met these two conditions for a world that
consists of blocks. We consider a subset of 4 of his labels, illustrated in
figure 3.5. The labels tell us whether a line segment is concave (such as
the inside step edge in figure 3.5) or convex, and whether it is an outside
edge of a block with the body of the block on its left or an outside edge
with the body of the block on its right. Following Waltz's notation, we
label these four types of edges using the symbols "+" and "−" for the
inside edges, and using arrows to indicate outside occluding edges.

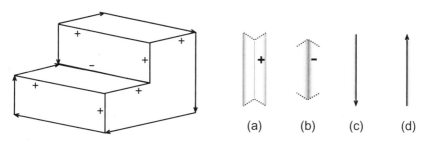

Figure 3.5
Illustration of a simplified line-labeling scheme. Labels specify the type of 3D edge that corresponds to each line in the 2D image. Labels (a) and (b) refer to convex and concave edges, respectively. Labels (c) and (d) refer to outside occluding edges with the block being on the left or on the right, respectively (using a "left-hand rule"—if you place your thumb in the direction of the arrow your left hand will wrap around the outside edge of the block).

The labels are interpreted as follows: a "+" indicates that the edge in the scene is convex, a "−" indicates that it is concave, and arrows on the line indicate that it is an outside edge (using the left hand rule which says that placing your hand around the line with your thumb in the direction of the arrow results in your fingers wrapping around the outside edge of the block). In the original Waltz labeling scheme there were 11 different edge labels (figure 3.4 also shows an S label for "shadow," an SS label for "self-shadow" where the shadow is cast by the same black as the one on which it falls, and a C label for a "crack" or edge where two objects would separate if moved apart). Notice that the lines we are labeling are *image* lines, so that at the beginning of this analysis we don't know what their 3D interpretation will be. What we must do is label them with all possible labels and hope that as the analysis proceeds, we will be able to eliminate some of the labels (this is the same general process as used in grammatical analysis of sentences: we begin by assigning all possible parts of speech to words and then as the analysis proceeds, we use grammatical rules to pare them down to the permissible ones).

The parsing system begins by assigning labels to lines that form a vertex (i.e., it labels the edges that terminate at a junction). Each type of 2-line image vertex can mathematically have 4×4 or 16 combinations, and each type of 3-line image vertex can logically have 64 possible combinations of labels in our simplified 4-label system. Three distinct types of trihedral junctions are recognized as part of the labeling scheme (referred to as Y, T, and arrow junctions), making a total of 192 trihedral junction labels and 16 dihedral junction labels. What makes the analysis possible is that *most of these label combinations cannot occur in the physical world.* The physically possible combinations (assuming we are only dealing with a world of blocks) are shown in figure 3.6 for the four types of vertices we have considered. Waltz's contribution was to identify 11 different edge labels and then by brute force to enumerate all the physically possible vertex types. He did this for dihedral and trihedral vertices by imagining a cube cut into 8 cubic regions (octants) and then considering what each of the corners would look like from every distinct perspective when one of the octants was filled with a solid square, then when two octants were filled, and so on up to seven octants being filled. The octant process allowed Waltz to enumerate all possible junctions for every possible configuration that creates dihedral or trihedral junctions in a world of rectilinear blocks. The result of this inventory actually turned out to be a relatively small list that includes the 18 junction labels shown in figure 3.6, out of a logically possible 208 junctions based on this set of labels. Notice that a very large number of junc-

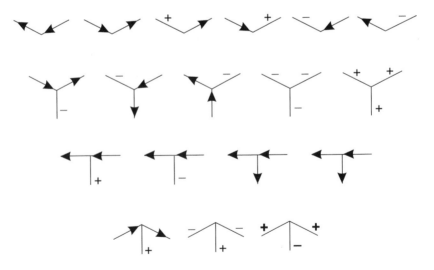

Figure 3.6
This figure shows a subset of all the physically possible Waltz vertex types that can occur in a blocks world.

tion labels simply cannot occur in a real world of blocks (of course, they can occur if we expand the world to include other kinds of shapes, which is why the Waltz technique is of limited value in real vision, except to illustrate the principle of natural constraints and label propagation). Notice that an L junction between two lines cannot be due to a part of a scene in which the two edges are of the type labeled "−". That would require a situation with no other edge in view at the junction—a situation that is physically impossible in a blocks world. When the inventory of possible vertices is complete, we end up with the L, Y, T, and arrow vertices shown in figure 3.6.[2]

The way these line and vertex labels are used in assigning a labeling to the figure is by considering all possible labels at a vertex and then tracing each line to a second connected vertex. Notice the central role that tracing plays here, and has played in our appeal to label propagation to explain some of the human vision phenomena that we encountered in chapter 1. We assume that a line must have the same label at each end; i.e., since a line corresponds to a particular real physical edge, it cannot change from, say, being concave to being convex with no intervening junction. Such an assumption is a typical "natural constraint," and constraints such as these play an important role explaining the apparently "intelligent" nature of vision. To apply the technique known as "label propagation" (or sometimes "constraint propagation"), we need to consider each pair of connected junctions and ask whether the line label that one of them allows for a particular line is a label allowed at the other junction. In other words, we trace a line from one junction to another and check whether the junction at either end prohibits that label (i.e., whether the line label in question occurs in both of the vertices, as identified in figure 3.6). If it is not, then that particular label is eliminated from the candidate labels for that particular edge. Thus the pair of vertices shown in figure 3.7 cannot occur if they are to share a common edge, since that line would have to be labeled "+" according to

2. This is a highly simplified version of Waltz's labeling scheme. In this version, only 4 types of line labels (illustrated in figure 3.5) are used, and some vertex types (e.g., those that include 4 edges, such as the K vertex) are omitted. The complete Waltz set includes over 50 line labels. These can generate over 300 million logically possible junctions, of which only 1790 are physically possible (see Waltz, 1975).

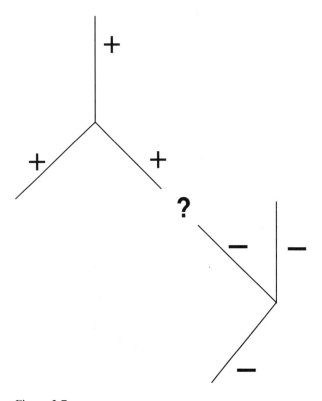

Figure 3.7
The top vertex shares a line with the bottom vertex, but the labels given to the connecting line at each end are incompatible. In a world consisting of blocks it is not physically possible to have an single edge with two different labels chosen from the set shown in figure 3.5. This pattern is then ruled out by the consistency constraint so one or the other vertex has to be relabeled using some other Y or Arrow label from figure 3.6.

the top left vertex, whereas the label "+" is prohibited on the corresponding edge of the bottom right vertex. Hence the putative labels assigned to the connecting line by one or the other vertex must be eliminated by going back to the list of vertex types in figure 3.6 and choosing another possible label for that vertex type (Y or arrow vertex) from the permissible list. This elimination can then be iterated and will result in the elimination of other line and vertex labels. If we are lucky, the effect propagates through the network of vertex and line labels in a domino effect until only one consistent set of labels remains. At that point the diagram has been successfully analyzed within the limits of the set of labels provided by the technique.

Such a constraint-propagation technique, when used in conjunction with a richer set of line labels (Waltz, 1975), generally results in the elimination of all but the perceptually admissible labels for the figure. Ambiguous figures, such as the Necker cube, end up with two permissible *consistent* labelings, and certain impossible figures (such as the devil's pitchfork in chapter 1 and the impossible triangle illustrated in figure 3.2) end up with no consistent set of labels. A similar story could in principle be told for a world other than the blocks world: perceptually ambiguous stimuli (such as the Necker cube shown in figure 3.8) have at least two labelings not prohibited by some "natural constraint." The consistent labeling that remains after this constraint propagation allow us (in some cases with the addition of other grouping principles) to figure out which lines go together to form faces and which faces occlude other faces, and so on.

The set of labels described above invariably allows for multiple interpretations not only of figures such as the Necker cube, but also of figures which our visual system interprets as univocal and free of ambiguities. One of Waltz's discoveries is that if the set of line labels is judiciously expanded to include shadow edges and cracks, which are edges that would become outside edges if the abutting blocks were moved apart, then the range of interpretations is decreased, even though the number of possible vertex labels in greatly increased. By combining these various types of edges, one gets about 50 different kinds of edge labels (instead of the 4 we used in figure 3.8) and also increases the number of vertex shapes from 4 to about 10, thereby increasing the combinatorially possible vertex labelings from the 208 we had to over 3 billion! Yet despite the large number of logically possible alternative labels for each vertex, the number of physically possible labelings only increases from 18 to around 1790. An enormous increase in the fineness of distinctions leads to an increase in number of labeling, as expected, but provides more opportunity for natural constraints to be felt. Indeed, Waltz discovered that the stronger constraints allow almost any blocks-world scene to be given a unique parsing (except for those cases where we too would see the scene as ambiguous, as well as a few other cases where the constraints fail to provide a unique analysis).

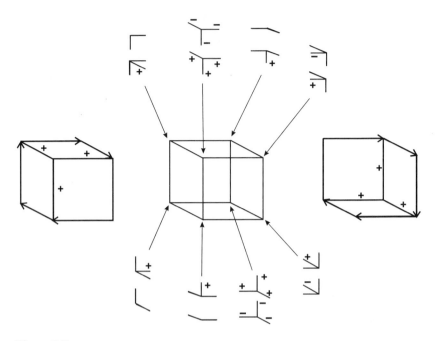

Figure 3.8
Labels of possible vertices for a Necker cube lead to two distinct sets of consistent labels, corresponding to the two interpretations shown here.

The application of constraints in this example works much as a computer spreadsheet (such as Excel) works. A set of requirements that must be met among rows and columns is provided (often in the form of equations) and each time one of the entries changes, the spreadsheet attempts to alter the contents of specified cells so that the constraints hold. In the case of vision, however, the constraints have to be discovered in nature and tested against the visual system to determine whether the candidates are indeed ones that the visual system respects. We will see later that not every constraint in the world is embedded in the visual system, and in fact many extremely strong (and common) real-world constraints are not mirrored by visual-system constraints, so that we can end up seeing things we know are impossible (two examples of physically impossible situations that we readily perceive are sketched in figures 3.16 and 3.17).

Other constraints: the "rules" of visual analysis   In a delightful book, Donald Hoffman (1998) lists 35 of these constraints, which he calls rules.

Here are a few of them (notice that they rely on the assumption that the image property in question is "nonaccidental," which means that it will continue to hold despite small changes in viewpoint):

1. Interpret a straight line in an image as a straight line in 3D.
2. If the tips of two lines coincide in an image, then interpret them as coinciding in 3D.
3. Interpret lines collinear in an image as collinear in 3D.
4. Interpret elements nearby in an image as nearby in 3D.
5. Interpret a curve that is smooth in an image as smooth in 3D.
6. Interpret a curve in an image as the rim of a surface in 3D.

What is perhaps most surprising is how powerful these simple principles are: they can make the 2D-to-3D inverse mapping univocal in most naturally occurring circumstances, resulting in an unambiguous 3D interpretation of an image. What is also important is that the principles are not determined by either geometry or physical law—they can easily be violated, as figure 3.3 shows. Rather, they are principles that frequently apply in a world populated by solid coherent objects—a world in which most visual elements (say bits of texture) are on surfaces and so when they are close together, they remain close together even when one changes one's viewpoint slightly or when the object moves. Similarly, because most of what we see in the world (unlike what fish see) consists of the surfaces of objects, only a very small percent of each image consists of outer edges, and these appear as contours at just the point where the surface "turns the corner" or presents a rim. This is why we can usually get a great deal of information about an object's shape from its profile (as specified by rule 6). This rule, by the way, is one of a series of remarkable closely related principles, discovered by Jan Koenderink (1990) and others, that can be shown mathematically to hold, given certain assumptions about the nature of objects that are common in our particular kind of world, and in particular, given the assumption that the image property is nonaccidental. These principles allow one to reconstruct 3D shapes when given both outside contours (profiles) and inside contours (concave and convex dimples and mounds).

The principles are not only concerned with properties of projective geometry. Some principles depend on facts that are true of our world and might not hold of other physically possible worlds. One such

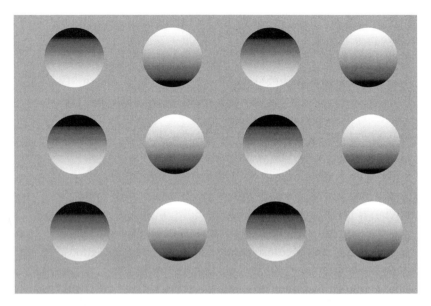

Figure 3.9
This figure shows both craters and mounds. The selection of which is seen is sensitive to the direction of light and shadows, as can be seen by turning the page upside-down, which generally reverses the craters and mounds. (Based on figures shown in Ramachandran, 1988.)

principle concerns the direction of light. Since we travel primarily on the surface of the earth with the sun overhead, the direction of light is invariably from the top. This simple fact allows certain kinds of ambiguities to be resolved. This can be seen from figure 3.9, where both mounds (bumps) and dimples (depressions) can be seen. How we tend to see this picture depends on the fact that the visual system acts as though it tacitly assumes that the light comes from above. This can be seen by turning the figure upside-down: doing so inverts the perception of mounds and dimples.[3]

Examples of natural constraints that apply to more general situations are based on the fact that matter is predominantly coherent and that

3. V. S. Ramachandran has pointed out to me that the orientation dependence of this percept is body-centered, so you can get the change in concavity-convexity by standing on your head. So, remarkably, the wiring of this particular natural constraint assumes not only that light tends to come from above, but also that you tend to be right-side up.

most substances tend to be opaque. Together these lead to the principle that neighboring elements on an image, as well as elements that move with a similar velocity, tend to arise from points on the surface of the same object. Another closely related constraint that has been used in computing depth from pairs of stereo images includes the (frequently, but not universally valid) principle that for each point on one retina, there is exactly one point on the other retina that arises from the same distal feature, and the principle that neighboring points will tend to have similar disparity values. These principles allow a unique interpretation of a pair of stereo images (see Marr, 1982, pp. 111–159) because they provide guidance in solving a central problem in stereo-image analysis known as the correspondence problem: which element in the left image should be paired with which element in the right image? Clearly, we should pair those elements that arise from the same element in the 3D scene, but how do we know which pairs have that property? Principles such as those sketched above provide a basis for solving this problem in a way that is *usually* correct (in our kind of world).

The rigidity constraint in apparent motion: the correspondence problem
Another example of the use of a constraint such as rigidity is the model that Michael Dawson and I (Dawson and Pylyshyn, 1988) developed to explain why successive presentations of visual elements are seen as one pattern of apparent motion rather than another. Although one can implement many different ways of pairing an element in the first display with some particular element in the second display, it is important that this be done in a principled way, and also that it be done in a way that respects any known neurophysiological constraints. This means appealing to a general constraint that holds in the world (a natural constraint), and it also suggests that the implementation should use only local information and compute correspondences based on local interactions. Since the computations in early vision tend to be done in parallel, they tend to be based on retinally local information and connections. In our model, each pair of logically possible correspondences between one of the 4 elements in image 1 and one of the 4 elements in image 2 is considered (there are 4! or 24 of these, not counting correspondences in which several objects collapse into one). The relative (vector) motion of each candidate pair is compared with the relative motion of its neighbors.

These potential pairings are each given weights by an iterative process. The more similar the relative motion of a particular pair is to that of its neighbors, the greater the weight given to it. In the end, the correspondence pairs left with the greatest weight represents the winning correspondence. This scheme is a direct reflection of the rigidity constraint, since it favors correspondences that constitute motions most like that of its neighbors, which is what one would expect if the elements were on the surface of a rigid object. Moreover, this scheme relies on only local comparisons. The correspondences computed by this relaxation scheme bear a close relation to those actually observed with human subjects. For example, figure 3.10 shows two different correspondences, out of a possible 24 noncollapsing correspondences, each of which represents a different possible perceived motion. The two curves show apparent motions that correspond to a rigid movement of the group of 4 objects, but only one of these, the one shown as a solid line, is computed based on local interactions. This solid line also corresponds to how observers tend to perceive this motion. In these cases, as well as a variety of others, the

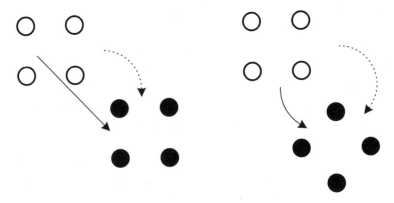

Figure 3.10
Illustration of the apparent motion predicted by a model that favors the interpretation corresponding to the elements being on the surface of a rigid object. Open circles are the configuration at time 1 and filled circles are the configuration at time 2. The solid and dotted curves are two possible correspondences between elements in the two frames that maintain the rigid configuration of four elements. The solid ones are the paths actually seen by observers. In each case they are the ones that favor correspondences in which the vector displacements of elements are most similar to that of the vector's neighbors. (Based on the description in Dawson and Pylyshyn, 1988.)

motion prediction based on a local implementation of a rigidity constraint is the one actually observed.

This way of solving the correspondence problem is closely related to the way I suggested that the visual system solves the problem of providing a 3D interpretation of a 2D pattern, despite the fact that the 3D-to-2D mapping is logically indeterminate. The solution to both these problems involves assigning an interpretation that favors some general property that holds in our world. This process involves principles quite different from those assumed in Bruner's and Helmholtz's analyses. The latter approach claims that the visual system infers the perceived shape (or motion) by hypothesizing, say, that the elements lie in a certain particular 3D configuration, and then attempts to verify this hypothesis. This way of dealing with the indeterminacy problem relies on expectations of what is likely in the particular scene being viewed. Consequently, if the observer had reason to believe that the points did not lie on the surface of a moving rigid object, that hypothesis would not be entertained, or at least would be given low credence. But this is patently false of our visual system. For example, experiments on the kinetic-depth effect are generally carried out on a flat surface, such as a computer monitor or projection screen, which observers know is flat, yet they continue to see the patterns as moving in depth. By contrast, the natural-constraint view says that the visual system is so constructed (through evolution) that a certain sort of rigid interpretation will be the one automatically given (independent of knowledge of the particular scene; indeed, even despite knowledge to the contrary) whenever it is possible, that is, whenever such a representation of the distal environment is consistent with properties of the proximal stimulus. Since in our world (as opposed to, perhaps, the world of a jellyfish) most moving features of interest do lie on the surface of rigid objects, this constraint will generally lead to veridical perception.

The idea that early vision embodies, but does not explicitly represent, certain very general constraints that require vision to derive representations that are often veridical in our kind of physical world, has become an important principle in computer vision. The notion of "our kind of world" includes properties of geometry and optics and includes the fact that in visual perception the world presents itself to an observer in certain ways (e.g., projected approximately to a single viewpoint). This basic insight has led to the development of further mathematical analyses and to a field of study known as "observer mechanics" (Bennett, Hoffman, and Prakash, 1989). Although there are different ways to state the constraints—for example, in terms of properties of the world, in terms of the use of "general purpose models" of objects (Lowe, 1987; Zucker et al., 1975), or even in terms of some world-independent mathematical principle, such as "regularization" (Poggio, Torre, and Koch, 1990)—the basic assumption remains that the visual system follows a set of intrinsic principles independent of general knowledge, expectations, or needs. The principles express the built-in constraints on how proximal information may be used in recovering a representation of the distal scene. Such constraints are quite different from the Gestalt laws (such as proximity and common fate) because they apply not to properties of the proximal stimulus, but to how such a stimulus is interpreted or used to construct a representation of the distal perceptual world. In addition, people (like David Marr) who work in the natural-constraint tradition often develop computational models that are sensitive to certain general neurophysiological constraints. For example, the processes tend to be based on "local support"—or data that come from spatially local regions of the image—and tend to use parallel computations, such as relaxation or label-propagation methods, rather than global or serial methods (Dawson and Pylyshyn, 1988; Marr and Poggio, 1979; Rosenfeld et al., 1976).

3.1.2   On "intelligence" and "problem-solving" in vision

There are other cases of apparently "intelligent perception" that differ from the cases discussed above because they seem to involve more than just 2D-to-3D mapping. These include many examples that are reviewed in the important book by Irvin Rock (1983), where a strong case is made that vision involves "intelligent perception" or even "problem solving." In what follows, I argue that these cases represent the embodiment of the same general kind of implicit constraints as those studied under the category of natural constraints, rather than the operation of reasoning and problem solving. Like the natural constraints discussed earlier, these constraints frequently lead to veridical percepts, yet as in the amodal completion examples discussed earlier (e.g., section 2.3.2), they often also appear to be quixotic and to generate percepts that do not bear any rational connection to the rest of the scene nor to what might rationally be expected in the scene. As with other natural constraints, the principles are internal to the visual system and are not sensitive to beliefs and knowledge about the particulars of a scene, nor are they themselves available to cognition.

Paradigm examples of "intelligent perception," cited by Rock (1983), are the perceptual constancies. We are all familiar with the fact that we tend to perceive the size, brightness, color, and so on, of objects in a way that appears to take into account the distance of the objects from us, the lighting conditions, and other such factors extrinsic to the retinal image of the object in question. This leads to such surprising phenomena as different perceived sizes of afterimages when viewed against backgrounds at different distances (retinal images, such as produced by an afterimage, appear larger when viewed against a more distance background—following a principle known as Emmert's law). In each case it is as if the visual system knew the laws of optics and of projective geometry and took these into account, along with retinal information from the object and from other visual cues as to distance, orientation, the direction and type of lighting, and so on. The intelligent way that the visual system takes these factors into account is striking. Consider the example of the perceived lightness (or whiteness) of a surface, as distinct from the perception of how brightly illuminated it is. Observers distinguish these two contributors of objective brightness of surfaces in various subtle ways. For example, if one views a sheet of cardboard half of which is colored a darker shade of gray than the other, the difference in their whiteness is quite apparent. But if the sheet is folded so that the two portions are at appropriate angles to each other, the difference in whiteness can appear as a difference in the illumination caused by their different orientations relative to a common light source. In a series of ingenious experiments, Gilchrist (1977) showed that the perception of the degree of "lightness" of a surface patch (i.e., whether it is white, gray, or black) is greatly affected by the perceived distance and orientation of the surface in question, as well as by the perceived illumination falling on the surface (the last was experimentally manipulated through a variety of cues, such as occlusion and perspective).

Rock (1983) cites examples such as the above to argue that in computing constancies, vision "takes account of" a variety of factors in an

"intelligent" way, following certain kinds of "rules." In the case of lightness perception, the rules, he suggests, embody principles that include
"(1) that luminance differences are caused by reflectance-property differences or by illumination differences, (2) that illumination tends to be
equal for nearby regions in a plane . . . and (3) that illumination is
unequal for adjacent planes that are not parallel" (Rock, 1983, p. 279).
These are exactly the kinds of principles that appear in computational
theories based on natural constraints. They embody general geometrical
and optical constraints, they are specific to vision, and they are fixed and
independent of the details of a particular scene. Lightness constancy is a
particularly good example to illustrate the similarities between cases that
Rock calls "intelligent perception" and the kind of natural-constraint
cases we have been discussing, because there are at least fragments of a
computational theory of lightness constancy (more recently these have
been embedded within a theory of color constancy) based on natural
constraints that are similar to the principles discussed above (see, for
example, Maloney and Wandell, 1990; Ullman, 1976).

Other examples are cited by Rock as showing that perception is not
only "intelligent" but involves a type of "problem solving." I will
examine a few of these examples in order to suggest that they bear a
striking resemblance to the natural-constraint examples already discussed. The examples below are also drawn from the ingenious work of
Irvin Rock and his collaborators, as described in Rock (1983).

Chapter 1 (figures 1.15 and 1.16) described perception through an
anorthoscope, or what some people call the Zollner-Parks phenomenon
(sometimes also called the eye-of-the-needle phenomenon). In these
studies, a form is shown through a narrow slit as the slit moves back
and forth across the form, producing a (somewhat impoverished) percept
of the entire figure. But when the line segments that are visible through
the slit stop short of the edge of the slit (so that it no longer looks like
the form is seen *through* the slit), a percept of the form does not occur.
Rock (1981) constructed an apparatus (shown in figure 3.11) that presents the same view to an observer that would have occurred in a genuine
anorthoscopic presentation (shown on the left), but also allows the line
segment seen through the slit to stop short of the edges of the slit (shown
on the right). In this case the perception of a shape behind the contour
does not occur, which suggests that the visual system takes into account

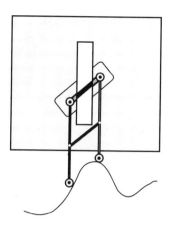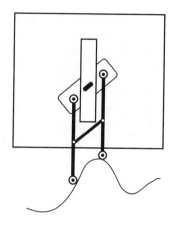

Figure 3.11
A trick version of the anorthoscope presentation. In both these illustrations the line segment is made to move just as it would if it were a view of a larger form seen through a moving slit in an opaque screen (regular anorthoscope presentations are shown in figures 1.15 and 1.16). In the panel on the right, however, the contour segment seen through the apparently moving slit does not reach the edge of the slit, so no occlusion cues are present. In this case no percept of the entire form occurs. (Adapted from Rock, 1981.)

the evidence that the moving slit does not in fact present a view of a stationery form behind it.

Another example uses a familiar phenomenon of early vision in which the perception of motion is created in certain flicker displays—so-called apparent or phi motion. In these displays, when pairs of appropriately separated dots (or lights) are displayed in alternation, subjects see a single dot moving back and forth. The conditions under which apparent motion is perceived have been thoroughly investigated. From the perspective of the present concern, one finding stands out as being particularly interesting. One way of describing this finding is to say that if the visual system is visually provided with an alternative "reason" for why the dots are alternatively appearing and disappearing, then apparent motion is not seen. One such "reason" could be that an opaque object (such as a pendulum swinging in the dark) is moving in front of a pair of dots and is alternately occluding one and then the other. Experiments by Sigman and Rock (1974) show, for example, that if the alternation of dots is accompanied by the appearance of what is perceived to be an opaque surface in front of the dot that has disappeared, apparent motion is not seen (figure 3.12B). Interestingly, if the "covering" surface presented over the dots is perceived as a transparent surface, then the apparent motion persists (figure 3.12A). Moreover, whether or not a surface is perceived as opaque can be a subtle perceptual phenomenon, since the apparent motion can be blocked by a "virtual" or "illusory" surface, as in figure 3.13A (since the opaque surface moving back and forth "explains" why the dots are not seen at that location), though not in the control figure 3.13B.

There are many examples showing that the visual system often appears to resolve potential contradictions and inconsistencies in an "intelligent" manner. For example, the familiar illusory Kanizsa figure, such as the rectangle in figure 3.13A is usually perceived as a number of circles with an opaque (though implicit) figure in front of them that occludes parts of the circles (circles with slices cut out of them are often used in illusory contours that form Kanizsa figures; they resemble creatures in the

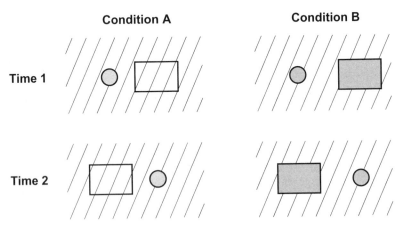

Figure 3.12
In the left figure (A), the texture seen through the rectangle makes the rectangle appear to be a transparent frame, so the circle is seen as appearing and disappearing in alternation in the two locations and apparent motion is perceived. In the figure on the right (B), the distinct texture on the rectangle makes it appear to be opaque, so the appearance/disappearance of the circles is compatible with the assumption that they continue to be present but are successively covered by an opaque moving rectangle. Consequently the circles in this case are not seen as undergoing apparent motion. (After Sigman and Rock, 1974.)

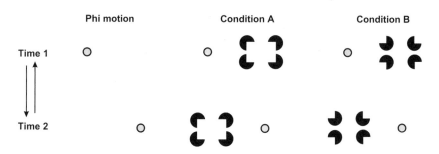

Figure 3.13
When an object such as the circle appears and disappears alternating in two locations it is usually seen as moving back and forth (in what is called apparent motion or Phi motion). In the figure on the left (A), the illusory rectangle is seen to be opaque since it cuts off a pie-shaped segment of each black circle. Thus when the configuration alternates between the top and bottom patterns (labeled time 1 and time 2), the opaque rectangle appears to alternately cover the two dots, providing an "explanation" for why the dots appear and disappear. Consequently apparent motion is not perceived in that case. By contrast, there is no moving opaque rectangle in the display on the right (B) to explain the circles' disappearance and reappearance, so apparent motion of the circles is perceived. (After Sigman and Rock, 1974.)

early computer game Pacman). The figure is thus seen as closer, brighter, and opaque, so that it hides segments of the circles. (For other examples, see Kanizsa, 1976.) However, that very same stimulus will not be seen as an illusory figure if a texture is seen through it (as in the figure on the right in figure 3.14), since this provides counterevidence to its opacity, and thus there is no opaque illusory figure to explain the missing segments in the three circles.

On the other hand, if the figures are presented stereoscopically or in 3D, with the observer free to move and thus to see that the texture is actually in front of the Kanizsa figure, there is no longer a contradiction: subjects see the illusory opaque figure, as it is normally seen, but this time they see it through what appears to be a transparent textured surface (Rock and Anson, 1979). Figure 3.15 shows a schematic of the two situations. Notice that for the Kanizsa figure to be seen (as in the situation on the right), the observer has to *visually perceive* that the circles with cutouts are on a layer behind the texture. It is not enough that the observer know that this is how they are located in 3D. So, for example, if the observer has an opportunity to observe the experimental layout by walking around

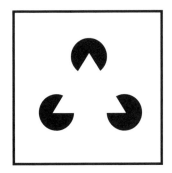 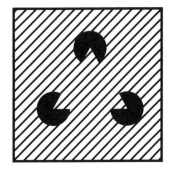

Figure 3.14
A Kanizsa triangle appears vividly in the figure on the left, but it is not seen as clearly (is not as stable) if there is conflicting evidence that the triangle is not opaque, as in the case on the right where the background texture apparently can be seen through it.

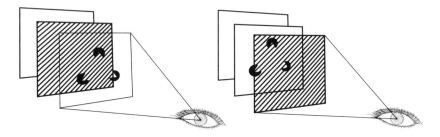

Figure 3.15
Two ways of displaying in 3D the figures that make up the situation depicted in figure 3.14. The one on the left shows the Kanizsa triangle, viewed so as to show it as being in front of the textured surface (the layer nearest the viewer is a transparent sheet with a Kanizsa triangle painted on it, the next layer is a sheet with textured lines). Since seeing the textured lines is incompatible with seeing the triangle as opaque, the triangle is not seen, only the three circles with slices cut out. On the right the viewer (who is examining the figures in 3D) sees that the textured surface is in front of the Kanizsa triangle (the layer closest to the viewer is a transparent texture, the second is the Kanizsa triangle), which does not contradict seeing the triangle as opaque, so the triangle is seen. (Adapted from Rock and Anson, 1979.)

it and then looks at it monocularly through a peephole (so no depth cures are available—either stereo-disparity cues or parallax-motion cues), the display will still be perceived like the figure on the right of figure 3.14— without the vivid Kanizsa triangle.

Examples such as these are sometimes interpreted as showing that how we perceive parts of a scene depends on making some sort of coherent sense of the whole. In the examples cited by Rock, the perception of ambiguous stimuli can usually be interpreted as resolving conflicts in a way that makes sense, which is why it is referred to as "intelligent." But what does "making sense" mean if not that our knowledge of the world is being brought to bear in determining the percept?

What distinguishes a function that embodies natural constraints from one that draws inferences from general knowledge is the following: (a) The natural constraints do not influence any processes outside of the visual system (e.g., they do not in any way inform the cognitive system). Even if one views the visual system as possessing implicit knowledge, this knowledge would have to be recognized as special, inasmuch as it is not used freely to draw inferences about the world—it is not what Stich (1978) calls "inferentially promiscuous." (b) The visual process itself does not respond to any other kind of knowledge or new information related to these constraints, for example, the constraints show up even if the observer knows that there are conditions in a certain scene that render them invalid in that particular case. For example, even if the observer knew that the textured surface was in front of the Kanizsa triangle, it would make no difference to what is seen: in general, only visually present collateral information can influence what is seen. What this means is that no additional regularities are captured by the hypothesis that the system has knowledge of certain natural laws and takes them into account through "unconscious inferences." Even though in these examples the visual process appears to be "intelligent," it may be carried out by prewired circuitry that does not access encoded knowledge. Notions such as knowledge, belief, goal, and inference give us an explanatory advantage when sets of generalizations can be captured under common principles such as rationality or even something roughly like semantic coherence (Pylyshyn, 1984a). In the absence of such over-arching principles, Occam's Razor and Lloyd Morgan's Canon dictate that the simpler or lower-level hypothesis (and the less powerful mechanism) is preferred. This is also the argument advanced by Kanizsa (1985).

3.1.3 Constraints do not reflect high-frequency or physically permissible real-world principles

Are natural constraints just a reflection of what we frequently see, or what usually occurs in the world? Given the empiricist tradition that has colored the past half-century of psychology and biology, one might expect this to be so. But it turns out, perhaps surprisingly, that the constraints embodied in vision do not reflect what frequently occurs in the world. The visual constraints that have been discovered so far are based almost entirely on principles that derive from laws of optics and projective geometry. Properties such as the occlusion of features by surfaces closer to the viewer are among the most prominent in these principles, as are principles that are attributable to the reflectance, opacity, and rigidity of bodies. What is perhaps surprising is that other properties of our world—about which our intuitions are equally strong—do not appear to share this special status in the early-vision system. In particular, perceptual conflicts are rarely resolved so as to respect such physical principles as that solid objects do not pass through one another. Consequently, some percepts constructed by the visual system fail a simple test of rationality or of coherence with certain basic facts about the world known to every observer.

Take the example of the Ames trapezoidal window, which, when rotated about a vertical axis, appears to oscillate rather than rotate through a full circle. When a rigid rod is placed inside this window (at right angles to the frame) and the window-and-rod combination is rotated, an anomalous percept appears. The trapezoidal window continues to be perceived as oscillating, while the rod is seen to rotate—with the result that the rod is seen as passing through the rigid frame (figure 3.16).

Another example of this phenomenon is the Pulfrich double-pendulum illusion (Wilson and Robinson, 1986). In this illusion two solid pendulums constructed from sand-filled detergent bottles and suspended by rigid metal rods swing in opposite phase, one slightly behind the other. When viewed with a neutral-density filter over one eye (which results in slower visual processing in that eye), one pendulum is seen as swinging in an elliptical path, while the other one is seen as following it around, also in an elliptical path but lagging behind (figure 3.17). As a result of

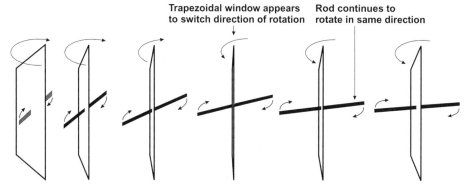

Figure 3.16
When a trapezoidal window rotates about a vertical axis it is seen as swinging back and forth about that axis. When a rod is placed through it, the rod is not subject to this illusion, so it is seen to rotate through 360 degrees. As a result, at certain points in the rotation it is seen to penetrate the solid frame. (Described in Rock, 1981.)

these distinct trajectories the rigid rods are seen as passing *through* one another. From a certain angle of view, the bottles also appear to pass through one another, even though they also appear to be solid and opaque. Interpenetrability of solid opaque objects does not seem to be blocked by the visual system, even though it is clearly at variance with what we know about how things inevitably happen in the world.

To repeat the moral of this section, many cases in which our visual system provides unambiguous (and usually veridical) percepts, despite the inherent ambiguity of the 2D image, can be explained without having to assume that the visual system draws inferences from general knowledge regarding what the 3D scene is likely to contain. Although the *beliefs* we come to have about what is in the scene invariably take into account what we know, the output of the early-vision system, or to put it loosely (though I believe correctly), *how things look,* does not take into account such knowledge. The visual system is so constructed, presumably because it has become tuned over eons of evolutionary history, that the range of interpretations it is able to make is severely restricted. This range of alternatives is specified by principles (or "rules") such as the 6 discussed on page 107 (and others discussed by Hoffman, 1998; Marr, 1982; Richards, 1988). These principles are invariably associated with spatiotemporal and optical properties, rather than with physical

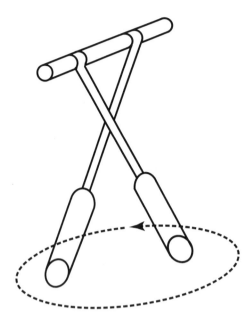

Figure 3.17
The "Pulfrich double pendulum," described by Wilson and Robinson (1986). When a pendulum is viewed binocularly, with one eye covered by a neutral density (gray) filter, it appears to swing in an ellipse (possibly because the weaker signal to one eye is processed more slowly). When there are two such pendulums, they appear to swing out of phase, and consequently would have to be seen as passing though one another. The visual system has no problem constructing such a physically impossible percept. This and many other examples show that vision does not incorporate physical constraints, even ones as obvious as the impenetrability of solid objects.

properties. Consequently, they do not appear to reflect high-frequency properties of the world we live in so much as those critical spatial properties that all animals need to survive as mobile agents.

3.2   What Is Computed by the Encapsulated Early-Vision System?

The last chapter argued that the essential, or uniquely visual, part of the visual system, called "early vision," is isolated from the rest of the cognitive mind. As a consequence, cognition has only two loci of potential control over what we see. These lie in the *attentional selection* that occurs before early vision and in the *interpretation and memory-based recog-*

nition that occurs after early vision. The latter may also include a cognitively mediated postperceptual selection. According to this proposal, the visual system may generate several logically possible interpretations, and the alternative that best fits with the system of beliefs and expectations may be selected as the most plausible interpretation, with the others decaying rapidly in time. (This sort of process has been proposed for language understanding, where the language-specific syntactic module provides several simultaneous analyses from which the most plausible is selected [see, e.g., Swinney, 1979].)

While I have defended the claim that early vision is isolated from thought, I have said very little about what goes on within this encapsulated visual system. If what is encapsulated ends up being simple sensory transduction—the conversion of light patterns on the retina to neural patterns on a one-to-one basis—then the thesis that this part of vision is cognitively impenetrable is neither surprising nor interesting: few people believe that the rods and cones of the retina and their immediate successors (e.g., the cells with limited retinal receptive fields) are subject to direct control by the cognitive system. What would be more interesting—and what was implied by the discussion in the last chapter—is that the encapsulated function is much more complex and covers much more of the total process that we call visual perception than was generally believed (at least by the psychologists of the past half-century). Indeed, the implication of the last chapter is that the early-vision system starts at the point where focal attention zeroes in on relevant aspects of the scene and extends to the construction of the sort of percept that we might have of a totally unfamiliar scene. For example, I assume that early vision would allow you to make out the individual objects and the spatial layout of a totally unfamiliar scene, such as the landscape of an alien planet where nothing is recognized as familiar. The questions of what constitutes the inputs and outputs of the visual system, and what mathematical function is computed by the visual system, are thus of paramount importance to understanding how vision works, since they demarcate the scope of early vision.

So far I have also said nothing about the nature of the processes that go on within vision, except that they are not what would normally be called *inference*, at least not of the sort that is carried out in cognition, where there are no principled restrictions on what knowledge can be brought to bear.[4] It is important to see that even though the processes of vision are distinct from the processes of reasoning, they are nonetheless highly structured and made up of distinct stages and submodules. These stages may generate intermediate representations in the course of computing the final output. Some of these representations are sufficiently rich and sufficiently different from one another that many vision scientists have suggested that there may be more than one distinct visual system. In the following sections, I will address the nature of the early vision system in somewhat greater detail, beginning with a consideration of its inputs and outputs and then moving on to an examination of the various subprocesses that make it up.

3.2.1 What are the inputs to the visual system?

David Marr (1982) pointed out rather forcefully that to understand vision we need to first understand what function the visual system computes. For Marr, this meant specifying not only the input-output function (in the mathematical sense—i.e., what function it computes), but also how computing that function, rather than some other, supports the organism's needs. Thus Marr analyzed the visual function in terms of what it was for. One need not accept the tenet that vision needs to be analyzed in terms of some teleological specifications in order to recognize the need to characterize vision in terms of more general functions of an organism. Indeed, this rejection of the tenet is implicit in the discussion above about natural constraints. But in characterizing the function computed by the visual system, we need to be concerned with what exactly constitutes the input to this system. A number of radically different approaches to understanding vision, such as the approach taken by Gibson (1979) and by newer variants of the Gibsonian program (e.g., O'Regan and Noë, 2002), have taken as their point of departure the claim that traditional vision science has misconstrued the nature of the

---

4. This is, in part, a terminological point. There are those (e.g., Fodor, 1983; Fodor and Pylyshyn, 1981) who refer to any process that constructs a representation that goes beyond what is in the incoming information as an inference (although it is no easy matter to explicate what it means to "go beyond the incoming information"). I prefer to reserve the term "inference" for a process that Stich (1978) calls "inferentially promiscuous"—i.e., that is not restricted in a principled way to what information it can use.

input to vision. In this section I will only sketch these approaches in the most cursory manner (for a more thorough treatment, the reader is invited to read Fodor and Pylyshyn, 1981; Pylyshyn, 1984a). The question of what constitutes the proper input and output of vision is important because it has a direct bearing on the thesis that vision is independent of cognition (the "modularity of vision" thesis). If we do not constrain what is to count as the input or the output of visual processing, we will find that vision includes all of cognition, and the study of vision can become intractable.

When we talk of the visual system, it is obvious that in the first instance we are referring to the system that interprets information coming in through the eyes. This system starts with optical information and eventually produces either the phenomenological experience of seeing or some relevant observable consequences, such as visually guided action or visual memories or some of the objective psychophysical observations that I alluded to earlier (e.g., those discussed in chapter 1). There are many reasons to believe that information other than optical stimulation to the two retinas may play some role in vision. Several different types of input to the visual system have been proposed. One kind of input comes from other sensory modalities, from sense organs other than the retina. I will briefly survey some of these extraretinal influences below. They include not only the modulation of vision by such related modalities as the vestibular system and proprioceptive signals from the head and neck muscles, but also information from audition. All these influences may play a role in the perception of such properties as spatial location and orientation.

Some researchers have also pointed to the fact of *synesthesia*, in which information coming in from one modality is experienced in a different modality (such as when people experience sounds as different colors) as showing that the visual system can, under certain conditions, be stimulated by nonvisual inputs. I will touch on this sort of evidence briefly below and will suggest that it does not threaten the thesis that early vision is an independent encapsulated system.

A more problematic proposal has been the widely held view that the input to the visual system can also include what are called "mental images," or visual information retrieved from memory or generated as a consequence of certain problem-solving activities (e.g., reasoning with the aid of mental imagery). Although it is not inconceivable that an encapsulated visual system might take pictorial inputs generated by cognition, I will later argue that the evidence suggests that this does not in fact take place in the human mind/brain. The case against the view that cognition generates pictures that the visual system interprets will be discussed in the last third of this book. Suffice it to say at this point that the proposal is fraught with difficulties, both conceptual and empirical. The notion of a "pictorial" form of representation that "depicts" rather than "describes" is so ill defined as to make the question difficult, if not impossible, to answer. Moreover, the strong intuition that invites one to think that there are "pictures" in the mind, which the "mind's eye" can examine, is illusory, just as the parallel case of postulating mental pictures in visual perception was found to be illusory (as argued in chapter 1).

Cross-modal visual processing   There is some evidence that information from other modalities can modulate vision in systematic ways even early along the visual pathway. For example, inputs from the vestibular system appear to affect the perception of orientation, and proprioceptive and efferent signals from the eye and head can effect perception of visual location (Howard, 1982). These findings suggest that certain kinds of spatial information may have an effect across modalities, and therefore that in certain cases nonoptical sources of information may have to be included among "visual" inputs. Most of these cases concern spatial location, where there is even evidence that acoustical information may affect where objects are visually perceived to be located. Various sources of evidence (e.g., Radeau, 1994) suggest that perceived location may be determined by a fusion of information from several senses, with vision contributing an important share. Whether this is a case of fusion of postvisual information or a modulation of vision itself does not affect the principle of dissociation of vision and cognition, though it does affect whether we view, say, certain proprioceptive information from the eye muscles as constituting visual input. There is no a priori requirement that visual input consist only of information from the eyes, though that is certainly the prototypical form of input.

There are other sources of evidence of cross-modal influences on visual perception. For example, the perception of certain aspects of speech can be affected by vision and vice versa. In particular, it appears that in speech, what we see and what we hear both form part of the input to an encapsulated speech-perception system. Interestingly, it appears that this applies both to the recognition of the phonetic shape of the signal and also to its location in space (for an extensive discussion, see Radeau, 1994, and the commentaries published with it).

There is evidence to suggest that the domain of visual perception may not be coextensive with a single sensory modality. There is also intriguing evidence that the visual system itself may be taxonomized longitudinally, as an encapsulated process that runs from the sensors through to some specific motor subsystems—and consequently that in certain cases the module should be viewed as a *visuomotor* system, rather than as a strictly *visual* system. This evidence (which has been persuasively presented in Goodale, 1988, and Milner and Goodale, 1995) comes from neuroanatomy, from clinical reports of patients with visual agnosias and related neurological deficits, from psychophysical studies of perceptual-motor coordination, and from studies of animal behavior. I review this evidence in section 3.4 below, where I discuss the general question of what the visual system outputs to the rest of the mind/brain.

Synesthesia: Cross-modal perception?   It has long been reported that some people experience sensations that they identify as belonging to one modality, say color sensations, when they are in fact being stimulated by a different modality, say by sounds. Such phenomena are known as synesthesia.

Some writers (e.g., Baron-Cohen et al., 1993) have taken the existence of synesthesia to suggest that vision may not be encapsulated, as I have claimed. These writers feel that synesthesia shows that the visual system can sometimes be rather indiscriminate as to where it gets its inputs from, since there are cases where the input appears to come from other sensors in other modalities. But the fact that color sensations can be triggered by sound (or sound sensations by touch) does not imply that vision itself, or what I have been calling the early-vision system, can take its inputs from sound or other sensory receptors. The reason that the existence of synesthesia does not imply the failure of the boundary of visual perception is of some interest, since it helps to clarify what I mean by the "visual system."

A variety of cases of synesthesia have been examined in recent reviews. These include reviews of case studies (Cytowic, 1989, 1993) and experimental studies (Baron-Cohen and Harrison, 1997). The following facts about synesthesia are relevant to the boundaries of the visual system:

• The cross-modal sensations in synesthesia are not true percepts in a number of respects. Cytowic (1997) describes such sensations as being "generic" rather than "pictorial." Even when the generic sensations are perceived as deriving from a source in extrapersonal space, the sensations do not displace the perceptual content of the primary modality. Synesthetes do not see notes as colored *instead* of hearing them as forming a melody; rather, they hear the melody and they also have sensations of color. In fact, it seems correct to say that what they perceive to be out there in the world is melodies, the perception of which happens to be accompanied by sensations of color. The "perceptions" that they have are very different from both veridical perception *and* from perceptual illusions: people who have synesthetic experiences do not mistake melodies for a sequence of colored objects, as people who may be subject to a visual illusion might mistake the illusion for the true situation.

• The connection of synesthesia with conscious sensation is problematic in several ways. While visual perception may be generally associated with a certain sort of conscious experience, the experience itself may be neither necessary nor sufficient for vision. In general, what I have been calling visual perception need not itself be accompanied by *any* conscious sensations or other experiential content. Sometimes visual percepts, in the sense of the term that may be the most relevant to visual science, may not have an experiential content. They may, instead, have other kinds of objectively measurable consequences that signal their presence. Examples of these have been given earlier; they include clinical phenomena in which accurate visually guided action is observed in the absence of visual awareness (the most dramatic of which is the phenomenon referred to as blindsight, in which people report no vision in certain parts of their visual field yet are able to reach for objects in the blind field) and experimental cases of subliminal perception (the clinical cases will be discussed on pp. 153–156). It remains an open question how such cases of visual perception should be treated, but at present it seems at the very least premature to confine vision solely to processes that eventuate in conscious sensations. Conversely, the occurrence of visual experience in and of itself need not always indicate that the visual system is involved. In the case of visual experiences arising from hallucinations, dreams, and direct brain stimulation, it is not obvious that any visual information processing is occurring, or even that what I have called the early-vision system is directly involved (I will have much more to say about this question in chapters 6, 7, and 8).

• Even if we stipulated that visual sensations must arise from the visual system, this need only be true of a visual system in its normal mode of operation. If we produced visual sensations by cortical stimulation, this may or may not mean that we were stimulating the early vision system as we understand the term in the present discussion. We could in fact be bypassing the visual system and stimulating structures that mediate sensations rather than those that compute visual representations. Similarly, if something like the "sensory leakage" theory of synesthesia (Harrison and Baron-Cohen, 1997) were correct and the phenomena were due to leakage across neural pathways that lead, say, to visual sensations, it would still not necessarily mean that inputs to the visual system itself came from the auditory system.

There is a great deal we don't know about where, if anywhere, sensations reside in the brain, and it may well be that visual sensations do *not* arise from what many people consider the anatomical counterpart of what I have been calling early vision—cortical area V1 (Crick and Koch, 1995). Indeed, there is even doubt that an answer to the question of how (or where) the brain produces conscious experiences, including visual sensations, can be formulated in the vocabulary of contemporary psychology and neuroscience. Our current state of understanding of consciousness is such that we are far from warrant even to assume that sensations are the sorts of things that are "produced" or that "occur" in certain places, since there are good reasons to think that they may not be among the "functional properties" of the mind in the usual sense (i.e., properties that have an information-processing role). The question of whether conscious experience must have some "functional" consequences is a deeply perplexing problem that has been explored, with widely differing answers, by Block (1995); Block, Flanagan, and Guzeldere (1997); Chalmers (1996); Dennett and Kinsbourne (1992); McGinn (1999); and Searle (1995).

Given all these problems and unknowns, it seems prudent not to draw conclusions about how the visual system is functionally organized on the basis of data from synesthesia or other conscious contents, despite the fact that vision science must begin with facts about how things look to us.

The message so far is that what constitutes the input to the visual system cannot be prescribed in advance of the development of adequate theories of vision, nor can we appeal to our conscious experience of seeing to tell us whether some input is to count as *visual* input. Such questions about the fundamental functional taxonomy of the mind can only be answered as the science develops. Similarly, the question of what the visual system delivers as output also can not be prejudged. There is, however, already some interesting evidence bearing on that question, which I take up on page 133.

Should "visual input" include actual and potential motor actions?   We saw on page 126 that visual inputs could be modulated by proprioceptive signals. But the effect of motor activity goes beyond just modulating inputs. In fact, there are those who equate the content (or even experience) of vision with the set of possible stimulus-action contingencies (recent statements of this position can be found in O'Regan and Noë, 2002; Thomas, 1999). Such a point of view can be traced to the influential work of J. J. Gibson (1979), who took the position that visual perception is an organism's active responding (or, as he put it, "resonating") to the information available in its environment or in the "optic array." Such information, according to Gibson, does not just passively impinge on the sensors (if it did, our perception would be filled with illusions and ambiguities). Rather, the organism has to actively explore the optic array, just as, in the absence of sight, we would have to actively explore a shape using our tactile (or more generally, haptic) senses. The idea of vision as an *activity* has seen a recent revival, both in vision science and in artificial intelligence. This approach, versions of which are sometimes referred to as "situated vision" or "embedded cognition," has helped to correct a long-standing failure of vision science (and cognitive science in general) to pay sufficient attention to how cognition and the world share the responsibility for determining intelligent action.

Herb Simon (1969) gives the following example of how a cognitive process and the world together determine patterns of behavior. If we observe an ant on a beach from high above, we will see that the ant is executing a very complex path. To explain the path, we might be tempted to hypothesize a very complex cognitive process. But the truth is much simpler: the ant is following a very simple algorithm (e.g., keep at a certain angle to the sun, and refrain from climbing any steep slopes) applied to a complex environment of hills and valleys in the sand.[5] So it is with many other cognitive activities, including doing arithmetic and perceiving the world: the environment plays an important and often neglected role. I will have more to say about this concept of situated vision in section 5.4.

This perspective raises the question of whether we might not provide a better analysis of how vision works by describing vision as an active interaction between an organism and an environment. Gibson believed that the difficult problems of explaining visual perception could be avoided if we described the visual function appropriately, which for him meant shunning the vocabulary of optics and instead using a vocabulary closer to perceptual experience and action. For example, instead of describing the inputs to vision in terms of their proximal projections on the retina, he would have us describe them in terms of what things in the world are perceived *as*, such as objects, surfaces, layouts, and so on, and what potential actions they are perceived as permitting, which Gibson called their *affordances*. The latter category brings the study of visual perception into closer contact with the action-based approach advocated by those who view the function of perception as being primarily for allowing us to act on the world. While this is a commendable tempering of an overly zealous cognitivism, it runs in the face of much that has been learned about the intentionality of the mental.

It's true that explaining visual perception or other cognitive phenomena entirely on the basis of inferences carried out over mental representations will not do. In chapter 2 we saw some reasons for rejecting the traditional approach of treating vision as an extension of reasoning, and in chapter 5 (especially section 5.4) we will discuss other reasons why viewing vision solely as the construction of representations has to be augmented. However, there are three essential properties of a cognizing mind

5. This too is an oversimplification. As it turns out, the ant's internal navigation system is much more complex and sophisticated since it has to compute by dead reckoning, which entails measuring distance and time and integrating the component of the vector distance in the intended direction, while taking into account the movement of the sun over the course of the trip (Gallistel, 1990)—a far from trivial bit of computing. Mammals use an even more complex process to get where they want to go (Gallistel, 1994; Gallistel and Cramer, 1996).

that makes representations indispensable. It is beyond the scope of this book to consider these in detail here (they are discussed at length in Pylyshyn, 1984a) so I will only summarized them for reference.

• The equivalence classes of stimuli over which behavioral regularities have to be stated are semantically defined: stimuli (e.g., sentences) that have the same or similar meanings (e.g., are synonyms or paraphrases), or that have similar interpretations, play the same or similar roles in causing behavior.

• Intelligent behavior is largely stimulus-independent. You cannot predict the behavior of an intelligent cognizing agent solely by describing its environment (even including its past environments). This point was made so forcefully in Noam Chomsky's review of Skinner's attempt to characterize linguistic behavior in a behaviorist framework (see Chomsky, 1957) that it should never have to be raised again.

• Any cognitive (informational, as opposed to physical) regularity or rule can be overturned by additional relevant information. Some portion of any intelligent behavior is always *cognitively penetrable*.

These properties are among the reasons why representations are essential for explaining human cognitive behaviors, and therefore why even a sophisticated psychology of perceptual-motor contingency, or a psychology of environmentally determined behavior in any form, will eventually run into trouble. The active-vision position is often presented as the claim that vision should be characterized in terms of its potential for action, rather than its role in thought, and that when this is done, we find that representations become less important. It's true that what we see is determined to some extent by how we might potentially act toward the perceived world and also in part by the sensory-motor contingencies we expect from such potential actions as eye movements (see, for example, O'Regan and Noë, 2002). It has long been known that how the eye moves provides important information about the shape of objects and contours (e.g., Miller and Festinger, 1977) and even accounts for some illusions (see pp. 337–340). It is also true that if an object has a certain shape, the organism expects certain sensory patterns to hold as the eye moves. If the eye moves and these expectations go unfulfilled, perceptual discordance results. The discordance can lead to changes in perception, as it does in the case of perceptual adaptation to distorting lenses. All this is true and important. So vision depends not only on the proximal visual stimulus (i.e., the retinal projection) but also on patterns of perceptual-motor inputs and even on patterns of expectations of these inputs. One can accept this without giving up on the notion that what vision does is to construct visual representations that then serve in motor planning and cognition as beliefs generally do, by entering into inferences that may or may not lead to plans based on goals (i.e., old-fashioned beliefs and desires).

Preparing for action is not the only purpose of vision. Vision is, above all, a way to find out about the world, and there may be many reasons why an intelligent organism may wish to know about the world, apart from wanting to act upon it. The organism may just be curious: even rats and pigeons will respond for nothing more than information about when some non-reward-contingent light will come on, and will do so with greater vigor than for food (e.g., Blanchard, 1975). In the case of humans, it is pretty clear that vision can serve many functions, including purely aesthetic ones. Indeed, so powerful is the human drive for knowledge for its own sake that it led George Miller (1984) to characterize humans as primarily "informavores."

3.2.2   What are the outputs of the visual system?
The visual output: Categories and surface layouts   The other important question about vision concerns the nature of the output of the early-vision system. This is a central issue because the entire point of the independence thesis is to claim that early vision, understood as that modular part of the mind/brain devoted specifically to processing visual information, is both independent and complex, beyond being merely the output of transducers or feature detectors. And indeed, the examples we have been citing all suggest that the visual system so-defined does indeed deliver a rather complex representation of the world to the cognizing mind.

As we saw in chapter 2, the new-look view, as espoused by Bruner (1957), assumes that we perceive in terms of conceptual categories. Thus, according to this view, the visual system does not provide us with raw experiences of the visible world; it interprets these experiences in terms of the categories of cognition, which may be learned or culturally determined. Consequently, our knowledge and expectations influence what we see by altering what Bruner called the "readiness" or availability of different perceptual categories. Hence the output of vision, according to this view, is categories of experience. It is important to be clear what the discontinuity or independence thesis, set out in chapter 2, claims about perceptual categorization. The discontinuity thesis does not claim that our readiness and willingness to categorize something in our field of view as a so-and-so is independent of our expectation that there are so-and-sos in our field of view. That is because, as I have already noted, what we believe is in our field of view clearly does depend on such factors as our prior beliefs, as it should if we are rational agents. Nor does the discontinuity thesis claim that the visual system does not divide the perceived world up into equivalence classes, which is another way of saying that it divides the world into some kinds of categories. The fact that the mapping from the distal 3D environment to a percept is many-to-one entails that the visual system fails to distinguish certain differences. Another way of saying this is that by collapsing certain differences, the visual system partitions the visual world into "equivalence classes." But these kinds of classes are not what Bruner and others meant when they spoke of the categories of visual perception. The perceptual classes induced by early vision are not the kinds of classes that are the basis for the supposed enhancing effect of set and expectations. They do not, for example, correspond to meaningful categories in terms of which objects are identified when we talk about "perceiving as," e.g., perceiving something as a face or as Mary's face, and so on. To a first approximation, the classes provided by the visual system are shape classes, expressible in something like the vocabulary of geometry.

Notice that the early vision system does not *identify* the stimulus, in the sense of cross-referencing it to the perceiver's knowledge, the way a unique descriptive label might (e.g., "the girl next door," or "my car"). This sort of identity or labeling is inextricably linked to past encounters and to what one knows about members of the category (e.g., what properties—both visual and nonvisual—they have). After all, identifying some visual stimulus as your sister does depend on knowing such things as that you have a sister, what she looks like, whether she recently dyed her hair, and so on. But, according to the view I have been advocating, computing what the stimulus before you looks like—in the sense of computing some representation of its shape sufficient to pick out the class of similar appearances,[6] and hence to serve as an index into visual memory—does not itself depend on knowledge.

So far I have spoken only in very general terms about the nature of the stimulus classes picked out by vision. These classes could well be coextensive with basic-level categories (in the sense of the term adopted by Rosch et al., 1976), but the visual system itself does not label the output in terms of the name of a category, for reasons already alluded to above. It also seems reasonable that the shape classes provided by vision are ones whose names could be learned by ostension, i.e., by pointing or holding up an example of the named thing, rather than by providing a description or definition. Whether or not the visual system actually parses the world in these ways (i.e., into basic-level categories) is an interesting question, but one that is beyond the scope of this book. I have also not said anything about the form and content of the output beyond the claim that it contains shape classes. I will return to this issue below.

For the time being, we have the very general proposal that the visual system might be viewed as generating a set of one or more shape descriptors, which in many cases might be sufficient (perhaps in concert with other contextual information and presumably along with other information about the objects) to identify objects whose shapes are stored in memory. This provisional proposal is put forward to try to build a bridge between what the visual system delivers, which, as we have seen, cannot itself be the identity of objects, and what is stored in memory that enables identification. Whatever the details of such a bridge turn out to be, I still have not addressed the question of how complex or detailed or articulated this output is. Nor have I addressed the interesting question of

6. The question of what constitutes "similarity of appearance" is begged in this discussion—as is the related question of what makes some things appear more similar than others. We simply assume that the capacity to establish something like similar-in-appearance is given by our cognitive architecture—i.e., that it is built into the nervous system. Whether it is explicitly recognized or not, every theory of vision (and of concepts; see Fodor, 1998) assumes such a capacity. Objects that are "similar" in appearance are typically taken to be ones that receive similar (or in some sense "overlapping") representations in the output of the visual system. This much should not be problematic since, as I remarked earlier, the output necessarily induces an equivalence class of stimuli and this is at least in some rough sense a class of "similar" shapes.

whether there is more than one form of output, that is, whether the output of the visual system can be viewed as unitary or whether it might provide different outputs for different purposes or to different parts of the mind/brain. Below I will return to this idea, which is related to the "two visual systems" hypothesis.

The precise nature of the output in specific cases is an empirical issue that we cannot prejudge. There is a great deal that is unknown about the output, for example, whether it consists of a combinatorial structure that distinguishes individual objects and object parts, and whether it encodes nonvisual properties, such as causal relations, or primitive affective properties, like "dangerous," or even some of the functional properties that Gibson referred to as "affordances." In principle, the early-vision system could encode any property whose identification does not require accessing general memory, and in particular that does not require inference from general knowledge. So, for example, it is possible in principle for overlearned patterns—even patterns such as printed words—to be recognized from a finite table of pattern information compiled into the visual system. Whether or not any particular hypothesis is supported remains an open empirical question.[7]

Although there is much we don't know about the output of the visual system, we can make some general statements based on available evidence. We already have in hand a number of theories and confirming evidence for the knowledge-independent derivation of a three-dimensional representation of visible surfaces—what David Marr called the 2.5D sketch (since a full 3D representation would also contain information about the unseen back portion of objects). Evidence provided by J. J. Gibson, from a very different perspective, also suggests that what he called the "layout" of the scene may be something that the visual

7. One of the useful consequences of recent work on connectionist architectures has been to show that perhaps more cognitive functions than had been expected might be accomplished by table-lookup, rather than by computation. Newell (1990) was one of the first cognitive scientists to recognize the important trade-off between computing and storage that a cognitive system has to face. In the case of the early-vision system, where speed takes precedence over generality (see, e.g., Fodor, 1983), this could take the form of storing a forms table or set of templates in a special intrasystem memory. Indeed, I have already suggested that this sort of compiling of a local shape-table may be involved in some perceptual learning and in the acquisition of visual expertise.

system encodes (Gibson would say "picks up") without benefit of knowledge and reasoning. Nakayama, He, and Shimojo (1995) have also argued that the primary output of the independent visual system is a layout of surfaces in depth. Their data show persuasively that many visual phenomena are predicated on the prior derivation of a surface representation. These surface representations also serve to induce the perception of the edges that delineate and "belong to" those surfaces. Nakayama et al. argue that because of the prevalence of occlusions in our world, it behooves any visual animal to solve the surface-occlusion problem as quickly and efficiently as possible, and that this is done by first deriving the surfaces in the scene and their relative depth.

Nakayama et al. were able to show that the representation of surfaces in depth, and therefore the occlusion relations among surfaces (i.e., which ones are partially behind which other ones), is encoded in the representation very early—in fact, even before shapes have been derived. The priority of surface derivation over the derivation of other features of a scene was shown by placing information about edges and shapes in conflict with information about relative distances of surfaces from the viewer. The demonstrations are very impressive, but unfortunately, they require displays presented as stereographic images in order to provide the depth information independently of the other form information. Without a stereoscope, many people find it difficult to obtain a stereo effect from a printed page. Doing so requires "free fusing," and it can be achieved with some patience.[8] The results can be spectacular.

Consider the display shown in figure 3.18. It consists of what appear to be Is and Ls. In a two-dimensional display the Is form a cluster and tend to "pop out" as a distinct region. If the figure is fused so it appears three-dimensional, the dotted regions appear in front of or behind the

8. To achieve the stereo effect, try one of the following two methods (called parallel fusion and crossed fusion). For parallel fusion, bring the figure close to your face and try staring *through* the page into the distance (let your eyes go out of focus at first). Then back the page away while watching the pair on the right until the plus signs merge (the X pairs are for crossed fusion and the U pairs are for uncrossed fusion). For crossed fusion it is better to start with the page farther away and to look at a pencil placed about halfway between the eyes and the page. Look at the pencil and line it up with some feature of the pair of figures on the left side of the display. With practice you will be rewarded with the sudden appearance of the clear impression of depth in these pictures.

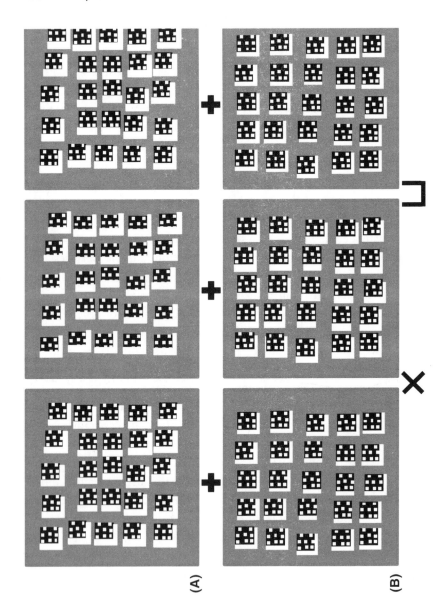

white regions. He and Nakayama (1994) showed that the outcome of the clustering process depends on the prior computation of depth and occlusion. The two rows of figure 3.18 show the two alternatives. If the Ls and Is are seen as *in front of* the dotted region, then we get the expected easy popout of the region of Is from the region of Ls. But if the Is and Ls are seen as *behind* the dotted regions, the visual system interprets them as the visible parts of a white square—so we see a field of squares partly occluded by the dotted regions, rather than a field of distinct Is and Ls. These alternative perceptions of the elements of figure 3.18 are illustrated in figure 3.19 for clarity. Because texture segregation is known to be computed at a very early stage in vision—in fact, a typical operation of early vision—this shows that early vision takes into account not only depth but, more important, the occlusion relation among surfaces, and that therefore that such information is implicit in the output of the early-vision system.

The evidence generally favors the view that some depth-encoded surface representation of the layout is present in the output of the early-vision system. The evidence also shows that the representation is not complete and uniform in detail—like an extended picture—and that intermediate representations are computed as well. I have already devoted considerable attention to the first of these claims in chapter 1 and have argued that the visual system certainly does not generate a complete picturelike representation in the mind. With regard to intermediate representation, there is evidence that several types and levels of representation are being computed, yet there is no evidence that these intermediate levels and outputs of specialized subprocesses are available to cognition in the normal course of perception. So far the available evidence suggests that the visual system is not only cognitively

Figure 3.18
When properly fused, the top row (A) shows the L and I elements as being in front (so they are represented as actual Is and Ls would be—see figure 3.19 for a graphical exposition). In the bottom row (B) the white elements are seen as being in back of the dotted figures, so they all look like partially occluded squares. In the top row the I elements pop out from among the Ls and form a cluster, while in the bottom example, the clustering has to be done deliberately and with difficulty. This shows that the automatic preattentive clustering process makes use of depth and occlusion information. (From He and Nakayama, 1994.)

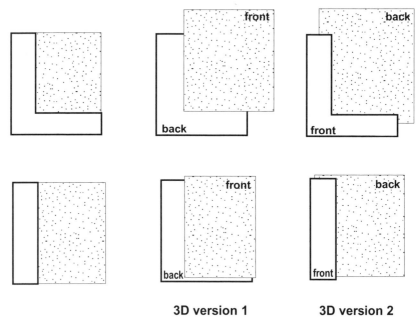

3D version 1   **3D version 2**

Figure 3.19
This helps to visualize how the individual elements of figure 3.18 are perceived as either Is or Ls, depending on the perceived depth of the white and textured regions. This figure shows how the items are seen in depth: in version (1) the white regions are seen as behind and so are visually completed as squares, whereas in version (2) the white regions are seen as in front and so are perceived as I or L.

impenetrable, but is also opaque with respect to the intermediate products of its processes (see section 3.3).

A phenomenon that may illustrate the opacity of early-vision processes is called the "word-superiority effect." It has been shown that it is faster to recognize whole words than individual letters, even when deciding which word a given word is *requires* having recognized the individual letters. For example, it is faster to distinguish WORD from WORK, than it is to distinguish the individual letter D from the letter K, despite the fact that differentiating WORD from WORK logically requires differentiating a D from a K. One possible explanation is that the D (or K) is recognized early in the word-recognition case but the information is not directly made available to the cognitive system, yet it is made available to the word-recognition system, which can then respond with the correct word and can also infer (after some delay) that there was a D (or K) present, on the basis of which word was recognized. This is even clearer in the case of phonemes, which every native speaker uses to make linguistic distinctions. Yet it requires special training to be able to detect the presence of a particular phoneme in speech (which is why making phonetic transcriptions of a foreign language is very difficult). It may be that a representation of a letter or phoneme is computed but the intermediate representation is not available except to the word recognition system, and therefore it can only be inferred from knowing what word was spoken or written.

In commenting on my paper in *Behavioral and Brain Sciences* (Pylyshyn, 1999), in which I argue for the impenetrability of early vision, Hollingworth and Henderson (1999) suggest that a "presemantic" match between memory and the description generated in the course of early vision may take place within early vision itself, allowing access to information about the object type. They base this proposal on the finding that when you control for the effect that context might have in focusing attention to certain locations, recognizing an object is not aided by the semantic congruence between the object and its scene context—it is just as easy to recognize a toaster or a chicken whether they are shown as being in a kitchen or in a farmyard (see Hollingworth and Henderson, 1998). Since semantic congruity does not help recognition, it cannot be mediated by semantic factors or by such semantically sensitive processes as reasoning. However, this result is compatible (as Hollingworth and Henderson recognize) with the idea that the early-vision system simply outputs what I have called a canonical shape or shape category (which I assume is very close to their notion of "presemantic" recognition). On the other hand, as I have argued, such a presemantic categorization need not involve matching anything to memory—it could simply be the structured description corresponding to an equivalence class induced by early vision. Of course, to recognize this class (which might have an internal name, say Q374) *as* a toaster (with all that this implies about its functional and conventional properties) *does* require making contact with a knowledge base, and this requires not only lookup but perhaps also various inferences (e.g., that it is usually found on the kitchen counter). Therefore, this sort of recognition lies outside the province of early vision. So I agree with Hollingworth and Henderson's proposal but do not see it as requiring memory lookup, except when it is associated with a judgment such as, for example, that the object is something that has been seen before or that it has a certain name. Once an appropriate canonical-shape description is constructed, it may be a relatively simple matter to match it to a knowledge base of names. In fact, what the Hollingworth and Henderson experiments show is that the step between achieving a shape description and locating its name is, at least in the case of simple objects, fast and direct and not enhanced by semantic congruence or degraded by semantic incongruence of the context.

One important question concerning visual processing that has not yet been explicitly addressed is the question of whether vision is a single uniform process or whether it consists of distinct subprocesses—or even whether there are distinct visual systems that operate in parallel or in different contexts. I have suggested that there are stages in visual processing, for example, the stage of computing depth precedes the stage at which shape is computed. The question of stages is also raised by a wide range of evidence suggesting that what is available to phenomenal experience may not be what is available to other processes. There is also strong evidence that the ability to make visual discriminations, the ability to localize and combine visual properties, and the ability to recognize familiar objects can be dissociated from the ability to act on the basis of visual information. These issues are discussed below.

3.3 Some Subprocesses of the Visual System

I have already suggested several ways in which the phenomenology of vision is seriously misleading. Another misleading impression is that vision happens suddenly, with little intervening processing. The experience of seeing appears to be so automatic and instantaneous that it is hard to believe that there may be different subprocesses involved, or that the visual system might inform different parts of the mind/brain in different ways or about different things. Like an inner screen, the phenomenological impression we have of vision is that of a unitary and virtually instantaneous process. But this impression is far from providing a valid characterization of what goes on in vision.

Since percepts are generally built up in the course of scanning the eye about a scene, it is obvious that vision typically involves an incremental process in which a representation is constructed over a period of time, during which the scene is scanned and various aspects are noticed. What may be less obvious is that visual percepts are built up incrementally even when they do not involve eye movements, that is, even when they result from a single fixation. Evidence from human psychophysics shows that the perception of simple patterns from a single fixation does not proceed by a single undifferentiated process but involves distinct stages and subprocesses. For example, there is evidence of intermediate stages in the computation of a depth representation. Indeed, the time course of some of the processing has been charted (e.g., Calis, Sterenborg, and Maarse, 1984; Reynolds, 1981; Schulz, 1991; Sekuler and Palmer, 1992), and there are computational reasons why earlier stages may be required. For example, Marr's analysis of early vision has room for at least a retinotopic representation called the raw primal sketch, as well as a full primal sketch, which groups together related edge-detector results and labels edges as to how sharp they are and so on, before the system produces a 2.5D representation and then finally an object-centered representation. Also, there is now considerable evidence from both psychophysics and clinical studies that the visual system consists in a number of separate subprocesses that compute color, luminance, motion, form, and 3-D depth, and that these subprocesses are restricted in their intercommunication (Cavanagh, 1988; Livingstone and Hubel, 1987). In other words, the visual process is highly complex and articulated, and there are intermediate stages in the computation of the percept, during which various sorts of information are available in highly restricted ways to certain specific subprocesses.

Much evidence suggests that there are severe restrictions on the flow of information among the many subsystems involved in visual perception. Indeed, the division between cognition and vision, with which I was concerned in the previous chapter, turns out to be an instance of a general property of many parts of the cognitive system. Partitioning into subsystems extends to many functions within vision itself. For example, there appear to be subsystems within vision with restricted access not only to general world knowledge but also to the outputs of their sister systems. Conversely, many of these subsystems do not provide information to the general cognitive system, but only to specific subsystems, such as certain motor subsystems. For example, the visual system appears to make certain information available to the motor system involved in reaching and grasping, but not to the general cognitive system. The visual system also appears to process some classes of features (e.g., color) independently of other classes (e.g., motion).

An impressive demonstration of the latter is to watch a display of moving blue/yellow or red/green bars (or sine-wave gratings) while the relative luminance of the pairs of colors is varied (so that the red or green bars become more/less bright). As the luminance of the two colors approaches subjective equality, the perceived speed of motion slows down and may even drop to zero, *despite the fact that you can clearly see that over time the gratings are in successively different locations!* Perceived speed of motion, it seems, is sensitive to luminance and much less to color information, even though the color information is sufficient to allow you to see where the gratings are. Similarly, it has been argued (but also contested) that luminance information alone does not contribute to stereo, at least in the case of nonfigural (random dot) stereograms. There is also evidence suggesting that color and luminance function differently in determining the perception of size and orientation.

Perhaps even more interesting are the findings concerning the role of different early analyzers in determining three-dimensional form percepts. In particular, when luminance or color or texture provides the sole input, the visual system may construct different percepts, even when the information defines the same 2D contours. For example, figure 3.20 shows that if contour information is provided in terms of luminance differences, then the contours may be interpreted as shadows, and the outlines and surface relief of the depicted objects may be reconstructed, whereas the same interpretations do not occur when the contours are presented by equiluminant contrasts (e.g., when contours are the borders between different equiluminant textures, as show here, or between regions of different colors, different relative motions, or binocular disparity). Figure 3.21 shows that information based on luminance contrast can allow the construction of so-called subjective contours, whereas the same information provided without luminance contrast does not. These examples show that information that is in some sense the same (e.g., they all define the same contours) but that arises from different analyzers at one stage in the visual process may nonetheless not be interpreted in the same way by the next stage in the visual process. In other words, certain analyzers

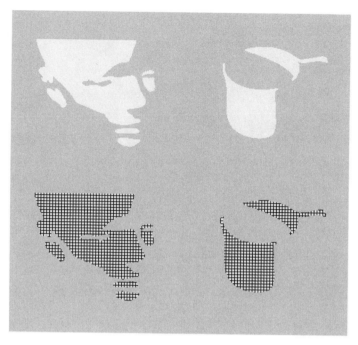

Figure 3.20
Figures with real and shadow contours produced by regions that differ in their luminance (top pair) or by regions that are approximately equiluminous (bottom pair). Although the regions and their outlines are equally visible in the two cases, perception of the figures as three-dimensional objects with shadows occurs only when the regions differ in luminance. (From Cavanagh, 1988.)

at stage *n* may not feed information to particular analyzers at stage *n* + 1, even though the equivalent information from a different stage *n* analyzer *is* used by the stage *n* + 1 analyzer.

In another series of demonstrations, Livingstone and Hubel (1987) showed that depth cues, such as occlusions or converging perspective lines, lose their potency for invoking depth in displays where the cues are presented as color features that are equiluminant with the background. Similarly, figure-ground discrimination and other low-level "Gestalt" phenomena disappear when the image features are presented in the form of color alone, i.e., as lines or edges with the same luminance as the background. Livingstone and Hubel develop an elegant neurophysiological story, based on the existence of different pathways and different types of neural cells, to account for these observations, and these

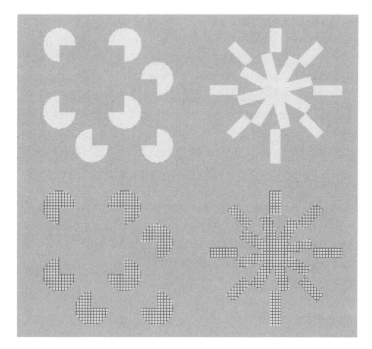

Figure 3.21
Figures with real and subjective contours produced by nonequiluminous regions (top pair) and by approximately equiluminous regions (bottom pair). Once again the perception of surfaces in three dimensions requires that regions have different luminance values. (From Cavanagh, 1988.)

help to anchor the taxonomy in biological data. From our perspective, we may conclude that there are subsystems in vision that compute their function independently of one another and that communicate the results of their analyses in a restricted manner to each other and to subsequent stages in the analysis. Figure 3.22 shows an example of a flow diagram of visual stages based on such an analysis.

3.3.1 Stages in early vision: The microgenesis of vision
I have already discussed the analysis of vision into stages, with attention allocation, early vision, and decision or judgment marking important distinctions within what is informally called vision. We also saw that within early vision, processes such as those that compute color, stereo, contour, motion, and three-dimensional layout have restricted intercommunica-

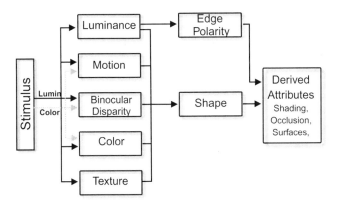

Figure 3.22
Some of the pathways in early vision, showing that color information (simulated in figures 3.20 and 3.21 by different textures) feeds into binocular disparity analysis, and to a lesser extent into motion analysis. Shape, as defined by explicit contours, can be determined by any pathway. Yet shape that is defined by subjective (or illusory) contours can be determined only by the luminance pathway, which, in turn, requires all the edges to have the same light-dark or dark-light polarity. (From Cavanagh, 1988.)

tion among each other and with higher cognitive systems. It also appears that within early vision a percept may involve a set of operations that are applied in sequence. Although not a great deal is known about such sequences, since they happen rapidly and unconsciously, there is evidence that some perceived properties take more time to construct than others, even when the construction does not involve appeal to memory and knowledge. Examples include the construction of illusory contours or other illusions (Reynolds, 1981; Reynolds, 1978; Schulz, 1991; Sekuler and Palmer, 1992), as well as higher-order visual processes such as involved in the perception of faces (Bachmann, 1989; Calis, Sterenborg, and Maarse, 1984; Hagenzieker, van der Heijden and Hagenaar, 1990). Although the stages described in the previous section may take time, I am not aware of any published studies concerning the time-course of these processes, despite the fact that it is known that some of these stages must precede other stages, as illustrated in figure 3.22. A few detailed empirical studies have been carried out, however, and have established the time course of certain operations applied to the visual input, providing evidence for what has become known as the microgenesis of vision.

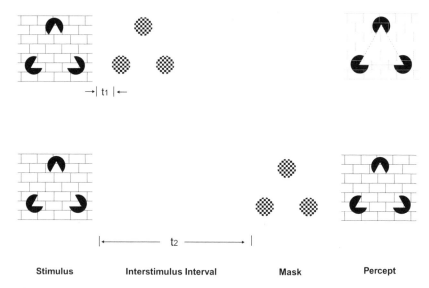

| Stimulus | Interstimulus Interval | Mask | Percept |

Figure 3.23
This figure illustrates that it takes time to integrate cues before a percept emerges. When insufficient time is available (top figures), the conflict between two sets of cues does not have an opportunity to operate. When an illusory Kanizsa triangle comes in conflict with cues that contradict the assumption that the triangle is opaque (as it does in figure 3.14), the triangle percept can be inhibited. But if there is insufficient time for the conflicting texture cue to be processed (in the top figure $t_1 < 150$ ms), the Kanizsa triangle is perceived. When more time is available (bottom figure) the conflict between perceiving the triangle as opaque and perceiving the background texture through it results in a diminution of the illusory Kanizsa triangle. (Adapted from Reynolds, 1981.)

For example, Reynolds (1978) showed that it takes some time for certain illusions to develop, and that the interactions responsible for such illusions as the Ponzo, Zollner, and rod-and-frame illusions occur only after about 150 ms of processing time. Reynolds (1981) also showed that it takes time for illusory contours to be constructed, and that early masking of the stimulus can disrupt this construction.[9] For example, figure 3.23 illustrates that under normal viewing conditions, or with a

9. Parks (1994) failed to replicate this result and cast some doubt on the experimental procedure used by Reynolds (1978). However, Parks (1995) subsequently developed a different technique and was able to confirm Reynolds's conclusion that construction of different aspects of a percept does indeed take time.

long interstimulus interval prior to masking, observers do not perceive an illusory triangle because perceiving the bricklike background is incompatible with perceiving the triangle as opaque—as required in order to see the illusory triangle covering the three black circles. If, however, the circles are masked after only a short interval, the illusory triangle is perceived because the incompatibility does not have time to interact with the perception of the background.

Using a different experimental paradigm to study the time course of constructing visual percepts, Sekuler and Palmer (1992) showed observers partially occluded figures or the corresponding visible fragments of figures or the whole figures. After each presentation, observers judged whether pairs of figures were identical. A judgment task such as this is speeded up when it is preceded by a brief exposure to the figure being compared—a phenomenon referred to as visual priming. The priming figures are show in row (a) of figure 3.24, and the figures involved in the subsequent judgment task are show in row (b). Sekuler and Palmer showed that in such a situation, a partially occluded figure (such as shown in the first column of figure 3.24) acts more like the completed figure (shown in the second column) than like the figure fragment that is actually present (shown in the third column and fourth columns). For example, presenting a partially occluded circle, such as in the first

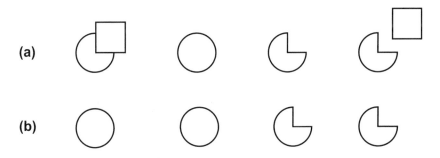

Figure 3.24
When primed with a figure such as in row (a), the effect on a subsequent comparison task is as if the viewer had been presented with the figure directly below it in row (b), providing that the time between the prime task and the comparison task is at least 200 ms (adapted from Sekuler and Palmer, 1992). Thus it appears that it takes time for the "amodal completion" of the missing parts of the figure to be constructed.

column of row (a), primes a subsequently presented figure-comparison task involving a circle, just as it would have if the actual circle had been presented (as shown in column 2). However, if just the fragment is presented (as in column 3), it will only prime a fragment figure, as show below it in row (b)—even if the same elements are present, as in the control case shown in column 4. The important additional finding was that the completed-figure priming effect (the one shown in the first column) is observed *only* if the occluded figure is viewed for at least 200 ms; otherwise it is the fragment that is primed, and not the whole figure partially hidden behind the occluding surface. It thus appears to take at least 200 ms for the occluded figure to be completed.

This study shows that the phenomenon known as "amodal completion" (discussed in chapter 1) does not just affect how something appears, but has real consequences for information processing (in this case for priming). Nonetheless, the completion of a figure takes time, and before the complete figure has been constructed by the visual system, only the fragment appears to be available.

3.4 Visual Control of Action: An Encapsulated System?

So far I have been speaking as though vision has as its sole purpose to provide us with knowledge of the world—an important aspect of which is to recognize objects—thereby providing a connection between the current scene and past experience. Vision is indeed the primary way that most organisms come to know the world, and such knowledge is important in that it enables behavior to be detached from the immediately present environment. Such visual knowledge can also be combined with other sources of knowledge for future use in inference, problem solving, and planning. But this is not the only function that vision serves. Vision also provides a means for the immediate control of actions and sometimes does so without informing the rest of the cognitive system—or at least that part of the cognitive system that is responsible for recognizing objects and issuing explicit reports describing the perceptual world. Whether this means that there are more than one distinct visual system remains an open question. At the present time the evidence is compatible with there being a single system that provides outputs separately to the motor-control functions and to the cognitive functions. Unless it is shown that the actual process is different in the two sets of functions, this remains the simplest account of the operation of the visual system. So far it appears that for both types of functions the visual system computes shape descriptions that include sufficient depth information to enable not only recognition, but also reaching and remarkably efficient hand positioning for grasping (Goodale, 1988). The major difference between the information needed for the two type of functions is that motor control primarily requires quantitative, egocentrically calibrated spatial information, whereas the cognitive system is concerned more often with qualitative or categorical information, with relative locations (Bridgeman, 1995), and with viewpoint-independent representations.

The earliest indications of the fractionation of the output of vision probably came from observations in clinical neurology (e.g., Holmes, 1918), which will be discussed on page 153 below. However, it has been known for some time that the visual control of posture and locomotion can make use of visual information that does not appear to be available to the cognitive system in general. For example, Lee and Lishman (1975) showed that posture can be controlled by the oscillations of a specially designed room whose walls were suspended inside a real room and could be made to move slowly. Subjects standing in such an "oscillating room" exhibit synchronous swaying even though they are totally unaware of the movements of the walls.

3.4.1 Evidence from studies of eye movements and reaching

The largest body of work showing a dissociation between visual information available to general cognition and information available to motor function involves studies of the visual control of eye movements as well as of reaching and grasping. Bridgeman (1992) showed a variety of dissociations between the visual information available to the eye-movement system and that available to the cognitive system. For example, he showed that if a visual target jumps during an eye movement, and so is undetected, subjects can still accurately point to the correct position of the now-vanished target. In earlier and closely related experiments, Goodale (1988) and Goodale, Pelisson, and Prablanc (1986) also showed a dissociation between information noticed by subjects and information to which the motor system responds. In reaching for a target, a subject first makes a saccadic eye movement toward the target. If during the saccade the target undergoes a sudden displacement, the subject does not notice the displacement because of saccadic suppression. Nonetheless, the trajectory of the subject's reaching shows that his or her visual system did register the displacement, and that the motor system controlling reaching is able to take this into account in an on-line fashion and to make a correction during flight in order to reach the final correct position.

Wong and Mack (1981) and subsequently Bridgeman (1992) showed that the judgment and motor systems can even be given conflicting visual information. The Wong and Mack study involved stroboscopically induced motion. A target and frame both jumped in the same direction, although the target did not jump as far as the frame. Because of induced motion, the target appeared to jump in the opposite direction to the frame. Wong and Mack found that the saccadic eye movements resulting from subjects' attempts to follow the target were in the actual direction of the target, even though the perceived motion was in the opposite direction (by stabilizing the retinal location of the target the investigators ensured that retinal error could not drive eye movements). But if the subjects' responses were delayed, their tracking saccades followed the perceived (illusory) direction of movement, showing that the motor-control system could use only immediate visual information. The lack of memory in the visuomotor system has been confirmed in the case of eye movements by Gnadt, Bracewell, and Anderson (1991) and in the case of reaching and grasping by Goodale, Jacobson, and Keillor (1994). Another asymmetry is that size illusions affect judgments (Aglioti, DeSouza and Goodale, 1995) but not prehension (Milner and Goodale, 1995). Also demonstrating the apparent insensitivity of the visuomotor system to certain illusions are some findings concerning the Müller-Lyer illusion. A surprising finding with this illusion is that the location of the endpoints of the lines can be judged very accurately under conditions where the line length shows a strong illusion (Gillam and Chambers, 1985; Mack, Heuer, Villardi and Chambers, 1985). The apparent dissociation between judgment of position and judgment of length is of particular interest in the present context because the location judgment was provided by motor gestures, while the length judgment was verbal. The location of the endpoints in these cases are indicated by making motor gestures toward the display. In the Gillam and Chambers experiment it was indicated by placing a dot under the endpoints, and in the Mack et al. experiment the response involved actually pointing to the endpoint. The pointing was free of bias even when the hand was hidden from view.

3.4.2 Evidence from clinical neurology

Clinical studies of patients with brain damage provided some of the earliest evidence of dissociations of functions, which in turn led to the beginnings of a taxonomy (and information-flow analyses) of skills. One of the earliest observations of independent subsystems in vision was provided by Holmes (1918). Holmes described a gunshot victim who had normal vision as measured by tests of acuity, color discrimination, and stereopsis, and who had no trouble visually recognizing and distinguishing objects and words. Yet this patient could not reach for objects under visual guidance (though it appears that he could reach for places under tactile guidance). This was the first in a long series of observations suggesting a dissociation between recognition and visually guided action. The recent literature on this dissociation (as studied in clinical cases, as well as in psychophysics and animal laboratories) is reviewed by Milner and Goodale (1995).

In a series of careful investigations, Milner and Goodale (1995) reported on a remarkable case of visual dissociation. This patient, known as D.F., shows a dissociation of vision-for-recognition and vision-for-action, illustrating a clear pattern of restricted communication between early vision and subsequent stages, or to put it in the terms that the authors prefer, she shows a modularization that runs from input to output, segregating one visual pathway (the dorsal pathway) from another (the ventral pathway). D.F. is seriously disabled in her ability to recognize patterns and even to judge the orientation of simple individual lines. When asked to select from a set of alternatives a line orientation that matches an oblique line in the stimulus, D.F.'s performance was at chance. She also performed at chance when asked to indicate the orientation of the line by tilting her hand. But when presented with a tilted slot and asked to insert her hand or to insert a thin object, such as a letter, into the slot, her behavior was in every respect normal—including the acceleration/deceleration and dynamic orienting pattern of her hand as it approached the slot. Her motor system, it seems, knew exactly what orientation the slot was in and could act towards it in a normal fashion.

Another fascinating case of visual processes providing information to the motor-control system but not the rest of cognition is shown in cases of so-called blindsight, discussed by Weiskrantz (1995). Patients with this disorder are "blind" in the region of a scotoma, in the sense that they cannot report "seeing" anything presented in that region. Because they don't "see" in this sense, patients never report the presence of objects or of any other visual properties located in their blind regions. Nonetheless, such patients are able to do some remarkable things that show that visual information is being processed from the blind field. In the case of D.B. (Weiskrantz et al., 1974), the patient's pupilary response to color and light and spatial frequencies showed that information from the blind field was entering the visual system. This patient could also move his eyes roughly towards points of light that he insisted he could not see, and D.B. performed above chance in reporting the color and motion of the spot of light. D.B. was also able to point to the location of objects in the blind field while maintaining that he could see nothing there but was merely guessing. Yet when asked to point to an object in his normal blind spot (where the optic nerve leaves the eye and no visual information is available), D.B. could not do so.

I defer until section 3.5 the question of whether these facts should lead us to conclude that there are two distinct visual systems, although it is clear from the results sketched above that there are at least two different forms of output from vision and that these are not equally available to the rest of the mind/brain. It appears, however, that they both involve representations that have depth information and that follow the couplings among perceived properties or the perceptual constancies (see Rock, 1997).

3.4.3   Evidence from animal studies

Inasmuch as human brains share many brain mechanisms and organizational principles with the brains of other animals, it is of interest to ask about perceptual processes in other organisms. Not surprisingly, there is a great deal of evidence in animals for a distinction between the vision-for-recognition and vision-for-action functions discussed earlier. The subdivision of the visual output by the functions it is used to perform, goes even further when we consider animals like frogs, where behavior is more stereotyped. In the case of the frog, Ingle (1973) and

Ingle, Goodale, and Mansfield (1982) found evidence for the separability of visual outputs for feeding, for escape, and for avoidance of barriers. Similar fractionation has also been found in the gerbil, whose visuomotor behavior is not as stereotyped as that of the frog. Goodale (1983) and Goodale and Milner (1982) found that in the gerbil, visual guidance of head turns (toward food), escape reactions, and navigation around a barrier could be dissociated by lesions.

In addition to the dissociation of visual output in terms of the type of motor-control functions that they inform, another remarkable type of dissociation was demonstrated by Cheng (1986) and Gallistel (1990). This dissociation led them to postulate what they refer to as a geometrical module in the rat's visuomotor system. This module seems to receive only visual information relevant to its function of computing orientation relative to the shape of a global environment and cannot take into account identity information. When a rat discovers the location of buried food in a rectangular box and is then disoriented and allowed to relocate the food, it can navigate back to the location of the food by using geometrical cues, where by geometrical cues I mean relative location information, such as "The food is near the corner that has a long wall on the left and a short wall on the right." What it cannot do, however, is navigate towards the food by using easily discriminable but nongeometrical visual cues, such as the color or texture or odor of nearby features. But since a rectangle is congruent with itself when rotated 180 degrees, there are actually two locations with the same "geometrical" properties. For this reason, if a rat is placed in a rectangular box where it previously had seen food, it will be indifferent as to which of two geometrically congruent locations it goes to, even if the correct location is clearly marked by distinctive color, texture, or odor cues. As Gallistel says,

The organ that computes congruence between perceived shape and remembered shape appears to be impenetrable to information about aspects of surfaces other than their relative positions. The congruence computation takes no account of the smells emanating from the surfaces, their reflectance or luminance characteristics, their texture, and so on. It takes no account of the nongeometrical properties of the surfaces, even when the relative positions of the perceptible surfaces do not suffice to establish unambiguously the correct congruence. (1990, p. 208)

This is an example of a function computed by the brain of a rat and other animals that uses only certain restricted information in the course of carrying out its task (in this case, navigation), even though other information would help to eliminate certain ambiguities, and even though the sensory system of the animal is fully capable of detecting the other information and of using it in different tasks. This is a classic case of the encapsulation of, or restricted information flow among, visual subprocesses that characterize a modular organization. It is also a case of the visual system being selective in which information it provides to which postperceptual system.

3.5   Interactions among Modular Systems

We have seen that the general phenomenon called "vision" has many subparts. These parts work together to produce the visual percept and perhaps also the phenomenology of visual perception. This fractionation of vision into subparts is, in fact, typical of complex systems and, as Simon (1969) and others have argued, is well motivated both from an evolutionary perspective as well as from a functional perspective. The discussion in this chapter has been about the organization of these parts, or what is often called the "architecture of the visual system." The notion of architecture is central to understanding the mind, and I have devoted considerable attention, here and elsewhere (e.g., Pylyshyn, 1984a, 1996), to what it means, why we must study it, and what we know about it. Some of this discussion will appear again in chapter 6 (especially section 6.3) and in chapter 7, where it becomes an essential part of understanding claims about the use of the visual system in mental imagery. What I have discussed so far in this and the previous chapter are certain large-scale structural properties of the visual system. In this chapter I argued that the evidence shows that vision (or early vision) forms a distinct module of the mind, that is, that the architecture of the mind has vision as a separate component interacting with the faculty of reasoning in certain restricted ways. In the present chapter I argued that vision itself exhibits further modular structure, inasmuch as it consists of a number of functional components with restricted lines of communication among them.

   In addition to the question of how a system divides into component parts, we can ask how the parts interact with one another. For example, given visual information that is inherently ambiguous, vision seems to come up with an analysis or a "solution" that is very often veridical, and in doing so, it appears to take into account factors that imply a faculty of intelligence of some sort. If the visual architecture is fixed and not malleable by what the organism knows, how does vision manage so often to produce an intelligent analysis of its input? The answers we have explored in this and the previous chapters are threefold. First, apparently intelligent perception can occur because of the constraints that the visual system imposes on all perceptual interpretation—not just the perception of certain likely or expected outcomes. These have often been called natural constraints. Second, cognition does intervene at two special loci: prior to the operation of early vision and after early vision has generated one or more outputs. These interventions take the form of selection. Prior to the operation of early vision, selection occurs through the mechanism of visual *attention*. After early vision, cognition is able to select the most likely interpretation from those provided by early vision, and is able to further interpret the information that vision provides in order to establish beliefs about what has been seen. I have said very little about these two types of selection except that, unlike early vision itself, cognition is able to make selections at these two loci based on any criterion (rational, heuristic, adaptive, statistical, etc.) that bears on the likelihood of certain situations occurring in the world or the likelihood of certain interpretations being veridical. In what follows, I will look in more detail at how the preselection can occur by examining the nature of visual attention, viewed as a way in which cognition can affect what is visually perceived.

4

Focal Attention: How Cognition Influences Vision

The last two chapters defended the view that a significant part of the visual system, referred to as *early* vision, is encapsulated so that its operation is unaffected by cognitive processes, including inference from general knowledge. But clearly, early vision does not function passively for the organism; rather, it exists in the service of other activities, including cognition and motor action. Even though cognition may not affect how early vision operates, it does exert some control over *what it operates on*, and it also makes judgments about what in fact might have caused certain perceptual experiences. Chapter 2 suggested that focal attention provides one of the two primary means by which the cognitive system can influence vision (postperceptual recognition and decision processes are the other), and that it does so by selectively directing the visual process to certain aspects of the perceptual world. Clearly, it is important to constrain what can serve as the object of attentional focus. If *anything* could count as a possible focus of attention, then the idea of attention would be devoid of explanatory value, since we could always explain why two people (or the same person on different occasions) see things differently by claiming that they were "attending" to different aspects of the world, which comes to pretty much the same claim as that vision is cognitively penetrable. The following sections will elaborate on the role that a suitably constrained notion of attention can play in allowing cognition to have certain specific sorts of effects on visual perception. Then in the next chapter I will develop these ideas further and show that certain mechanisms involved in visual attention also serve a quite different, and in many ways more fundamental, role—that of linking parts of the percept to the *things in the world* to which they refer.

4.1   Focal Attention in Visual Perception

One of the ways in which the cognitive system can influence perception is by choosing *where* or *to what* to direct the visual process. We obviously affect what we see when we choose *where to look*. Indeed, changing our direction of gaze by moving our eyes is one of the principal ways in which we selectively sample the visual world. But there is much more to the notion of selectively attending than directing one's gaze. For example, it is known that we can also direct our attention without moving our eyes, using what is referred to as "covert" attentional allocation (see section 4.3). In addition, attention can also be directed to certain properties rather than particular places in a scene. Indeed, there is reason to believe that at least some forms of attention can only be directed at certain kinds of visible objects and not to *unoccupied places* in a visual scene, and that it may also be directed at several distinct objects. In what follows, I will examine some of this evidence and its implications. Whatever the detailed properties of attention and whatever kinds of mechanisms it presupposes, we will see that what is called *selective* or *focal* attention represents the primary locus of cognitive intervention between our perception and the physical world we perceive.

There are a number of far-reaching implications of this way of understanding attention. It suggests that focal attention determines what we "notice," and therefore ultimately what we see. We take it for granted that there is always more that *could have been noticed* than actually was noticed. And that, in turn, is an informal expression of the view that visual processing is limited and therefore has to make choices about how to allocate its limited resources. This is indeed the basic idea behind the last 50 years of study of focal attention (but see Kahneman and Treisman, 1984, for an early recognition that this is a limited perspective). In addition to determining which aspects of the world will get processed, the allocation of focal attention also determines how visual perception carves up the world into distinct things—how the world is "parsed." As suggested in chapter 2, because of its key role as a gatekeeper between vision and the world, the allocation of attention is also one of the main loci of perceptual learning. Moreover, as we will see in chapter 5, some mechanisms of early vision closely related to attention may also determine how our percepts and concepts are connected to the world. And because it provides the principle interface between cognition and vision, focal attention also plays an important role in mental imagery, since generating and processing visual mental images appears to share properties with both vision and cognition. This will be the topic of chapters 6 and 7. First some background on visual focal attention.

4.2 Focal Attention as Selective Filtering

Attention is an ancient and ubiquitous concept. The term has been used to refer to a wide range of phenomena, from simply having an interest and motivation toward some task (as in "paying attention"), to the filtering function that was widely studied in the 1950s, owing in no small measure to the seminal work by Colin Cherry (1957) and Donald Broadbent (1958). These different senses of "attention" share, at least by implication, the assumption that the cognitive system cannot carry out an unlimited number of tasks at the same time, and therefore must choose or select the tasks to which it will direct its limited resources. Beyond this general idea, the notion of attention has been treated quite differently by different researchers and different schools of psychology. Regardless of the approach and the emphasis placed on different aspects of attention, the centrality of its role in visual perception has always been recognized. In the early twentieth century the main focus was on how attention increases the awareness or clarity of attended aspects of the perceptual world. Later the emphasis turned to the selectivity of perception and to the properties that enabled some information to be passed while other information (the unattended aspects of the world) was filtered out. Broadbent's "filter theory" played a major role in these discussions (which are summarized in Broadbent, 1958; as well as in Norman, 1969).

The importance of filtering rests on the assumption of limited processing resources. One of the most fundamental and widely accepted assumptions about human information processing is that, however it works in detail, its resources are limited. For example, there are limits on its working-memory capacity, on the speed and reliability with which it can carry out operations, on the number of operations it can carry out at one time, and so on. The assumption of limited processing resources leads immediately to several important questions:

If information-processing is limited, along what dimensions is it limited? How does one measure its limits? This is a deeper and more fundamental problem than might appear at first glance. In the 1950s the dimension of limitation was sometimes referred to as the "range of cues utilized" (Easterbrook, 1959). But under the widespread influence of information theory in psychology, it was common to look for limitations in terms of bandwidth, or entropy measures (i.e., in terms of number of bits per second). In a classical paper (1956), George Miller argued, however, that the limit of short-term memory (now often called "working memory") was not in the amount of information it could hold, as measured in information-theoretic terms (such as in the number of "bits" of information), but in the number of discrete units of encoding or what Miller termed "chunks." This was a very important idea and had an enormous influence on the field, despite the fact that what constitutes a "chunk" was never fully spelled out and that this lack of specificity has always remained a weak point in the theory. Another proposal (Newell, 1972), similar to the idea of limited working memory but differing in details, is that there are limits on how many arguments could be bound in evaluating cognitive functions or subroutines. A variant of this proposed, introduced later by Newell (1980a), is that rather than assuming a fixed limit on the number of arguments allowed, one might hypothesize that there are certain costs associated with each variable bound to a chunk, which leads to the well-known speed-accuracy trade-off in performance.

While the notion of resource limits is well entrenched, there is no general agreement on the nature of the information-processing "bottleneck" in visual information processing. The theoretical position that will be describe in chapter 5 provides one view of where the bottleneck resides in vision: it resides in the number of arguments in a perceptual function or predicate that can be bound to visual objects.

Limited-capacity information processing implies that a decision has to be made about where (or to what elements, properties, or more generally, "channels") to allocate the limited capacity. How and on what basis is this decision made? The first part of the question asks what properties (or perhaps what entities) can be the target of selective attention. This question cannot be given a simple univocal answer. In chapter 2, I discussed some evidence that attention may be directed to certain properties or a range of properties of a stimulus. For example, it has been shown that people can focus their attention on various frequency bands in both the auditory domain (Dai, Scharf, and Buss, 1991) and the visual spatial domain (Julesz and Papathomas, 1984; Shulman and Wilson, 1987), and under certain conditions, also on such features as color (Friedman-Hill and Wolfe, 1995; Green and Anderson, 1956), local shape (Egeth, Virzi, and Garbart, 1984), motion (McLeod, Driver, Dienes, and Crisp, 1991), and stereo-defined depth (Nakayama and Silverman, 1986). There must, however, be some principled restrictions on what can serve as the basis for selective attention; otherwise the notion would be of no use as an explanatory construct: we could (vacuously) explain why some people (e.g., Bernard Berenson) are experts in identifying paintings by Leonardo DaVinci by saying that they have tuned their visual systems to attend to the particular visual properties characteristic of DaVinci paintings. This issue is closely related to the reason why such properties as those that James Gibson (1979) called "affordances" (which includes properties such as being edible, graspable, or suitable for sitting on) cannot be the subject of attending, at least not in any explanatorily useful sense of this term. In Fodor and Pylyshyn, 1981, we noted that if properties such as being a particular recognizable object (such as a shoe), or being a particular "affordance," could be the basis of primitive selection or, as Gibson put it, could be *directly picked up*, then there could not be *misperception* of such properties—which is patently false, since it is easy enough to make something *look like* it had a certain affordance even though it doesn't (it could, for example, be a hologram). For this and other reasons we concluded that only a highly constrained set of properties can be selected by early vision, or can be directly "picked up." Roughly, these are what I have elsewhere referred to as "transducable" properties (Pylyshyn, 1984a, chap. 9). These are the properties whose detection does not require accessing memory and drawing inferences. Roughly speaking, visually transducable properties are either optical properties or are defined in terms of such properties without reference to the perceiver's knowledge or beliefs; they are functions of the architecture of the visual system, in the sense discussed in several places in this book (especially chapter 3 and section 6.3.1), as well as in Pylyshyn, 1984a. Detection of such properties is sometimes referred to as being *data-driven*. They clearly exclude properties such as *being edible* or *being a genuine da Vinci painting*, since detecting these properties depends on what you know about the world, including what you have learned from books. Properties that cannot be visually transduced in this sense cannot serve as a basis for filtering.

The view that attention is a selective filter whose function is to keep perceptual resources from being overloaded raises another serious question. If the role of attention is to filter out certain visual information in order to prevent overloading, then the information filtered out in this way cannot have any influence on perception. If it did, then attention would not have accomplished its goal, inasmuch as the visual system would have had to process all the information anyway. A great deal of research has been done on the question of whether unattended (i.e., filtered-out) information is completely eliminated from the perceptual system. Some of the earliest investigations were carried out on the auditory system by Broadbent (1958) and Treisman (1969). They generally found that the more simply a property could be characterized in terms of basic physical dimensions, the more readily it could be filtered out. For example, it is easier to filter out a speech stream defined by pitch or by which ear it is presented to than by which language it is in. And which language it is in is, in turn, an easier basis for filtering than is the topic of the speech. Distinguishable properties of a class of signals are often referred to as "channels," and the simpler the physical specification of the channel, the better the filtering. Despite the large amount of accumulated evidence showing the operation of channel filters, the research also shows that even when certain information appears to have been filtered out (e.g., observers are unable to report it), it nonetheless still has measurable consequences. Norman (1969) and Pashler (1998, chap. 2) describe a large number of experiments illustrating the "leakiness" of such filters. For example, a common paradigm involves presenting different information to the two ears (the so-called "dichotic presentation" method). These studies showed that information that was apparently filtered out (and could not be reported by observers) could nonetheless be shown to have consequences. Information in the "rejected" channel could even affect the interpretation of signals in the attended channel. For example, if the attended channel contained a lexically ambiguous word (e.g., the word "bank," which can mean either an institution or the land bordering on a river), the rejected message affected which reading was more frequently given to it (e.g., Lackner and Garrett, 1972, showed that if the rejected message was on a financial topic, the institutional sense of "bank" was reported more often in the attended channel). Also, the extent to which the presence of material in the rejected channel disrupted the material in the attended channel depended on whether the observer could understand the message in the rejected channel (e.g., if it was in a different language, the amount of disruption depended on whether the observer understood that language [Treisman, 1964]). This presents a puzzle for a pure filter theory, since the criterion of being able to understand the language presupposes that the rejected information was available after all. The next section provides other examples from vision showing that apparently ignored information can have important and long-lasting effects.

Despite a number of different ways of attempting to reconcile these findings within a pure filter theory of attention, the results have generally been inconclusive.[1] It seems as though for each putative channel or filtering property P, there are experiments showing (a) that items in the rejected channel (or items lacking property P) are in fact being processed, and (b) that the determination as to whether an item has property P is often made after the stage at which filtering needs to have occurred in order to ease the processing load. Also, it seems that the term "attention" often refers more to what we are consciously aware of than what is actually processed by the brain. This relates to the observation in chapter 1 that the phenomenal content of vision is an unreliable basis for concluding whether some visual information has been processed. The fact that an observer may be unaware of certain "unattended" information does not mean that such information has not been processed and has not had an effect on the rest of the cognitive (or motor) system. And, as we have also seen, the converse is also true: what we subjectively experience in vision may provide a misleading basis for concluding what information has been assimilated or encoded.

1. For example, it does not help to assume that the signal in the rejected channel is merely attenuated, rather than completely filtered out. That just makes it more surprising that the content of the attenuated signal has an effect on analysis of the attended channel.

4.3   Allocation of Visual Attention

Since the 1980s, the study of visual attention has tended to emphasize the role of spatial location in determining how visual information is processed. The major impetus for this tradition was the discovery that to shift attention in a particular direction, it is not necessary to move one's gaze in that direction. Such attention movement was referred to, rather enigmatically, as a "covert" movement of attention. Many investigators (e.g., Shulman, Remington, and McLean, 1979) showed that attention moved continuously through space under either "endogenous," or voluntary, control or "exogenous," or involuntary event-driven, control. Shulman et al. used the endogenous method, instructing subjects to move their attention in a given direction, and found that the detection of a faint stimulus was enhanced at various intermediate places along the path of attention movement. Subsequently, Posner (1980) used exogenously controlled attention movement and undertook a systematic analysis of what he referred to as the orienting of attention. He (and many other investigators [Tsal, 1983]) showed that if attention was automatically attracted towards a point in the periphery of the visual field, then stimuli along the path were more easily discriminated at various intermediate times. Figure 4.1 shows one such experiment, for example, using what is called a "cue-validity" procedure. A brightening of a spot either to the right or to the left of fixation provides a cue as to where a target will be on 80 percent of the trials. When the target does appear at the cued location, the time it takes to detect it is faster than when it appears in the invalid cue location. Moreover, the time by which the cue signal precedes the target determines how effective the cue will be. The time lapse for maximum effectiveness (shortest relative reaction time) provides an indication of how long it took for attention to arrive at that location. From measurements such as these, various researchers estimated the rate at which attention moves across a scene in such automatic, gaze-independent (or "covert") situations. These estimates cover a wide range: 4 ms/degree (Posner, Nissen, and Ogden, 1978), 8.5 ms/degree (Tsal, 1983), 19 ms/degree (Shulman et al., 1979), 24–26 ms/degree (Jolicoeur, Ullman, and MacKay, 1985). But the idea that attention does move through empty space was widely accepted.

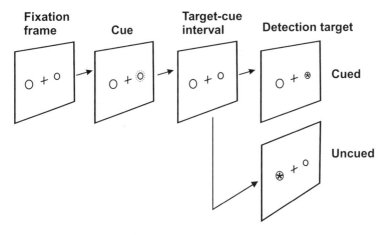

Figure 4.1
An example of an experiment using a cue-validity paradigm for showing that the locus of attention can travel without movement of the eye (so-called covert attention movement). By adjusting the target-cue interval for optimal detection it is possible to obtain an estimate of the speed of covert attention movement (described in Posner, 1980).

The study of such covert movements of attention occupied a great deal of research effort during the 1980s. Various mechanisms were proposed to account for this apparent movement of attention, including the widely cited "spotlight" metaphor (Posner, 1980). Also proposed were mechanisms not involving a discrete moving locus, such as proposals involving increasing and decreasing activation at two loci, which results in a spreading pattern that can appear as a moving maximum of attention (Hikosaka, Miyauchi, and Shimojo, 1993; McCormick and Klein, 1990; Schmidt, Fisher, and Pylyshyn, 1998; Sperling and Weichselgarter, 1995). For example, Sperling and Weichselgarter (1995) defend an "episodic" theory that assumes that attention decreases at the point of origin and both increases and spreads at the new focal point. They showed that from this assumption one would predict that at various times after the occurrence of the detection target (as in the rightmost panel of figure 4.1) the sensitivity at intermediate locations would follow the pattern found by Posner.

Regardless of the underlying mechanism, a large number of experiments showed that the locus of attention appears to move rapidly and continuously from place to place under either exogenous control or endogenous control. Exogenous control can be accomplished by presenting certain cues that reliably capture attention—the most robust of which is the sudden-onset of a new visual element—whereas endogenous control is typically obtained by providing cues that inform subjects in which direction to move their attention (e.g., using an arrow that appears at fixation). Although both types of attention-shifting cues show attentional enhancement at the cued location, there are differences in the type of enhancement and its time-course for these two sorts of attentional control. For example, a number of studies (e.g., Henderson, 1991; Van der Heijden, Schreuder, and Wolters, 1985) have shown that accuracy of discrimination is improved only by exogenous cues. Moreover, it has been shown (Mueller and Findlay, 1988; Mueller and Rabbitt, 1989; Nakayama and Mackeben, 1989; Shepherd and Mueller, 1989) that facilitation of response to exogenous cues appears earlier and is stronger than the facilitation due to endogenous cues. Attentional facilitation in response to exogenous cues is maximal approximately 100–150 ms after cue onset and fades within 300 ms after cue onset. Moreover, when such cues actually identify target locations to which subjects respond, the early facilitation peak produced by exogenous cues (but not by endogenous cues) is followed after about 500 ms by inhibition (so-called "inhibition-of-return"). Despite the difference between exogenously and endogenously triggered attention movement, and despite different theoretical interpretations of the various results, it is generally accepted that attention *can* be moved without eye movements. Indeed, it is widely held (Kowler, Anderson, Dosher, and Blaser, 1995) that a covert attentional movement *precedes* the overt movement of the eyes to certain locations in a scene, though such a covert movement may not be essential for an eye movement to take place.

In addition to covertly controlling the locus of spatially localized attention, it has generally also been held that people can control the extent or breadth of the focus of attention. For example, Eriksen and St. James (1986) have argued that observers can widen the scope of their focus at the cost of decreasing the level of attention allocated to certain regions. This so-called "zoom lens" view of attention has had detractors as well as supporters. In addition to the evidence that attention can be covertly moved and can be expanded or zoomed, there is also evidence that it can spread to certain shapes (such as bars or even letter-shaped templates) if some visible anchors for these shapes are available. In the latter case such shaped attention profiles can be used to facilitate the detection of brief stimuli on those forms. For example, Farah (1989) showed subjects the matrix on the left panel of figure 4.2, where 19 of the cells are colored a faint gray, and asked them to attend to the cells corresponding to either the H subfigure region or the T subfigure region (shown in the other two panels). When they did this, their sensitivity to detecting a dim flash of light within the attended region was enhanced, suggesting that they could spread their attention at will over a region defined by specific visible squares. Subsequent experiments (see p. 186) also showed that cuing part of a shape would spread to enhance sensitivity to the whole shape.

In a related experiment, Hayes (1973) showed that subjects are better at recognizing a certain pattern if they are first shown the exact shape, size, and location of pattern that they are to expect. Such findings have often been taken as evidence that subjects can project an image onto a visual display. However, these findings can easily be explained if one assumes that what subjects are doing is allocating attention to regions defined by certain simple visible objects (including simple texture elements) on the display screen, just as they did in the Farah study described above. Such an explanation also makes sense in view of other findings (e.g., the studies by Burkell and Pylyshyn, 1997, to be discussed on

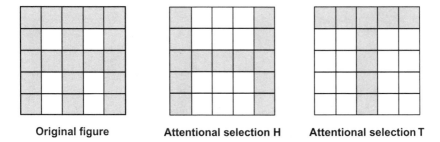

| Original figure | Attentional selection H | Attentional selection T |

Figure 4.2
Studies showing that people can allocate attention to certain well-defined regions (after Farah, 1989). Detection performance is increased throughout the region where observers were asked to attend (which was either the T- or the H-shaped region).

pp. 232–236) that show that a phenomenon generally associated with focal attention (namely, priority of access) can be split across several disparate objects in a display. Thus it appears that some form (or stage) of attention can be focused on larger areas and shapes and can be split across distinct elements. Later I will suggest that this form of attention is actually allocated to objects rather than to regions and that the multiple-object phenomenon is more primitive than what we generally understand by the term "attention."

Rock and Gutman (1981) showed that the patterns people attend to may be distributed over a relatively large area and can be kept separate from distinct overlapping regions. They showed subjects figures such as the ones in figure 4.3. Observers were asked to make aesthetic judgments about the shapes that were in a particular color (e.g., the green figures) while ignoring the other shapes in the display. After viewing about 10 such displays, the subjects were given a surprise recognition test. They were able to recall the items they had attended to with the same level of performance as if they had been presented alone, but their recognition of the rejected items was nearly at chance. Brawn and Snowden (2000) used a priming paradigm with overlapping figures (they used a figure like figure 4.19, except with circles added at each vertex) and showed that when observers saw the figure as two distinct shapes, their attention spread over the single primed figure and not the unprimed one.

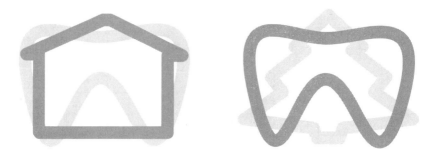

Figure 4.3
Figures similar to those used by Rock and Gutman (1981) to show that attention can be allocated to whole figures even when the figures are intertwined among other figures. Attended figures were later recalled but unattended ones were systematically ignored and not recognized later as having appeared in the experiment. (Adapted from Rock and Gutman, 1981.)

The Rock and Gutman study answers the question of whether an entire distributed shape can be attended even when it is entwined with another (often more familiar) shape. The answer is that at least for the purpose of entering into memory, entire shapes can be encoded to the exclusion of equally prominent overlapping shapes. But the study does not answer the question of whether the unattended shape is processed in any way. This question has received opposite answers in a number of studies. One important set of studies (reviewed in Mack and Rock, 1998a) found what has become known as *inattentional blindness.* These studies showed that shapes that are not attended to receive almost no processing and are unavailable to conscious awareness and recall. The demonstrations are quite dramatic. For example, Mack and Rock (1998b) showed that small squares presented unexpectedly right at fixation are not noticed if the observer is engaged in another more peripheral visual task and is not expecting them. Indeed, the evidence seems to suggest that when no new information is expected at particular marked locations, observers actually *inhibit* attention and encoding of information into memory, leaving an apparent blindness at those marked locations. If the location where the surprise event is to occur is not visually marked in some way, however, no inhibition of such an unoccupied location is observed (Mack and Rock, 1998a, 1998b). This finding is consistent with the view, to be developed below, that both attention and inattentional blindness are object-based, since it is not regions in space that are inhibited, but entire individual objects. The inhibition of nonselected shapes has also been demonstrated in search experiments by Watson and Humphreys (1997), so there appears to be some consensus on the role of object-based inhibition as a mechanism for shutting out information about irrelevant or unwanted objects.

Other studies, appear to show that *actively* ignoring objects has a strong long-term effect. A number of studies (see the review in Fox, 1995) asked subjects to identify or otherwise attend to certain figures—e.g., those in a given color—while ignoring other overlapping figures. At a later stage in the experiment one or more of the stimuli initially ignored (unattended) appeared as stimuli about which some judgment was required. When the figure had appeared earlier as one that had to be ignored, it took longer to identify (or otherwise respond to). This phenomenon, called "negative priming" has been the subject of a great deal of research, and a number of remarkable findings have been reported. For example, DeSchepper and Treisman (1996) and Treisman and DeSchepper (1995) used random shapes similar to the Rock and Gutman shapes of figure 4.3 in a discrimination task. Two figures were presented. The one on the left contained two overlapped figures, such as those on either side of figure 4.3. On the right was a single figure. Subjects had to judge whether one of the overlapped figures on the left, say the red one, was identical to the single figure on the right. The time it took to make this judgment was very sensitive to whether the test figure on the right had earlier appeared in a trial where it had been the nonattended figure on the left. If it had, the reaction time was significantly longer, even if the figures were totally unfamiliar and had never been seen before their first appearance in this experiment.

It seems that a representation of an individual shape is created even for figures that are ignored. DeSchepper and Treisman (1996) report that the negative-priming effect is robust enough to last through over 200 intervening stimuli and even to persist for as long as a month. It is apparent that unattended shapes are encoded somehow and leave a lasting trace, even though, according to both the Rock and Gutman (1981) and DeSchepper and Treisman (1996) studies, there is essentially zero explicit recall of them. Both the incidental recall study of Rock and Gutman and the negative-priming effect suggest that attention is paid to entire figures, even when the figure is extended and when it is intermingled with other figures that are ignored—and indeed, even when they appear to have been ignored as judged by explicit recall measures. (Additional related findings on the tendency of attended objects to refrain from attracting attention immediately after they have been attended to—so-called inhibition of return—will be discussed below on pp. 188–189.) The negative-priming results also suggest that the naive notion of attention as a focal beam that is necessary for memory encoding may be too simplistic. These findings fit well with a growing body of evidence suggesting that something like attention may be allocated to individual objects very early in the visual stream.

Although I have been concentrating on attentional selection from visual displays, the notion of object-based attention is not confined to static visual objects. Some time ago Neisser and Becklen (1975) showed that people can sometimes selectively follow one of several complex sequences of events—for example, they can selectively attend to one of two games superimposed on a video. There is also evidence that object-hood is a much more general notion and that it applies not only to spatially defined clusters, but also to clusters defined by other properties, as for example in various forms of "streaming" (to be discussed in greater detail later; see figure 4.14) that occurs not only in vision but also in audition. Auditory streaming (in which a series of superimposed notes may appear not only as single sequence of chords but also under certain conditions as two or more distinct overlapping melodies) is a well-studied phenomenon (Bregman, 1990; Kubovy and Van Valkenburg, 2001).

4.4   Individuation: A Precursor to Attentional Allocation?

4.4.1   Individuation is different from discrimination
The surprising negative priming result discussed above raises the question of whether what we intuitively refer to as "attention" is really a single process, or whether there are different stages in the process responsible for the phenomena we classify as "attention." In this section, as well as in chapter 5, I suggest that there are a number of reasons to believe that *individuation* of what, for now, I will call *visual objects*[2] is a primitive operation and is distinct from discrimination and recognition

2. In the context of attention studies such as those to which I alluded earlier, the elements in the visual field are typically referred to in the psychological litera-ture as "objects," where the exact referent of this term is deliberately left ambigu-ous. In particular, it is left open whether what is being referred to are enduring physical objects, proximal visual patterns, or other spatially local properties. The only property that appears to be entailed by the term in this context is that it endures over changes in location, so that when we call something an object we imply that it retains its individuality (or, as it is sometimes called, its "numeri-cal identity") as it moves about continuously or changes its properties over a wide range of alternatives. In every case considered here, "object" is understood in terms of whether something is perceived as an individual. Is it possible to have an objective definition of "visual object"? I will return to this issue later, but my conclusion will be that although something like "primitive visual object" can be defined by reference to certain theoretical mechanisms, it will remain a viewer-dependent notion (or, as philosophers would say, the concept is mind-dependent). Moreover, I confine my usage to *visual* objects, not to real physical objects, although, as we will see, the two are closely linked.

and, indeed, from what we generally call "attention." Individuation appears to have its own psychophysical discriminability function. He, Cavanagh, and Intriligator (1997) showed that even at separations where objects can be visually resolved, so that you can tell that there are several objects, they may nonetheless fail to be *individuated*, preventing individual objects from being picked out from among the others. Without such individuation one could not count the objects or carry out a sequence of commands that require moving attention from one to another. Given a 2D array of points lying closer than their threshold of individuation, one could not successfully follow such instructions as "Move up one, right one, right one, down one," and so on. Such instructions were used by Intriligator (1997) to measure what he called "attentional resolution" and what I refer to as "individuation." Figure 4.4 illustrates the difference between individuating and recognizing. It shows that you can distinguish between a group of objects and a single (larger) object, and even recognize the general shape of objects and yet not be able to focus attention on an individual object within the group (in order to, say, pick out the third object from the left). Studies reported in He et al., 1997, show that the process of individuating objects is separate and distinct from that of recognizing or encoding the properties of the objects. Perhaps, then, one must individuate objects even before one can attend to them.

Studies of rapid enumeration of small numbers of objects, a process known as subitizing, have also thrown some light on the distinction between individuation and other stages in visual processing. Subitizing has been studied for a long time, and it has generally been recognized that small and large numbers of objects appear to be enumerated differently: sets of 4 or fewer objects are enumerated more rapidly and more accurately than larger sets. The reason for this difference, however, has remained a puzzle. I will discuss some interesting findings concerning the important role that individuating plays in this process and will propose an explanation for the apparent difference between subitizing and counting in section 5.3.5. For present purposes I simply point out that items arranged so that they cannot be preattentively individuated can't be subitized either, even when there are only a few of them (Trick and Pylyshyn, 1994b). For example, items that can be individuated only by deploying focal attention serially to each in turn—cannot be subitized;

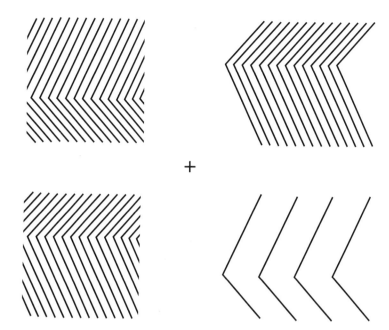

Figure 4.4
At a certain distance, if you fixate on the cross, you can easily tell whether there were many lines or just one gray region in each of the quadrants (so the lines are within your visual acuity). In fact, you can even recognize which groups consist of similar-shaped lines. But you can *individuate* lines only in the bottom right group: You cannot count the lines or pick out the third line from the left, etc., in the other three groups. The attentional resolution phenomenon was first described by Intriligator and Cavanagh (2001).

i.e., the rate of enumeration does not change when the number of objects exceeds around 4, as shown by the fact that the graph of reaction time as a function of number of items does not have a "knee." An example of elements arranged so that they can or cannot be individuated preattentively is shown in figure 4.5 (other examples will be discussed on pp. 239–240). When the squares are arranged concentrically (as on the left), they cannot be subitized, whereas the same squares arranged side by side can easily be subitized. Trick and Pylyshyn provided an explanation for this phenomenon that appeals to a theory that will be discussed at length in chapter 5. A critical aspect of the explanation is the assumption that individuation is a distinct (and automatic) stage in early vision and that when the conditions for automatic individuation are not

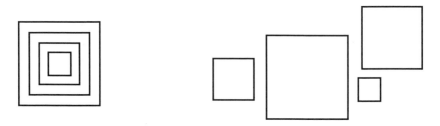

Figure 4.5
When squares are arranged so they are not atomically and effortlessly (i.e., preattentively) individuated (as on the left), they cannot be subitized (as described in the text), whereas the ones on the right are easily subitized. (Described in Trick and Pylyshyn, 1994b.)

met, then a number of other phenomena that depend on it, such as subitizing, are not observed. Notice that the individual squares are clearly visible and distinguishable in both versions of figure 4.5, yet in the figure on the left they are not automatically individuated and therefore are not easily counted or subitized.

4.4.2 Individuating an object is distinct from encoding its location or visual properties

It appears that under certain conditions there is dissociation between the detection of certain properties and the perception of where those properties are located. For example, Anne Treisman and her colleagues showed that when focal attention was directed at a particular item in a display, certain properties of other (unattended) items in the display could still be reported, but in that case combinations of those properties were frequently assigned to the wrong items in what are called "conjunction illusions." Treisman and Gelade (1980) and Treisman and Schmidt (1982) found that if attention was distracted by a subsidiary visual task (such as reading digits aloud), subjects frequently reported seeing the correct shape and color of items in a display like the one shown in figure 4.6, but with false combinations or *conjunctions* of color and shape (e.g., they reported that the display contained a red X and a green O when in fact it contained a green X and a red O). Moreover, when subjects were required to search for a particular target in a display, they were faster at scanning the display when they were looking for

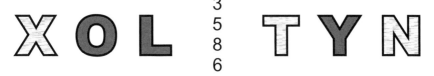

Figure 4.6
Displays leading to what are known as conjunction illusions (erroneous reports of conjunctions of color and shape). In experiments by Treisman and Gelade (1985), subjects read the numbers at the center of the display. Then, after the display is extinguished, they report the letters and their colors. Under these conditions, many incorrect letter-color combinations are reported. Read the vertical column of numbers, then close your eyes and report letters and colors (the dark letters are meant to indicate red letters, and light gray shapes indicate green letters).

disjunctions of properties (e.g., for either an X or a red figure in a field of both red and green Xs and Os) than when they were looking for conjunctions of properties (e.g., for the single red X in a field of both red and green Xs and Os). A large number of studies established a variety of further properties of such rapid search and led to what is known as *feature integration theory*, which claims that a major role of focal attention is to allow distinct features to be bound to the same item, solving what is called the binding problem for properties. This *attention-as-glue* hypothesis helps to explain a variety of findings and has played an important role in the development of current views of attention.

Illusory conjunctions appear with a large variety of properties including shape features, so that a display with \-shaped (left oblique) lines, L-shaped figures and S-shaped figures led to the misperception of triangles and dollar signs. It seems as though attention is required to bind properties together. Such findings may be interpreted as suggesting that when features are detected, their location remains uncertain until the feature is attended. Thus you might see that a display contains the letter X, but fail to correctly detect *where* it was located or "see" it to be at the wrong location (Chastain, 1995). There have been a number of discussions in the literature of the role played by the *location* (of objects or features) in the initial encoding of a visual scene. The idea that the location of features is subject to uncertainty serves as an assumption of several models that have been developed to explain certain aspects of the conjunction illusion, mentioned in the last paragraph. For example, contrary to the original claim made by Treisman and Schmidt (1982), it now appears that the frequency of conjunction illusions may depend on the distance between objects whose properties are erroneously conjoined, as well as on the similarities among the particular properties themselves. Ashby, Prinzmetal, Ivry, and Maddox (1996) have argued that the inherent uncertainties in both the features and their location, combined with various response-selection strategies, explains both the distance and similarity effects in the occurrence of conjunction illusions.

Ashby et al. (1996) present a detailed mathematical model that is able to sort out various types of response biases and noise sources in detection experiments. The Ashby et al. model, like all other theoretical discussions of the conjunction illusion, does not distinguish between *individuation* of a visual object (or recognizing something in the visual field *as* a particular individual object) and encoding its location. Thus, for example, the only sources of uncertainty that are considered are the uncertainty of the location and the features involved in the conjunction error. Yet even after one has encoded such properties as location, shape, and color, there is still the question of whether one has assigned these properties to a *particular individual object*, and if so, which one. This distinction is particularly cogent when all dimensions—including location—are changing. The question then is whether we make conjunction errors by misassigning properties to an individual object as it moves about, or whether we assign the detected properties to the location occupied by that property at some particular time but do so with a certain degree of error. Other alternatives are also possible. For example, it might be that there is no uncertainty about assigning properties to objects, but under certain conditions there is uncertainty in deciding when what appear to be two objects are actually two instances of the *same* object (e.g., the same object at two different times). I will return to these possibilities later when I discuss what is known as the *correspondence problem* in chapter 5. There I make the assumption that when an instance of a property is detected, it is detected *as the property of an individual object*. Distinguishing *which* object it is, is typically done by a preattentive and preconceptual mechanism that will be described in the next chapter.

Many investigators have claimed that, in contrast with the object-based view of property encoding presented above, detecting the location of an object *precedes* detecting its other properties and is the basis for conjoining or binding different properties together. This is the assumption made by Treisman in her feature integration theory (Treisman and Gelade, 1980). There have also been a number of studies (reviewed in Pashler, 1998) showing that in most cases where an object is correctly identified, its location can also be reported correctly, from which it is usually concluded (e.g., Pashler, 1998, pp. 97–99) that location is the basic property used for recovering other properties. What all these studies actually show, however, is that when some property of an object (e.g., shape or color) is correctly reported, its location is usually also correctly reported. This does show that there is a priority ranking among the various properties that are recorded and reported, and that location may be higher on the ranking than other properties. What it does *not* show is that *to detect the presence of a feature, one must first detect its location.*

In an attempt to provide a more direct test of this hypothesis, Nissen (1985) used a conjunction-detection task and compared the probability of correctly reporting an individual stimulus property (say shape or color), the probability of correctly reporting the location of that property, and the joint probability of correctly reporting the property and location. She found that accuracy in reporting shape and color were statistically independent, but accuracy in reporting shape and location, or color and location, were not statistically independent. In fact, the conditional probabilities conformed to what would be expected if the decisions were sequential, that is, if observers detected the presence of a particular conjunction of color and shape by using the detected (or cued) color to determine a location for that color and then using that location to access the shape.[3] From this Nissen concluded that detection of

---

3. The reason that the probabilities of reporting shape and of reporting location are not independent is that location is used to find shape. However, according to the theory, finding the location from the color cue and finding the shape from the location cue are done independently. Consequently, we can multiply their probabilities to get the probability of reporting both the location and the shape in the color cue experiment. In other words, we should find that $P(L \text{ and } S \mid C) = P(L \mid C) \times P(S \mid L)$, which was indeed what Nissen (1985) found.

location underlies the detection of the conjunction of the two other features, or, to put it slightly differently, that in reporting the conjunction
of two stimulus features, observers must first find the location that has
both features. This way of interpreting the results is also compatible with
how Treisman interpreted the slower search times for detecting conjunction targets. Treisman assumed that in searching for conjunction
targets, subjects had to first establish the location of one of the conjuncts
and then use the location to find the corresponding second conjunct by
moving focal attention serially through the display (or at least to all items
having the first conjunct property).

But notice that in all studies that examine the mislocation of properties, as for example in the case of conjunction illusions, location and
object identity (i.e., *which* object it is) are confounded, since the objects
have fixed locations: in this case *being a particular object O* is indistinguishable from *being at location X*. Because of this, the findings are
equally compatible with the view that individual objects *as such* are
detected first, before any of their properties (including their locations)
are encoded. Of course once an object is detected, then it may be that
among the first properties to be encoded is its location in some frame of
reference. The studies described in chapter 5 (dealing with multiple-
object tracking) suggest ways to separate the question of whether an
object's individuality (its identity as the same object) or the location of
a feature serves as the basis for property judgments.

Such a distinction requires that we have a more precise sense of what
we mean by an object, as such, being detected. I will attempt to provide
such a notion in terms of what I call "indexing," which I will explicate
in terms of the correspondence problem and will relate to the multiple-
object-tracking paradigm. The notion of indexing is close in spirit to
what others have called "marking" or "tagging." Indexing an object in
this sense is independent of whether any of its properties have been
detected and encoded. The theoretical position developed in chapter 5
entails that one can detect, or obtain access to, or *index* an object without
encoding any of its properties, including its location. The general position I will defend is that the early visual system possesses a mechanism
for detecting and tracking what I will refer to as "primitive visual
objects." It does so by keeping track of them *as individuals* rather than
as "whatever is at location *X*" or "whatever has property *Y*." Indeed,

we will see that there is evidence that people fail to notice properties or changes in properties of items that they are able to track, thus showing that keeping track of the individuality of an object is independent of encoding its properties. Before taking up the idea of indexing and of tracking objects as individuals, we will consider some evidence that bears on the question of whether attention might be directed at individuals or objects as such, rather than at whatever occupies particular locations. In recent research this issue has received considerable attention under the label of object-based attention.

4.5   Visual Attention Is Directed at *Objects*

The original understanding of focal attention assumed that it shares a number of critical properties with direction of gaze. For example, it was generally assumed that although attention may be allocated voluntarily or reflexively, may be allocated in a narrow or diffuse manner, and may be allocated to regions of some particular shape, it is always allocated in a spatially unitary manner, in other words, that it is not divided among disparate noncontiguous regions. Moreover, it was also assumed that, like direction of gaze, focal attention is directed in a certain *direction*, or to a certain *region* of the visual field. In addition, it was generally assumed that when attention is *focused*, it means that processing resources (or at least preferential access to such resources) is made available to the region on which attention happens to be focused. Many of these widely held assumptions will be challenged in what follows. In particular, I will discuss the following claims: (a) the claim that the evidence (some of which has already been discussed) suggests that the focus of attention is in general on certain primitive *objects* in the visual field rather than on unfilled *places*, and (b) the claim that there is a mechanism (which I call a visual index) that is deployed prior to focal attention being allocated, and that individuates objects and allows them to be addressed even before any of their properties have been detected. Claim (b) is the subject of chapter 5. In what follows, discussion will be confined to the first of these claims: the view that focal attention is typically directed at *objects* rather than at *places*, and therefore that the earliest stages of vision are concerned with individuating objects and that when visual properties are encoded, they are encoded as *properties of individual objects*.

4.5.1   The capacity of the "visual buffer"

It has been known for a long time that even for very short periods of time (less than a second) the amount of information that can be retained is limited. This idea of short-term memory had been investigated for many years (and led to the famous paper "The magic number seven . . ." [Miller, 1956], alluded to in section 4.2). In general, the consensus is that short-term memory is limited in the number of units or "chunks" it can store. However, the application of this idea to visual information had not been investigated in detail. Recently Luck and Vogel (1997) took up the question of what corresponds to a "chunk" in vision. They showed that visual short-term memory holds about 4 colors or shapes or orientations or other features of this sort over a brief period of time. Then they asked what would happen if the features to be recalled were associated with a single individual object. They found, rather surprisingly, that a much larger number of features could be retained so long as the number of individual *objects* was not more than 4. In fact, it seems that one can retain the conjunction of at least 4 features when they are associated with a distinct object, and one can retain 4 such individual objects—thus making 16 distinct features in all. The fact that visual information appears to be chunked according to individual visual objects suggests that encoding of visual information proceeds by objects, not by features. This in turn suggests that the attentional bottleneck operates over individual objects, and that what happens early on in the visual pathway is that objects are individuated or selected. This is an idea that has received considerable and varied support in recent years, and I shall examine the evidence in the following sections.

4.5.2   Extracting visual information from within and between objects

The notion that objects are detected as such and then visual properties are bound to them at a very early stage in visual perception has also received support from many studies showing that subjects are faster in reporting several features or properties if they are associated with the same object. Also features that are part of different objects interfere less in a search task. For example, Duncan (1984) and later Baylis and Driver (1993) showed that access to relational properties of two features (such as "larger than") is faster when the features in question belong to the same perceptual object than when they are parts of different objects, even when they are the same distance apart.

The original study (Duncan, 1984) sought to control for location as the basis for attention focusing by superimposing figures at the same location. Using overlapping figures such as those in figure 4.7, Duncan asked observers to make concurrent judgments about pairs of properties. These properties could both concern one object, or they could concern each of two objects. He found an advantage for pairs of judgments made concerning one object over those concerning two objects. This has become known as the single-object-superiority effect, or the two-object cost.

Duncan's choice of figures was not ideal in a number of respects. In particular, since the features do not cover precisely the same region in space, judgments might involve spatially focused attention. To counter this sort of criticism, Baylis and Driver (1993) used figures in which the stimuli for the one-object and two-object conditions were physically identical and the difference was in how the observer viewed or parsed the figures in the two cases. Examples of the figures Baylis and Driver used are shown in figure 4.8.

Figure 4.7
Figures used by Duncan (1984) to compare the time it takes to report pairs of concurrent judgments of properties of a single "object" and the time it takes to report pairs of concurrent judgments of the same properties belonging to two objects. The judgments were: solid vs. dashed line, left vs. right-leaning, small vs. large rectangle, and left- vs. right-side gap (adapted from Duncan, 1984). Results showed a single-object advantage—performance was better when pairs of judgments concerned the same object.

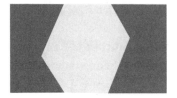 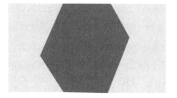

Figure 4.8
Like the patterns in figure 4.7, these stimuli were used to show that access to relational (two-feature) information is faster when both features are part of one object than when they are part of two objects. However, the stimuli were the same for the two experimental conditions; only instructions about where to attend were different. The two figures shown are shapes that can be parsed as one or two objects depending on whether observers are instructed to attend to red or green regions (shown here as dark gray or light gray). The task is to say whether the left vertex is lower or higher than the right vertex. When the vertices are seen as part of a single figure the judgment is faster. (Adapted from Baylis and Driver, 1993.)

When observers are asked to attend to the inner (or red) figure, their judgment of the relative heights of the convex vertices is a within-object judgment, whereas when they are asked to attend to the outer (or green) figure, their judgment of the relative heights of the two vertices is a between-object judgment. As predicted, Baylis and Driver found a faster reaction time when the elements of the judgment belonged to the same object. But as usual, there are refinements and qualifications to such experiments. For example, the "figures" in the two cases investigated by Baylis et al. differ in that the one involved in the single-figure case is convex whereas the ones involved in the two-object case are concave. Is that what makes the difference between the single-object and two-object conditions? Gibson (1994) argued that it does, but Baylis (1994) showed that the longer two-object reaction time remains even with equal convexity (row 2 of figure 4.9). But there are other possible confounds. For example, Davis, Driver, Pavani, and Shepherd (2000) showed that many cases of dual-object feature-report decrements are due to the increased area that has to be examined in the two-object case. The bottom row of figure 4.9 shows alternative displays designed to counter this particular alternative explanation for the single-object superiority effect. But it is also worth noting that many alternative ways of explaining the effect tacitly assume that the visual system has already parsed the scene into objects. So, for example, when one speaks of the "area" that has to be

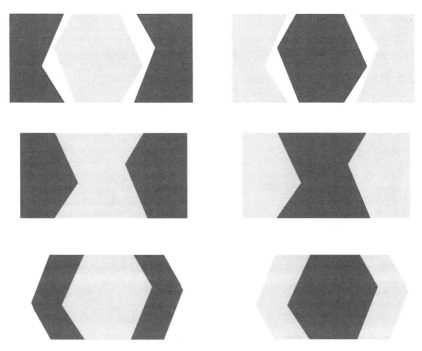

Figure 4.9
Additional figures designed to control for some possible confounds in the study described in figure 4.8. The first row shows that observers are able to selectively attend to the single figure in the original study by showing that the same results are obtained when the figures are separated. The second row controls for concavity/convexity, and the third row controls for overall area. (Adapted from Baylis, 1994.)

examined, one tacitly assumes that it is the area of the *relevant object*, not any area, that matters. The same is true of other ways of looking at what the visual system may be responding to (e.g., that vision responds to the trajectory of an objects' motion rather than to the object's identity). At the present time the object-based nature of attention allocation remains generally accepted, even if other factors (e.g., location) may also contribute.

Another approach to investigating the connection between access to information and objecthood is to examine the spread of attention using a priming method. Attention appears to spread through a region, and when that happens, it spreads more readily within an object than between two objects. For example, Egly, Driver, and Rafal (1994) showed that priming a location increases the detection speed at nearby places and does so more when the places lie inside one object than when they fall across two objects, even when their relative distances are held constant (as shown in the two top illustrations in figure 4.10). Moreover, Moore, Yantis, and Vaughan (1998) showed that this is true even when the objects are partially occluded, so that the spread follows perceived rather than geometrically defined regions, as shown in the bottom figures in figure 4.10.

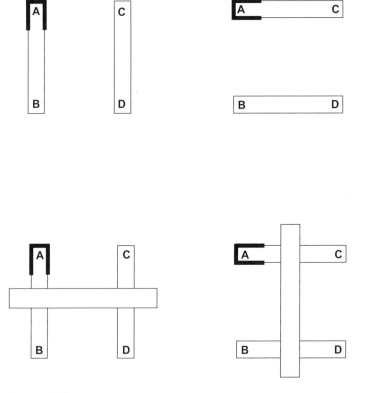

Figure 4.10
The top pair of figures illustrate that when a region such as that marked "A" is primed (by briefly brightening the contour in that region), detection is enhanced in regions within the same object, relative to equidistant regions that lie on another object. Moore et al., 1998, found that this holds true even when there is an occluding bar breaking up the region, as in the bottom figures. (Adapted from Egly et al., 1994.)

The basic idea that attention priming spreads more readily within objects appears to hold even when an "object" is not confined to a particular contiguous region. For example, Brawn and Snowden (2000) found that priming (measured in both detection and discrimination tasks) occurs within each of two overlapping objects (two triangles superimposed to form a "star of David" shape, similar to that illustrated in figure 4.19). Moreover, they found that the effect disappeared when the figure was not perceived as two distinct objects.

4.5.3   Endurance of object-based attention despite changes in the object's location

A number of different studies appear to point to the conclusion that once individuated, the identity of an object—its status as the *same object*—is maintained despite changes in its location or other properties, and that it is this enduring object that remains the focus of attention. One of the first demonstrations of this more robust location-invariant notion of objecthood is a series of studies we carried out on multiple-object tracking (described in section 5.3.1). Because I now view these studies in a somewhat different light, I will reserve discussion of these studies until chapter 5. I will, however, describe a series of studies by Kahneman, Treisman, and Gibbs (1992) that appear to show that both attention and access to the memory record of a visual scene (called an *object file*) is organized in terms of individual objects. Studies using the object file shown in figure 4.11, for example, show that the priming of letter-reading task follows the object in which the letter occured rather than the location where the priming letter had been presented. Observers were shown two squares or "boxes" (panel 1). A different letter was briefly flashed in each box. Then the boxes moved on the screen until each was in a position that was equidistant from the two original box positions (panel 3). A letter then appeared in one of the boxes (panel 4), and subjects had to report the letter as quickly as possible. Although either of the original letters was equally likely to occur in either box, subjects were faster in reporting the letter if it reappeared in the same box in which it was originally presented. But "same box" has to be understood in terms of the continuity or endurance of the box over time, since the boxes were identical in appearance and their locations changed. In some conditions, a box in which a different letter had been displayed ended up at the same

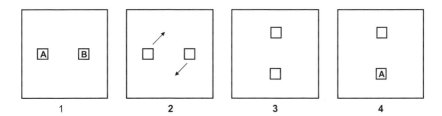

Figure 4.11
Studies by Kahneman et al. (1992) showed facilitation of the time it took to name a letter when the letter was primed by the previous occurrence of the same letter *in the same box*. Since there was an equal chance that either letter would occur in either box the identity of the letter was not predicted by where it had occurred earlier. It seems that the priming effect travels with the object in which it occurred.

location as the one in which the prime letter had been initially displayed. Yet it was the identical-box condition, and not the identical-location condition, that resulted in faster naming. The obvious conclusion is that a priming stimulus is most effective if it is seen to be part of the same object as the pattern it primes. This finding led to the theory that the presence of an object in the visual field (in this case, each of the boxes) leads to the creation of an *object file* in which properties of that object are stored (in this case, this includes the identity of the letter that was displayed in that box). This study can be viewed as extending the Baylis and Driver (1993) demonstration of object-based access to visual information, though now we see that when the object changes location while its identity remains the same, it is object identity that enhances reporting the constituents of the object. Another way of viewing this finding is that objecthood endures certain kinds of location changes, and when it does, it carries object-based effects along with it.

There are now many experiments showing that object-based effects travel with moving objects, including ones that use the phenomenon known as inhibition of return (described in Klein, 2000). Inhibition of return refers to the phenomenon whereby it is more difficult to reassign focal attention to a place that had been attended approximately 600–900 ms earlier than assign it to a new location. Recent studies have shown what is inhibited is not primarily the location that had been earlier attended, but the object that was at that location. It seems that the inhibition travels with the object as the latter moves (Tipper, Driver, and Weaver, 1991). Figure 4.12 illustrates this experiment: it appears to be the individual cued box, rather than its location, that is the locus of inhibition (though both can be factors, as was shown by Tipper, Weaver, Jerreat, and Burak, 1994).

Infants as young as 8 months of age also show object-based effects. Johnson and Gilmore (1998) found that when the inside of an object was primed and stimuli were presented equidistant from the prime, the infant looked significantly *less* often at the stimulus that was inside the same object as the prime than at the stimulus inside the other object. These results suggest that even for 8-month-old infants, entire objects are subject to an inhibitory or satiation effect. (This is opposite to the result reported by Egly, Driver, and Rafal, 1994, but the different time scale means that a different mechanism is involved. Such inhibition or habituation is often found in infant research.)

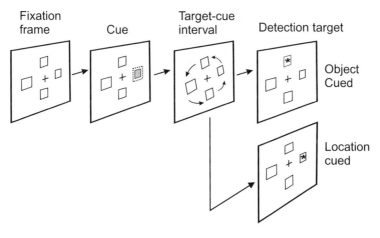

Figure 4.12
Illustration of an experiment showing that inhibition of return (IOR) is object-based. When a target is cued in advance (as shown in figure 4.1) detection is speeded up. However, if the target-cue interval is around 600–900 ms, it takes longer to detect a small stimulus that occurs on the object that had been cued—even if that object has moved to a different location. (Adapted from Tipper et al., 1991.)

4.5.4   Endurance of object-based attention despite temporal interruption

Another illustration of the endurance of objecthood is provided by Yantis (1995, 1998) and Yantis and Gibson (1994). These studies showed that object-based effects can not only withstand changes in the object's location but, under certain conditions, can endure despite a brief but total disappearance of the object from view. Yantis and Gibson argued that when an object suddenly disappears and then is followed by an identical object that suddenly appears in the same location, the second object can be seen as either the same object reappearing or as a new object, depending on certain conditions. For example, if there is a very short time between the disappearance and reappearance, the visual system treats the two as the same object. If the time delay is increased, they may be treated as different objects. The first two panels of figure 4.13 illustrate this point. They show a pair of dots displayed in sequence in an ambiguous display known as the Ternus configuration. The leftmost object in the bottom pair is located in the same place as the rightmost object of the top pair, but separated by some time delay. When the delay is about 50 ms or less, the middle dot is seen as remaining in place while the end one jumps over it: this is called the single-element-motion condition. When the delay is 100 ms or longer, the pair of dots are perceived as moving from left to right: this is the group-motion condition. Yantis and Gibson argued that the difference is that for short time intervals the middle dot is perceived to remain continuously in place, so it does not take part in the apparent motion. But when the interval is longer, this dot is seen as disappearing and reappearing, and hence is perceptually a different object in the two displays. This favors the perception of group motion. But even with relatively long delays the center (disappearing) dot may, under certain conditions, be treated as the same object. Yantis and Gibson showed that if an apparent occluding surface is inserted during the interval (as shown in the rightmost panel of figure 4.13), then even with the longer time interval (an interval that normally leads to group motion) single-element motion is perceived. Their explanation is that when an occluding surface is perceived as hiding the middle object, the object is perceived as persisting throughout the interval, even though briefly hidden by the occluding box. Under these conditions the display

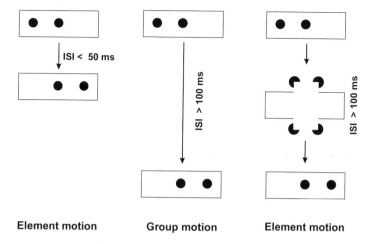

Element motion   **Group motion**   **Element motion**

Figure 4.13
The Ternus apparent-motion display. When the delay between frames is short (with an interstimulus interval less than about 50 ms) the middle dot is seen as remaining in place (it is perceived as a single enduring dot rather than a dot that disappears and is replaced by a new one), and so the outside dots are seen to jump back and forth over it (this is called single-element motion). When the delay is longer, the middle dot is seen to disappear and a new one appears in its place, resulting in "group motion" (where the left or right pairs of dots are seen as moving together). The panel on the right shows a condition in which the durations are the same as in the center figure (where we see group motion), but the appearance of a virtual opaque rectangle during the interval "explains" the apparent disappearance of the middle dot, so the percept is that of element motion as in the left figure (adapted from Yantis, 1995). This is similar to the finding illustrated in figure 3.13.

acts like the short-duration display, since the middle dot is seen not as disappearing and being replaced by a new object, but rather as being briefly hidden by an opaque surface.

In chapter 5 we will see other examples of the persistence of object-identity through changes in other properties and also through longer periods of disappearance from view—though the latter occurs only under conditions that, like the Yantis and Gibson example discussed here, provide cues to the presence of an occluding surface. These cases involve the multiple-object-tracking studies that will be discussed at length in chapter 5.

4.5.5   Object-based attention when "object" is not defined spatially

The most direct test of the idea that the single-object superiority effect does not require spatially distinguishable objects was reported by Blaser, Pylyshyn, and Holcombe (2000a, 2000b). Blaser et al. used two superimposed disks called Gabors. Gabors are patches of sign-wave-modulated color or intensity stripes that fade off at the edges according to a normal or Gaussian distribution. Each of the two superimposed Gabor patches changed continuously and independently over time along the dimensions of spacing (also called "spatial frequency"), orientation, and color. By rapidly alternating two continuously changing Gabor patterns (at 117 Hz), a display was created in which the pairs of figures are perceived as two overlapping transparent layers that change individually rather than as a single changing plaid texture. Figure 4.14 shows a sequence of such Gabor patches, rendered in black and white instead of in the original color. Blaser et al. showed that such "objects" could be individually tracked over time even though they do not move in spatial coordinates but "travel" through a three-dimensional "property space," as shown in figure 4.15. Blaser et al. also showed that performance in detecting discontinuities in pairs of properties (e.g., sudden small jumps in orientation and color) was better when the discontinuities occurred on the same "object" than when they occurred on different objects, even

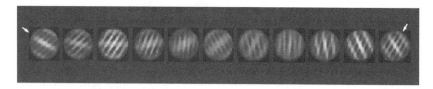

Figure 4.14
This figure shows a sequence of snapshots, taken every 250 ms, of overlapping, slowly changing pairs of striped patches, called Gabors. They are shown here side by side and in monochrome gray, rather than in the original two-color presentations varying in time. When presented in rapid succession they look like superimposed transparent pairs of gratings rather than as a plaid pattern. The two patches vary continuously in color, orientation, and spacing. Observers were asked to track them as two slowly changing individual "objects." They were able to do so and to indicate which of the two overlapping Gabor patches had initially been designated as "target" (from Blaser et al., 2000b). These patches act like general "objects" and show a single-object advantage effect when observers are asked to report sudden changes in two of their properties.

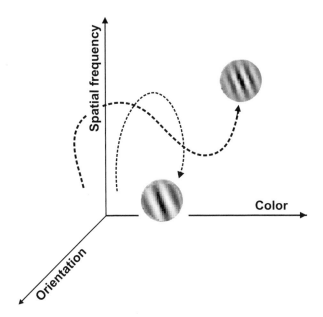

Figure 4.15
Graph of the above sequence showing it as moving through a three-dimensional "property space," while remaining fixed in spatial coordinates. (From Blaser et al., 2000b.)

though in this case the "objects" are perceptually defined in terms of their continuous motion through the property space. This demonstrates that whenever some set of properties is perceived as a unitary whole, the resulting whole has many of the properties of a perceptual "object," insofar as it can be tracked through continuous changes (in properties, not in space) and shows single-object superiority effects. It appears, therefore, that "objecthood" need not be defined in terms of spatial coherence or spatiotemporal continuity. This lends further support to the notion that in general the detection of objecthood need not proceed by the prior detection of location, or by the detection of something like property-*P*-at-location-*X*, where property *P* and location *X* are part of the initial encoding of the display.

4.6   Neuropsychological Evidence for Object-Based Information Access

4.6.1   How do the ventral and dorsal visual systems coordinate information?

There has also been considerable interest in recent years in what have been called "two visual systems." Ungerleider and Mishkin (1982) claimed that there are two streams of visual processing in the brain: a dorsal stream, which encodes *where* a thing is, and a ventral stream, which encodes *what* it is (its identity, in terms of some category stored in memory). Although it now appears doubtful that "where" and "what" are the proper way to characterize these two systems (Milner and Goodale, 1995, for example, have made a strong case that the ventral system is best characterized as concerned with recognition, while the dorsal system is concerned with the visual control of action), it remains generally accepted that the location of various features in space is computed relatively independently of their configuration or what they are recognized as. But if this is true, then the question immediately arises, *What* does the dorsal system compute the spatial location *of*, if it does not know *what* is at that location? A reasonable answer is that it computes the location of whatever it is attending to. Since there is reason to think that what the visual system attends to are objects, we might expect that both systems share an interest in properties of *objects*.

However one characterizes the two visual systems, it is clear that they must interact. In fact, Duncan (1993) has shown that this interaction can result in interference between judgments based on where and those based on what. Duncan showed observers displays, such as those illustrated in figure 4.16, each of which had two "objects" that are briefly displayed in unpredictable locations (an "object" consisted of 4 dots and a grid of parallel lines), and asked them to make two concurrent judgments. The two judgments could concern either the same object or different objects, and could involve either the same visual system or different visual systems (e.g., they might both concern location—such as which is to the left or above—or both concern some visual feature—such as the spacing, orientation, or length of the gridlines). Results showed that pairs of concurrent judgments made across different objects underwent strong interference, whether they involved the same or different visual systems. No interfer-

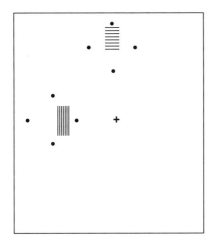 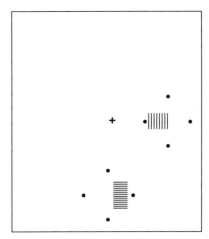

Figure 4.16
Two displays such as those used by Duncan (1993) to examine availability of "what" and "where" information from within one object and across two objects. Here "objects" are clusters of four dots and one grid, location information is assessed by a judgment of whether the grid is left or right or above or below the center of the object, and feature information is assessed by a judgment of high vs. low spacing, long vs. short grids, and horizontal vs. vertical orientation. Duncan showed that the two kinds of judgments (which neurophysiological evidence suggests are processed by different visual pathways) interfere with one another except when they concern the same object. (Based on examples in Duncan, 1993.)

ence between the two visual systems was observed, however, when both judgments concerned *the same visual object*. Duncan concluded, "The separate outputs of 'what?' and 'where?' processes can be used concurrently without cost, but only when they concern the same object" (1993, p. 1269). This suggests that coordination of "what" and "where" occurs at a stage after objects have been individuated and attended.

Neuropsychological evidence for the importance of the object-individuation stage in vision also comes from a number of characteristic dysfunctions of attention, chief of which is hemispatial neglect and the Balint syndrome, discussed below.

4.6.2   Visual neglect
Visual neglect or hemispatial neglect is a disorder that often went undetected in the past but has received a great deal of attention in recent

neurological studies (see the review in Rafal, 1998). So-called visual neglect patients, who usually have lateralized parietal lesions, appear to neglect information on the side of their visual field contralateral to their lesion. For example, they exhibit such symptoms as failing to eat food on half of their plate, failing to draw details of half a scene, and even failing to dress half their body. Recent evidence has suggested that rather than neglecting half of their visual field, such patients may neglect half of individual visual objects, regardless of the visual field in which the objects are presented—in other words, neglect may often be object-based. For example, Behrmann and Tipper (1994) tested left-neglect patients on a task that required that they detect targets presented in "dumbbells" consisting of two circles connected by a line. These patients were slower to detect targets presented on the left side of the dumbbell, as expected. But when they saw the dumbbell rotate through 180 degrees, they were then slower to respond to targets presented on the *right* side of the dumbbell. Tipper and Behrmann (1996) also showed that this reversal occurred only with connected pairs of circles (i.e., dumbbells), which were treated as a single object. When the line connecting the two circles was removed, subjects were always slower to respond to targets on the left side of the display, regardless of how they moved about. This suggests that these patients do not neglect half of their visual field (i.e., half of egocentric space), but rather half of the individual objects. In other words, it appears that in this case the frame of reference that characterizes their neglect is object-based, so that when the object is rotated by 180 degrees, the basis of their neglect rotates with it, resulting in the right side of the visual field (which now contains what was initially the left side of the object) becoming the neglected side. Behrmann and Tipper (1999) also showed that object-centered and body-centered neglect could occur at the same time. When stationary squares were added to the dumbbell display, as in figure 4.17, patients simultaneously neglected the stationary square on the left side of the display and the rotated dumbbell circle on the right side. This suggests that neglect can simultaneously operate in multiple reference frames. Body-centered neglect and object-centered neglect may also interact. Thus, for example, the primary axis of a slanted object may serve to *define* egocentric left and right for an observer, so neglect might still be considered as a primarily egocentric disorder, but with object-based contributions to the

Figure 4.17
Left visual neglect patients respond more quickly when detecting a brightening of the objects on the right of their visual field. But if dumbbell-shaped object-pairs are used and they are rotated as shown here while being observed, these left-neglect patients respond faster to the circle on the left—the one that had previously been on the right. If an unconnected pair of squares is also present at the same time, the one on the right of this pair continues to receive preferential responding (as shown by the dots around the figures), thus illustrating simultaneous object-based and egocentric-based neglect. (Adapted from Behrmann and Tipper, 1999.)

egocentric axis (e.g., Driver, 1998; Driver and Halligan, 1991). Other findings of object-based effects in visual neglect (and related disorders) are reported by Driver (1998); Driver, Baylis, Goodrich, and Rafal (1994); Driver and Halligan (1991); Rafal (1998); and Ward, Goodrich, and Driver (1994). Egly et al. (1994), Humphreys and Riddoch (1994), and Humphreys and Riddoch (1995) have also used neglect patients to explore attentional selection within and between objects. These studies have generally provided support for the notion that attention is directed at objects, and therefore that deficits of attention show up in an object-centered frame of reference.

4.6.3 Balint's syndrome
Additional neuropsychological evidence for the object-based nature of visual attention comes from the study of patients with Balint's syndrome, in which patients with parietal lesions (usually bilateral) exhibit surprising object-based deficits (see the review in Rafal, 1997). Patients with Balint's syndrome exhibit many different types of deficits, which may not all share a common cause. These deficits include near-complete spatial disorientation (including the inability to indicate an object by pointing

or even by verbal description), abnormal eye movements, optic ataxia (a disorder of visually guided reaching), and impaired depth perception. One of the most remarkable components of Balint's syndrome, referred to as *simultanagnosia*, is the inability to perceive more than one object at a time, despite otherwise normal visual processing, including normal acuity, stereopsis, motion detection, and even object recognition. Patients with this type of deficit fail even the simplest of tasks that require them to judge a relation between two separate objects (Coslett and Saffran, 1991; Holmes and Horax, 1919; Humphreys and Riddoch, 1993; Luria, 1959; Rafal, 1997). The object-based nature of Balint's syndrome (and especially of simultagnosia) was noted many years ago. Studying brain injuries after the First World War, Holmes and Horax (1919) noted that although Balint patients were unable to determine if two parallel lines were of equal lengths (as on the left of figure 4.18), they could tell whether a simple shape was a rectangle or a trapezoid (as on the right of figure 4.18), even though in the latter case the same two lines were simply connected to form a single shape. What seemed to matter was whether the judgment involved what the person saw as one or two visual objects.

In classical simultanagnosia, patients are typically unable to see two separate items, such as two circles, simultaneously, yet they are able to

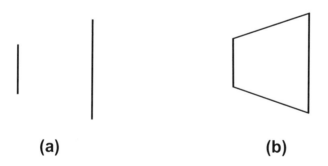

(a)   **(b)**

Figure 4.18
Simultagnosic patients have trouble judging whether the pair of lines (a) on the left are equal, but find it easy to judge that the figure on the right (b) is a trapezoid and not a rectangle. Although both involve judging the same pair of lines, in the example on the right they are part of a single object whereas on the left the judgment involves two objects. (These findings were described by Holmes and Horax, 1919.)

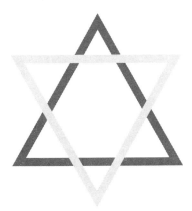

Figure 4.19
A two-colored star. Some simultanagnosic patients see only one triangle—although which one they see may switch over time as they shift their attention.

see a single dumbbell made up of the same two circles (Humphreys and Riddoch, 1993; Luria, 1959). It was even noted (Luria, 1959) that object-based percepts did not have to be localized, so that if the two overlapping triangles, composing a Star of David, were drawn in different colors, so they could be distinguished and attended to individually, simultanagnosic patients would often perceive only one of them (figure 4.19). The existence of simultanagnosia as a syndrome confirms once again that vision and visual attention operate over units that I have informally referred to as objects.

4.7 What Is Selected in Visual Attention?

It appears, then, that a variety of evidence strongly suggests that attention operates—at least in part—on whole objects, rather than on places or regions or any other spatially defined aspects. Such visual attention may be allocated voluntarily by an observer who wishes to devote extra processing capacity to the object, or it may be attracted automatically by events in the visual scene. Among the deeper puzzles that remain is, What happens to the information that is not selected? Some evidence suggests that after a brief delay, it is simply lost. But other evidence suggests that it may have a lasting effect even though it cannot be explicitly recalled. This effect can be either positive (as when recognition of the unattended information improves or "primes" subsequent recognition of related stimuli) or negative (as when unattended stimuli are inhibited so that it subsequently takes longer to respond to them). The exact conditions under which one observes positive priming, negative priming, or simply neglect of unattended information are not well established. Nonetheless, there appears to be converging evidence that whatever focal attention does, it appears to deal with entire objects (or sometimes with distinct parts of a larger object).

Because focal attention can be allocated voluntarily according to what the perceiver is trying to detect or recognize, it provides one of the few mechanisms by which cognition can influence visual perception, as we saw in chapter 2. When perceptual learning occurs, what is learned can almost always be formulated in terms of what aspects of a scene the person learns to attend to (an extreme case of which is when people learn *where to look*, as in the chicken-sexing example discussed on p. 86).

In the next chapter we will see that the idea that attention is object-based has far-reaching implications for how the visual system makes contact with the perceived world. That's because object-based attention is fundamentally directed at objects *in the world*, so it depends on being able to determine when two distinct visual elements arise from the same individual object in the world. The fact that visual attention is object-based and the objects it focuses on are enduring distal objects means that visual attention must compute same-object-hood. Computing when two proximal image features arise from the same distal object requires solving a recurrent problem in vision called the *correspondence problem*. To put it another way, the object-individuation mechanism discussed earlier is indifferent to the location or other visual properties of the objects but rather tracks individuals *qua* individuals. Solving the correspondence problem, tracking individual objects as individuals (as opposed to features that happen to occupy a particular location), and parsing the world into objects are three aspects of the same problem. It is to this fundamental and largely overlooked problem that we now turn.

5

The Link between Vision and the World: Visual Indexes

In this chapter I describe a theory of a mechanism in early vision that is related to focal attention but is more primitive and operates earlier in the information-processing stream. The theoretical idea, which I have developed over the past fifteen or more years, is called *visual-index theory*. It postulates a mechanism, called a visual index (sometimes referred to as a FINST [see note 3]), that precedes the allocation of focal attention and allows the cognitive system to pick out a small number of what I will call *primitive visual objects* or *proto-objects,* in order subsequently to determine certain of their properties (i.e., to evaluate certain visual predicates over them, perhaps by probing them). The theory is based on the recognition that to allocate focal attention, or to do many other visual operations over objects in a visual scene (e.g., encode their spatial relations, move focal attention to them, direct the eyes to them), it is first necessary to have a way to *bind* parts of representations to these objects. A less technical way to put this is to say that if the visual system is to do something concerning some visual object, it must in some sense know *which* object it is doing it *to*. This applies equally whether the activity is detecting a property, making a judgment, or recognizing a pattern among certain objects in the field of view. Detecting a property may be of little use unless that property can be assigned to something in particular in the perceived world. Properties are predicated of *things*, and relational properties (like the property of being collinear) are predicated of several things. So there must be a way, independent of the process of deciding which property obtains, of specifying which objects are being referred to (i.e., which objects have that property).

The usual assumption about how objects can be referred to is that they are referred to by some unique property that they have—in the most general case, by their *location*. But there are empirical reasons to reject this view, some of which have already been discussed in the previous chapter in connection with the evidence that attention is allocated to *objects*, and that the location of an object is independently detected, like any other property of the object. I take the view that *objects* are indexed directly, rather than via their properties or their locations.[1] The mechanism for binding visual objects to their representations is called a *visual index*. We will see later that this approach finds unexpected support in several disparate areas, including research into the cognitive capacity of infants as well as philosophical writings concerned with special ways of referring called *indexicals* or *demonstratives*. I will return to these issues when I examine the wider theoretical and philosophical implications of our approach. For now I will concentrate on the empirical arguments that derive from the study of visual attention and that led me and my colleagues to postulate the FINST binding mechanism. I begin by offering a description of the indexing idea and the motivation behind it.

5.1 Background: The Need to Keep Track of Individual Distal Objects

As a matter of history, the original context in which the present ideas developed was that of designing a computer system that could reason about geometry by drawing diagrams and "noticing" properties in these diagrams (some of this work is described in Pylyshyn et al., 1978). It soon became clear that it was unreasonable to assume that the entire fully detailed diagram was available in the visual representation, for reasons such as those discussed in chapter 1. So it seemed that the actual diagrams would have to be scanned by moving the fovea, or focal atten-

---

1. Note that this is independent of the question (discussed in the last chapter) of whether or not attention can be directed to locations as well as to objects. It is possible that attention can be moved through empty space to fall on unoccupied regions of the visual field, and yet, for location to play no special role in the individuation and detection of objects. Indeed, it is even possible (and likely) for the relational property *being at a different location* to play a central role in *individuating* objects without the actual locations playing a role in determining their identity or having a special role relative to other properties that are encoded for particular objects. See section 5.5 for an example of different properties being used for individuating and for identifying.

tion, to different parts of the diagram. Consider a diagram such as shown in figure 5.1, which may be drawn while proving some theorem or merely looking for some interesting properties of a construction.

If the figure is explored over successive glances, or even just over a stretch of time while various properties are noticed, there immediately arises the problem of maintaining a correspondence between objects seen on successive glances (as in figure 5.2) as well as between parts of the diagram and an evolving representation of the figure. The latter representation might even contain such nongeometrical information as what

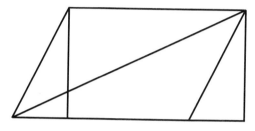

Figure 5.1
An example of a figure that might be drawn in the course of proving a theorem in plane geometry.

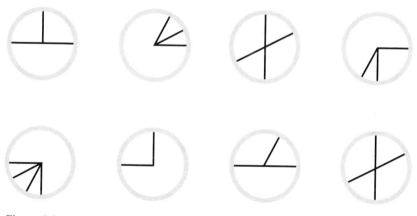

Figure 5.2
An example of the kinds of partial glimpses one might get in the course of examining figure 5.1. The problem is to keep track of which of these glimpses are of the same parts of the diagram. This is an instance of a ubiquitous problem in vision known as the "correspondence problem"—putting into correspondence different elements in the proximal (2D) image that arise from the same element in the distal (3D) scene.

the person had *intended* to draw (diagrams have to be viewed in terms of idealizing concepts like "line," "side of a triangle," or "bisecting angle" and so on, irrespective of exactly how accurately the diagram was drawn), as well as the interpretations already placed on the diagram by earlier perceptual analyses. In addition, there is the problem of recognizing parts of the diagram visited earlier in the scanning, that is, cross-visit correspondences have to be maintained in some way.

We have already come across the correspondence problem in earlier discussions (e.g., pp. 109–112). It arises because vision must build a representation of the distal 3D world from proximal (e.g., retinal) information. Because distinct token features in the proximal image may arise from a single individual object in the distal world, the visual system must treat some proximal elements as the same object in its representation; that is, it must solve a correspondence problem for proximal features. The correspondence problem arises in many situations: when objects move (whether the motion is smooth or apparent), when the eyes move, and when elements on the two retinas are fused into a 3D stereo percept, among others. These various instances of the correspondence problem have been studied extensively. The version raised in the discussion above is a particularly important one because it arises in every case of visual perception. This is because a visual representation is not constructed all at once, but is built up over time as various properties are noticed. Such discrete "noticings" may arise from eye movements, attentional scanning, the movement of objects in the scene, or simply how the visual representation is constructed over time (as we saw in the discussion of the microgenesis of vision on pp. 146–150). The incremental nature of visual processing always raises the correspondence problem, since the stages of construction of the representation have to be coordinated so that different tokens or time slices of the same object are not treated as distinct distal objects.[2] How does the visual system manage this? How can it put

2. It has sometimes been suggested that when the distal object moves slowly and continuously, no correspondence problem arises since one can "see" that it continues to be the same object. But the reason one can see that it is the same object is the same as the reason one sees the "same" object in cases of apparent motion, such as illustrated in figure 3.10, namely, that the visual system puts time-slices in correspondence to yield a single object-representation. No matter how fine the time slices may be, the option still exists to parse the world differently into objects. (See also note 10.)

distinct proximal tokens into correspondence to reveal the single distal object that is their common cause?

Most theories, both in cognitive science and artificial intelligence, treat representations as a type of description. As we saw in chapter 1, this makes sense because representations are conceptual in nature, and because the arguments for this form of representation as the basis for thought are very persuasive (Fodor, 1975). However, this form of representation creates difficulties in solving the correspondence problem, which arises from the incremental nature of constructing a visual representation. With this form of representation the obvious way to maintain correspondences is to assign a unique description to individual objects as they are encoded, and then to match descriptions each time a potentially new object is perceived. When a property F of some particular individual (token) object O is noticed or encoded, the visual system checks whether object O is already represented. If it is, the new property is associated with the existing representation of O. But if the only way to identify a particular individual object O is by its unique description, then the way to solve this correspondence problem is to find an object in memory with a particular description (one that is unique at the time). But *which description*? If objects can change their properties, we don't know under what description the object was last stored. Even if the objects don't change properties (e.g., in a static scene), the description under which it was stored may be different from that under which it is currently encoded. Finding a match with past descriptions is nontrivial. Perhaps we look for an object with a description that overlaps the present one, or perhaps we construct and record a description each time that somehow incorporates time, such as some space-time trajectory.

Even if it were otherwise feasible to solve the correspondence problem by searching for a unique past description, this would in general be computationally intractable (technically, matching descriptions is an NP-complete problem, where "NP" means nonpolynomial). In any case, it is unlikely that this is what our visual system does, for many reasons, for example, we do not in general find it more difficult to construct a representation of a scene that has many identical parts, as this technique would predict (since it would then be more difficult to find a unique descriptor for each object and the correspondence problem would quickly grow in complexity).

At minimum, this way of solving the correspondence problem would require keeping a rich and detailed representation of the scene (or at least of the relevant objects in it)—an unrealistic assumption for the human visual system (for reasons discussed in chapter 1 and below). Problems such as these led my collaborators and me to postulate FINSTs as a type of index or virtual finger that keeps track of particular objects in the scene currently in view and binds them to objects in the partial description already constructed from previous visits.[3] This indexing mechanism does not compute correspondences by making use of information stored in memory; rather, it maintains references to individual objects in a primitive causal manner by *tracking individuals qua individuals,* and not as things that have the same or even similar representations. The visual-indexing mechanism provides links between objects and representations, but it does not maintain the links by consulting contents of representations. This notion is one that is familiar to philosophers, since it corresponds to a particular kind of reference known as a demonstrative or an indexical. It also has strong similarities to recent work on the use of deictic reference in vision (Ballard et al., 1997) and in robotics (Lespérance and Levesque, 1995). Before discussing the broader ramifications of this idea, I will examine a variety of empirical studies that point to the need for such a mechanism.

The more general need for a mechanism such as an index became clearer as we considered what was involved in recognizing certain relational properties that held between different elements in a scene. It seemed clear that in such cases the visual system must have some mechanism for picking out and referring to particular elements in a display

3. This (perhaps unfortunate) name, originated as an acronym for "fingers of instantiation." It arose because we initially viewed this mechanism in terms of the metaphor of keeping "fingers" on certain objects, so as to be able to refer to them, direct inquiries to them, or to move attention to them. If you imagine the cartoon character "Plastic Man" sticking long flexible fingers on a number of objects, and imagine that the fingers themselves cannot sense any properties of these objects directly but allow the individuated objects to be queried by attending to them, this captures the basic idea behind visual indexes. The term "instantiation" connotes the use of the indexes to bind mental particulars (or symbols) to objects, which then "instantiates" the variables. But all that is a (mere) historical footnote; the notion has since gained its own independent foundation in the context of investigating multiple foci of attention and access.

in order to decide whether two or more such elements form a pattern, such as being *collinear*, or being *inside, on,* or *part of* another element, and so on. Shimon Ullman (1984) has argued that detecting certain of these relational properties requires, by the very nature of these patterns, that a serial process access or scan the scene in certain ways, visiting the elements in question in a serial fashion. These processes, constructed from such elementary operations, are called "visual routines." The question that immediately arises is how the visual system designates or picks out the objects over which the visual routines compute properties. The problem is even deeper than merely finding a unique way to specify which items the visual routine must visit; for example, suppose the visual system succeeds in detecting the patterns *inside* or *same contour* in figure 5.3. How does it specify *which* particular things these relations are true of? Clearly, it will not do to simply assert that the relation holds in the figure—if it holds at all, it must hold of particular individual *elements* in the figure. Asserting that it holds of elements meeting a particular unique description also will not do in general, as we will see in detail later (section 5.4). What the visual system needs is a way to refer to individual elements *qua* token individuals. Ullman, as well as a large number of other investigators (e.g., Ballard et al., 1997; Olivers, Watson, and Humphreys, 1999; Theeuwes, Kramer, and Atchley, 1998; Watson and Humphreys, 1997, 1998; Yantis and Jones, 1991) talk of the objects in question as being "tagged" (indeed, tagging is one of the basic operations in Ullman's theory of visual routines). Informally, the notion of a

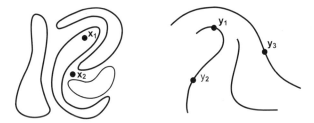

Figure 5.3
Examples of properties that Ullman (1984) suggests require serially applied "visual routines" for their detection. On the left the property to be detected is whether a dot (either x_1 or x_2) has the property of being *inside* a closed contour. On the right the property in question is whether the pair of dots y_1, y_2 or y_1, y_3 have the property of being on the *same contour*.

tag is intuitively appealing, since it suggests a way of placing a unique mark on individual objects for reference purposes. A tag provides a means for referring to objects, somewhat like giving them a *name*, except that it suggests two important additional properties. A tag suggests (a) that unlike a name, the reference is available only while the object is in view, and (b) that maintaining the reference link is externalized—the link is there because of the external tag and not because of some top-down conceptual process that depends on the perceiver remembering the unique properties of the objects in question, such as where they were located in the visual field.

However, the notion of a tag is also misleading for several reasons that help us understand why something like our hypothetical FINST index is needed. One of the purposes of a tag was to allow the visual system to revisit the tagged object to encode some new property (as is explicitly assumed in the theory of Ballard et al., 1997). Thus it does no good to place a tag on an item in the *representation* of the scene, since revisiting the *representation* does not, in general, allow new visual properties to be discovered, as the representation is unlikely to already have the properties being sought. Such an exhaustive representation is implausible on information-theoretic grounds and also, as we saw in chapter 1, on empirical grounds. But the problem would arise even if the representation were pictorially exhaustive. Tags are supposed to also serve as a reference for commands such as those resulting in moving one's focal attention or gaze to particular features in the scene. But one moves one's attention or gaze not to a *representation of an object* but to a real object in the world, so the reference that is needed is a reference to objects in the distal world. The visual-indexing proposal is intended to fulfill this function. A visual index is a reference to an individual object in the world. The reference to a particular individual depends only on certain conditions having been met for the initial assignment of the index, not on the object continuing to have particular properties that are encoded by the perceiver and used in the course of maintaining the reference to that object. In other words, one refers to an object not as something that has a particular property—for example, as the thing that is located at certain coordinates—but as the individual one has selected for certain reasons (such reasons to be discussed later).

The visual indexing proposal is a hypothesis concerning a possible mechanism for "picking out," or "individuating," distal objects in order to allow further visual properties of those objects to be detected or to allow motor actions (such as eye movements) to be directed at them. Thus it is more like the proposal that objects in the *world* are "tagged" in some way. Of course, unless we can write on the real objects in the world, this cannot literally be what happens.[4] But something close to a functional tagging can be accomplished by a mechanism related to focal attention. In what follows, I will describe this proposal and show that this type of mechanism not only has ramifications for how cognition is connected to the perceived world, but also has considerable empirical support in a wide variety of experimental contexts.

5.2   Visual-Index (or FINST) Theory

The idea of a *visual index* is closely related to Kahneman and Treisman's *object files* (Kahneman et al., 1992), described briefly on pages 187–188, except that visual-index or FINST theory emphasizes the mechanism that connects the representation with the objects in question.[5] Despite the simplicity of the indexing idea, it sometimes gets complicated in the

4. Even a literal labeling of distal objects would not help, since we would then need to search the scene for a particular label or else remember which object had which label, which would again require us to be able to refer to distal objects. For example, if you needed to move your eyes back to a certain vertex in figure 5.1 that you remember as being labeled, say, "A," you could not directly move your eyes there but would first have to search the entire figure to find the label, which does not appear to be what actually happens (see, e.g., Hayhoe, Bensinger, and Ballard, 1998).

5. The relation between visual index theory and object file theory is not entirely transparent, owing to the fact that the two theories arose in somewhat different contexts. Although they deal with similar phenomena, object file theory has emphasized memory organization and its relation to the objects from which the information originated. In that respect it is similar to Morton's "headed records" theory of memory organization (Morton, Hammersley, and Bekerian, 1985). Indexing theory, on the other hand, arose from the need for a mechanism to keep track of preconceptual (or unencoded) visual elements in order to keep them distinct and to attach information to them as such information becomes available. Consequently, indexing theory emphasizes the mechanism required for establishing and maintaining the connection between objects in the visual field and mental constructs (representations) of them. The discussion of the difference between individuation and recognition in chapter 4, as well as the experiments to be described in section 5.3, should help make this difference in emphasis clearer.

explaining because it requires making a number of distinctions that are conflated in such everyday terms as "tracking," "recognizing," "identifying," "locating," and so on. I will try to develop the relevant distinctions by sometimes introducing narrower technical terms and by trying to make the same points in a number of ways.

The assumptions that form part of the theory are listed in table 5.1 for easy reference. This list emphasizes, in outline, how the mechanism might work, rather than the function it computes. This (as well as the further discussion in section 5.6 and appendix 5.A) is laid out here to ward off concerns that a mechanism whose essential purpose is to *refer to* individual distal-object tokens leaves us in the dark about how such a function could possibly be implemented. In much of what follows, I will concentrate on the role that this indexing mechanism plays in providing a causally mediated referential connection between mental entities (i.e., concepts) and things in the world.

One major initial motivation for my postulation of indexes is related to assumption (7). Before any visual object can be identified, it must first get *picked out* from the rest of the visual field, and its identity as an individual must be maintained or tracked over movements of the pattern across the visual field. My proposal claims that this is done directly by binding some of individual objects through indexes, *not* by identifying the object in terms of a description (including one that refers to its location). What distinguishes an object as an individual, separate from the other features in a scene, is a purely causal sequence of events beginning with some property or combination of properties of the scene and eventuating in an index being grabbed from a pool of potential indexes. Until some piece of the visual field gets segregated and "picked out," or made accessible, in this way, no visual operation can be applied to it, since it does not exist as something distinct from the entire field. Thus, to recognize or otherwise analyze a visible object in the world, we must first distinguish it as a primitive individual thing, separate from the other clutter in the visual field. Without that, we would not be able to attribute any properties we had discerned to the thing that had those properties. There would be no "x" to which we could predicate some visual property $P(x)$.

According to the theory, this particular sort of picking out and indexing is essentially a causal process, rather than a cognitive or

Table 5.1
Some provisional assumptions of visual-indexing (FINST) theory

1. Primitive visual processes of early vision segment the visual field into something like feature clusters automatically and in parallel. The ensuing clusters are ones that tend to be reliably associated with distinct token individuals in the distal scene. I refer to the distal counterparts of these clusters as *primitive visual objects* (or sometimes just as *visual objects*), indicating my provisional assumption that the clusters are, in general, proximal (i.e., retinal) projections of physical objects in the world.

2. These clusters are activated (also in parallel) to a degree that depends on such properties as their distinctiveness within a local neighborhood, including their temporal (e.g., onset) properties.

3. Based on their degree of activation, these clusters compete for a finite pool of visual indexes (or FINSTs). These indexes are assigned in parallel and primarily in a stimulus-driven manner. Since the supply of indexes is limited (to about 4 or 5), this is a resource-limited process.

4. Although assignment of indexes is primarily stimulus-driven, there are certain restricted ways in which cognition can influence this process through voluntary allocation of attention. For example, attention might be serially allocated to items with certain discriminable properties, and an index may get assigned to objects selected in this way. (I will return to this issue on p. 229.)

5. An index continues to be bound to the same visual object as the object changes its properties, including its location on the retina (within certain limits). In fact, this is what makes it the "same" visual object. On the assumption that proximal clusters are reliably associated with real distal objects (objects in the world), the indexes can then functionally "point to" objects in a scene without identifying what is being pointed to.

6. It is an empirical question what kinds of patterns can be bound by indexes. Patterns need not be spatially local and punctate, although patterns larger than the fovea are likely unindexable. Current evidence also favors the view that the onset of a new visual object is an important index-grabbing event. Perhaps the appearance of a new object within focal attention is another type of event that results in the binding of an index (as in assumption 4).

7. Only indexed tokens can enter into subsequent cognitive processing; e.g., relational properties like INSIDE(x, y), PART-OF(x, y), ABOVE(x, y), COLLINEAR(x, y, z), . . . can be encoded only if tokens corresponding to x, y, z, . . . are indexed.

8. Only indexed tokens can be the target of an action, such as the action of moving one's gaze or focal attention to it.

conceptually driven process. This means that assignment of an index is not mediated by a description or by the prior encoding of the properties of the things indexed in this way, and that keeping track of the indexed objects happens without continually updating the object's properties and matching them to elements in the visual field. Recall that in a geometrical-reasoning task, the fovea moves here and there over the diagram, which requires that we keep track of elements that we have seen before (as illustrated in figures 5.1 and 5.2). The idea is to keep track without having to re-recognize features using a stored description. But how can we keep track of something without re-recognizing it as the same thing at distinct periods of time, and how can we do that unless we know what properties it has (i.e., unless we have a description of it)? This is where the idea of tracking as a primitive operation arose. Just as the separation of figure from ground is a primitive function of the visual architecture, so also is tracking. What I propose is not a full-blooded sense of identity-maintenance, but a sense that is relativized to the basic character of the early-vision system. In general, we cannot re-recognize objects as being the *same individuals* without some descriptive apparatus. But I claim that under certain conditions the visual system *can* track visual objects in a more primitive sense, by treating the sequence that is picked out over time as referring to the same primitive-object token. This what I earlier claimed about how the correspondence problem was solved. Whatever the basis for the solution to the correspondence problem in particular cases, the solution *defines* what counts as a primitive visual object for the visual system.

We know that certain conditions favor a solution to the correspondence problem (see, e.g., the Dawson and Pylyshyn, 1988, theory of apparent-motion correspondence, which I sketched on pp. 109–112). For example, if visual elements follow certain kinds of (perhaps smooth) space-time trajectories, they are more likely to be treated as the movement of a single individual object. Exactly what the conditions are for optimal maintenance of identity remains to be discovered by experimental investigation. It is quite plausible that these properties do not form a natural physical class—that the physical properties involved may well constitute a large disjunction of properties with no overarching general property except for their effect on the visual system. This is, after all, generally true of properties that the visual system treats as equivalent. Consider the variety of physical-optical properties that correspond to any percept (e.g., a shoe). As we saw in chapter 1 (especially in discussing figures 1.7 and 1.8), such property sets may be impossible to circumscribe in a closed physical description, since they are mechanism-dependent; they are defined in terms of their common effect on the human visual system. Of course, there must be *some* properties that cause index assignment and that make it possible to keep track of certain objects visually—they just may constitute a very heterogeneous set and may differ from case to case. In section 5.3, I will have more to say about some constraints on tracking primitive individual objects.

The idea that *indexes* pick out and keep track of objects without first encoding their properties is consistent with the findings of studies that explicitly ask what information is stored with an object (i.e., that is stored in what Kahneman et al., 1992, called an "object file") (see the discussion on pp. 187–188). For example, Gordon and Irwin (1996) used a priming paradigm to explore whether a moving object carried with it information about the shape, location, semantic features, or category membership of the token object. They presented words and examined whether a second word that occurred at the same location or associated with the same moving object was detected more rapidly. They found a priming effect for same location and same object, but little or no priming for items that had similar physical features or similar meanings (as indicated by common semantic features or similar category membership). From this they concluded that object files contained "abstract identity information," but neither physical form of, nor semantic information about, the object. This is precisely what I have been claiming about bare indexes, although in other contexts, other kinds of information may be stored in memory and associated with indexed objects. The priming methodology, it seems, was able to isolate the object-based information stored when the task did not require other information to be stored about the indexed objects.

Notice a certain similarity in the motivation behind the above assumptions about visual indexes and the assumptions of various "natural constraints" operating in early vision (as discussed in section 3.1.1). In the cases where I appealed to natural constraints, I was able to give a noninferential account of certain phenomena of visual interpretation (such as the perception of structure from motion) that might appear to require inference from world knowledge. In these cases we found that on closer examination the phenomena could be explained more simply by assuming that the visual system had become wired (presumably through evolution) in such a way that, even though it was unable to use relevant knowledge concerning a *particular* scene, its operation is restricted in certain ways that ensure that representations of the 3D layouts it computes are generally veridical in our sort of world. Similarly, in the present case I hypothesize a tracking mechanism that appears to maintain individual identity—a task that in general *would* require appeal to concepts, descriptions, and inference—yet does so without involving the conceptual system. As in the case of the natural-constraints examples, this task is accomplished by what one might call an evolutionary heuristic: we have evolved a basic mechanism whose function, within its domain of application (or its "ecological niche"), is close enough to that of identity maintenance that it can serve as a surrogate for full individuation and identity maintenance. Such a mechanism maintains the correct identity correspondences in most circumstances of importance to us—situations that are typical in our kind of world. Because such a mechanism operates without regard to knowledge and expectation, it is able to operate quickly. Given additional time, we can always supercede it by imposing rational cognitive processes—we can decide that two things perceived as the same are not the same distal object. We can decide that what we saw moving in a continuous trajectory was first a rocket, then a person, then a person with a parachute. What we cannot do is decide to *see* three different things, as opposed to a single thing that changed along the way.

What this means is that in this theory neither *picking out* nor *tracking* need be based on top-down *conceptual* descriptions, but may be given preconceptually by the early-vision system, and in particular by the FINST indexing mechanism. Moreover, the visual system treats the object so picked-out as distinct from other individuals, independently of what properties this object might have. If two different objects are individuated in this way, they remain distinct as far as the visual system is concerned. They remain distinct despite changes in their properties, particularly changes in their location. Yet the visual system need not know (i.e., need not have detected or encoded) any of their properties in order to implicitly treat them as distinct and enduring visual tokens. The theoretical claim is that to bind an object *x*, *in this primitive sensory manner*, there need not be any concept, description, or sortal that picks out each token instance of x by type. The individuals picked out in this way by the early-vision system (by a mechanism described in table 5.1 and illustrated in figure 5.4) I refer to here as *primitive visual objects*. I use this technical terminology to distinguish these primitive visual objects from objects in the more general sense, which might include invisible things, abstract things (like ideas), and other more usual kinds of objects, such as tables and chairs and people. This sense of "object," as philosophers like Hirsch (1982), Wiggins (1979), and others have argued, *does* require sortal concepts to establish criteria of identity. But our concern here will be with objects that are in the first instance defined in terms of the special sort of primitive nonconceptual category of objecthood induced by the early-vision system. We don't know in any detail what properties define this sort of primitive objecthood, or even whether it can be characterized in any way except in terms of the structure of our perceptual system. Thus, what we have so far is the claim that the early-vision system must be able to individuate and keep track of certain primitively detected and primitively segregated visual objects over time.[6]

The basic idea of the FINST indexing and binding mechanism is illustrated in figure 5.4. A series of optically mediated events lead from certain kinds of primitive visual objects, via fundamental mechanisms of the visual system (including retinotopic grouping processes), to the establishment of a link with certain conceptual structures (which we may think of as symbolic structures in long-term memory). This allows certain sorts of objects to *grab* or *seize* one of the small number of available indexes and thus provides a means whereby certain conceptual entities (i.e., the active nodes or the items in working memory) can *refer* to these visible objects in the world. The important thing here is that the inward arrows are purely causal and are instantiated by the nonconceptual

6. I have confined this discussion to the visual system as an interim measure, because the empirical data that we have are primarily concerned with the visual system. But it seems clear that this notion will have to be extended beyond vision to include other sense modalities. For example, there is considerable evidence that under certain circumstances we can preconceptually track distinct melodies embedded in other melodies or sequences of chords (Bregman, 1990) and that we can track the movement of several sound sources in a dark room. As we will see, we can also visually track objects of a more general nature, such as the spatially coextensive patterns described on pp. 192–193. Although these are all relevant to the notion of individuation, tracking, and indexing, an examination of nonvisual phenomena is beyond the scope of the present discussion.

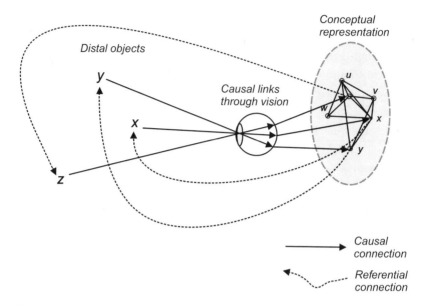

Figure 5.4
Sketch of the types of connections established by FINST indexes between primitive visual objects *x, o, z* and parts of conceptual (descriptive) structures.

apparatus of early vision. This apparatus guarantees that under certain conditions of change (some of which will be discussed later), the primitive objects that caused the link will maintain it in unbroken continuity, thus resulting in its counting as the *same link*. By virtue of this causal connection, the conceptual system can *refer to* the primitive visible objects. It can, for example, interrogate them to determine some of their properties, evaluate visual predicates (such as *collinear*) over them, move focal attention to them, and so on. How this can be done is illustrated in appendix 5.A, though merely to show that nothing mysterious is being assumed here. It is a straightforward problem of how to use a causally established link to send signals back to the original cause.

5.2.1 Some fine points about the properties involved in indexing
Before I turn to a discussion of the empirical support for the indexing hypothesis, two points of possible misunderstanding need to be cleared up. *First*, the reader may have noticed that there is a sometimes an ambiguity in the above discussion (e.g., in figure 5.4) as to whether the cause

of the index assignment—the primitive visual object—is a *proximal pattern* on the retina or a *distal* object in the world. Of course, both are involved, since they are links in the same causal chain from distal object to mental index. But it matters a great deal whether the index is taken (both by the theory and by the cognitive system being modeled) as pointing to a proximal or a distal object. There is typically no interest in pointing to a proximal (e.g., retinal) cluster, although it is a logical possibility. The essential function of indexes is to pick out and refer to *distal* objects. It is only when elaborating on the nature of the links in the causal chain that we may need to go into detail about the steps that intervene between the distal object and the visual index (as I do in table 5.1). We do this when we give a theory of how indexes are implemented in the brain or in a computer, or perhaps when we wish to explain certain deviations of the mechanism's behavior from pure cases of demonstrative reference. Of course, when the objects being indexed are marks on a computer screen, the situation remains ambiguous: the observer may be indexing clusters on the screen or, more likely, a virtual distal object, where only the part of the chain from the scene to the observer is real. This is like asking what a person sees when looking at a picture: is it a pattern on a 2D surface or a (possible) 3D scene in the world? Although some ambiguity remains (since the observer likely sees the scene as being pictured on a 2D surface and can decide to focus on the pixels or the pen strokes), the usual case is that the percept is of a (possible) 3D scene.

The *second* point of potential misunderstanding concerns what I mean when I claim that no concepts or encodings of properties of the objects are involved in assigning or in maintaining indexes. A reader might wonder how an index could be assigned—could be the outcome of a causal chain—if not by virtue of *some* property. My claim is not that no property is involved, but that no represented (or encoded) property is used in making the assignment of an index. But does not *some* part of the nervous system encode the property that causes the index to be assigned (or that causes the index to remain bound to the object)? This question merits some elaboration since it has led to considerable misunderstanding.

Properties responsible for indexing: A technical aside   This discussion requires that we distinguish between a property being encoded and a property causing some change of state to occur. Readers who take this distinction for granted or whose interest stops short of philosophical issues may skip this section.

The distinction between a property affecting a system by virtue of being encoded as opposed to affecting it in a purely causal manner may seem arcane, but in fact it is routinely made, especially in computational systems. Not every physical property impinging on a computer or on our nervous system is associated with, or results in, a representation of that property. Some years ago Uttal (1967) drew a distinction between *codes* and *signs* for just this reason. Uttal pointed out that the nervous system, *qua* physical system, may react to certain forms of energy arriving at its surface, yet the reaction may nonetheless fail to encode or to *represent* anything, in the sense that the change in the system's state may not be computationally relevant. Striking a computer with a hammer may change some things (e.g., its appearance, its position, the relative location of its parts, perhaps even the relative temperature or electrical properties of various parts) without the changes being computationally relevant. By contrast, events that are processed as data—even analog inputs, such as the movements caused by very same hammer blow—are said to be encoded if they take part in a computational process. Such processes, though they still depend on some causal sequence, are different from noncomputational physical changes, since to explain the effect they have, one would have to describe the computational process (the algorithm) involved. Similarly, a sudden onset of a visual object may cause an index to be assigned without the assignment either being based on prior encoding of the event *as an onset* or itself carrying the information that an onset occurred.

There are two issues here: (1) can a nonencoded property cause an index assignment or be responsible for tracking a moving object, and (2) can an index assignment fail to carry information about the nature of the property that caused it to be assigned? It is frequently the case that some property affects a system without being represented, either before or after the causal event. The occurrence of a loud noise or a flashing light may result in a person orienting his or her attention to the noise or light, even though the person need not have encoded the noise or light flash as such, either before or after it occurred. This is similar to what are called "interrupts" in computers (see the discussion of such issues in Pylyshyn, 1981a). Unlike inquiries or tests, interrupts occur not as a result of matching a description against an event, but as a result of the causal structure of the architecture itself. Moreover, an interrupt in and of itself need not carry any information about what caused the interrupt (in a computer, an interrupt usually leads to the execution of a routine that checks to see what caused the interrupt).

Similarly, the assignment of an index is like an interrupt: it happens because of the causal structure of the architecture of the visual system and the occurrence of a triggering event in the environment. As in the case of an interrupt, the assignment itself does not carry the information that a certain type of event occurred, in part because an unlimited number of different events or properties could have caused the index to be assigned.[7] The particular property that caused the assignment is typically not encoded. This also applies to the claim that objects are indexed without appeal to their location. The objects are, of course, at *some* location and have particular properties, and perhaps if they had not been at a particular location or had those particular properties, they would not have been indexed. But that does not mean that a property like location is encoded, or that indexing or tracking is carried out by means of detecting locations or trajectories.

But this leaves an apparent puzzle: how can a person or a robot carry out an action like pointing to or moving attention to a particular

---

7. The issue here is actually more complex than it appears, because "representing" or "encoding" involves a special kind of relation between the representation and what it represents. There is a many-one mapping between a representation and what it represents, as with the terms (codes) "morning star" and "evening star," which refer to the same thing, just as the codes "dog," "Mary's pet," "a fuzzy brown animal" may all refer to the same physical thing, and "unicorn" refers to no existing thing. A code does not just represent some particular object; it represents it *as having some property*, or as a member of a particular category. A term such as "chair" does not just refer to a chair, but refers to it *qua chair*, or as a member of the category *chair*. One might say that it refers to its "chairhood" and not to its color, size, shape, or any of an indefinite number of properties that the particular chair, *qua* object, might have.

The fact that encoding is a semantic relation means that what something is encoded *as* cannot be simply the result of a causal event; it is also a conceptual act. But I have claimed that index assignment is a purely causal event; consequently it differs from an encoding (thus, from this perspective, it is technically incorrect to call an index a deictic code as Ballard et al., 1997, do). Indexes, unlike codes, pick out things in the world to which they are related by a causal event, and they do not encode these things *as* something or other; indeed they do not encode them at all.

individual object, as I claimed in item (8) of table 5.1, unless it knows *where* the object is? This apparent puzzle rests on a misleading way in which the question is asked, since it assumes that knowing where the object is or pointing to or picking out requires knowing coordinates or some location code for the object. But in order to find or pick out a particular object, what you need is (a) an unambiguous way of referring to (or indexing) the object in question and (b) a way of using this index or this form of reference in a visual predicate or motor command. You need nothing more. In a computer you need the address of an object in order to operate on it, and the address is often (misleadingly) viewed as a location code. But the address is nothing more than a symbol that allows the computer to retrieve the contents associated with the symbol. Such a symbol is more like a name than a location. It works because there is a primitive operation in the architecture of all modern computers that, when given the "address" or name of some item in memory, retrieves the item associated with that name. To be sure, the individual bits of the stored item have a physical location, and that location is used by the electronics in retrieving the contents, but the location is not available outside the electronic level—it is not available as a location code at the level of the program. This sort of "location" is a property of the implementation and may be quite different in different implementations—in fact, in some possible implementations (e.g., holographic storage) there is no such thing as "the location of item X," since every part of the stored item is distributed throughout memory.

To see that you can uniquely specify an object without specifying its location (or any other property of the object), and that this way of specifying the object can be used in an argument to a motor command, consider the specification "what I am now looking at" or even simply "that." This is an exemplary deictic reference (sometimes called a demonstrative): It specifies something in a way that can be interpreted only within the context in which the reference is made.[8] Moreover, it does not

---

8. This is reminiscent of the way that variable binding occurs in programming languages, like LISP, that allow dynamic scope bindings. In such systems a particular variable binding exists only while the function within which it was defined remains active and may disappear (or change) when that function is completed, just as index binding does, according to the present theory, when the indexed object disappears from view.

provide an encoding of the location (or of time or of any intrinsic property of the object in question), yet it can be used to control the motion of a limb. Ballard et al. (1997) have shown that such a deictic reference provides a particularly efficient way of indicating (or referring to) the target of an intended action. As for the second requirement (that the form of reference be capable of serving as an argument in a motor command), specifying where to move a limb is best done by providing a deictic reference that binds the argument of a command such as MOVE(x) to an object. A command like MOVE(27, 408) cannot be executed without also knowing exactly where the agent is located, and that will keep changing as the agent moves. Notice that "what I am looking at" does not pick out an individual by its location, since its location is nowhere specified; it picks out the individual demonstratively, or directly without reference to any of the individual's properties.

The point of this example was simply to show that there is nothing mysterious about specifying objects using a deictic or indexical form of reference and in using this form of reference in a motor command. A robot that was simply told to move to the object of its gaze *could* just continue moving in a way that kept its gaze centered on the target, without ever knowing *where* the target was in terms of some allocentric frame of reference (nor, for that matter, need it know any properties of the target except that it was in its cross-hairs). It could do so because of the causal structure of the connections between head position and wheels and because the head position could be controlled by a simple feedback mechanism such as occurs in a servomechanism.[9] In such a mechanism one often controls a property that is not directly measured or encoded, simply by relying on some easily detectable correlates of the property. For example, to catch a fly ball, a baseball fielder moves so as to nullify the apparent curvature of the ball's flight, so it looks like it is descending in a continuous straight line (McBeath, Shaffer, and Kaiser, 1995).

9. The point here is not that one need not use coordinates or other magnitudes in specifying objects on which some action is to be performed. There may be good reasons why in certain cases you might use magnitudes such as distance, direction, time, etc. as the basis for implementing the execution of the MOVE(x) command. But these are details concerning the implementation level, not the "intentional level" at which objects are selected and at which they become the subject of intended actions. What I referred to as the implementation level has sometimes been called the "subpersonal" level.

Thus the property that the player wishes to control (the player's location at the time the ball is about to hit the ground) is nowhere represented, nor is any other magnitude of the ball's motion. The player simply monitors the deviation of the ball's trajectory from a straight path.

There are many examples where a physical magnitude has a causal effect on a process, yet is not encoded or represented. A car speedometer measures speed, defined as the rate of change of distance with respect to time, yet it typically does not represent either distance or time. Global Positioning System (GPS) satellite-navigation system, on the other hand, typically *does* measure (and represent) location, distance, and time in order to compute speed. Another example of a direct (causal) action of a property that is not encoded is the autofocus feature of many cameras. Autofocus does the equivalent of setting the focus ring on the camera to the appropriate distance. Yet insofar as the camera's mechanism can be considered to involve a computation, such autofocus mechanisms typically never actually *measure* distance directly, and consequently no distance measure is ever encoded. What the mechanisms measure may be time delay (sonar method), angle (triangulation method), intensity (infrared method), spatial spectrum (contrast method), or the phase difference between two sensors (phase-matching method). The measured quantities could be used to compute (and represent) distance, but they typically are not. The measurements usually enter into physical connections to the motor system for moving the lens, but the implied distance value need not be available as a distinct code in the camera's computer. Although the computed function may be properly characterized in terms of distance between camera and subject, no representation of distance need be involved in the process (even as an analog encoding) if the lens is moved as a function of other measured magnitudes.

Such examples show that there is nothing unusual about the claim that to move toward (or point to) an object, no location encoding is required, only a way of individuating and indexing the object, along with relevant motor commands to whose arguments such an index can be bound. Everything else is part of the implementation and can take many possible forms, depending on the available technology. (For more on the relevance of deictic pointers to robot control, see pp. 256–259.)

The idea of a visual index as a deictic reference can be made more concrete in the context of the experimental phenomena to which they have been applied. For this reason I now turn to the elucidation of the idea of a visual index by describing a number of experiments we have performed over the past fifteen or so years motivated by this theory. These studies (many of which are summarized in Pylyshyn, 1998, 2001a, 2001b; Pylyshyn et al., 1994) provide a wide range of support for the basic ideas introduced above and have the further virtue of making the nature of the indexing claim concrete and operational.

5.3   Empirical Support for Visual-Index Theory

5.3.1   The multiple-object-tracking (MOT) task

Perhaps the clearest way to see what is being claimed in the discussion above is to consider the first set of experiments to which these theoretical ideas were applied. The task involved is called the multiple-object-tracking (MOT) task and helps to make clear what is at issue. For this reason I will not only describe the basic experiments, but will also spend some time discussing what they mean in terms of plausible psychological mechanisms.

In a typical MOT experiment (illustrated in figure 5.5), observers are shown a screen containing 8 simple identical figures (e.g., points, circles,

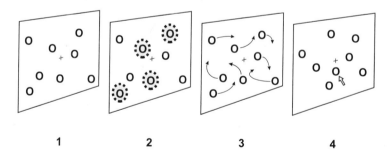

1   2   3   4

Figure 5.5
Illustration of a typical multiple object tracking experiment. A display of eight identical objects is shown (panel 1) and a subset of four are briefly flashed to make them distinctive (panel 2). Once the objects stop flashing this "target" set becomes indistinguishable from the other objects. All objects then move in a random fashion for about ten seconds (panel 3). Then the motion stops and the observer uses a computer mouse to indicate which objects had been designated earlier as targets (panel 4).

squares, plus signs, figure eights) that move in unpredictable ways, sometimes without colliding (because of a simulated barrier or "force field" between them) and sometimes (in more recent studies) with objects freely crossing over and occluding one another. At the start of each trial, a subset of these objects is briefly rendered distinct (usually by flashing them on and off a few times). The observer's task is to keep track of this subset of objects. At some later time in the tracking trial (say 5 to 10 seconds into the trial) all the objects stop moving and the subject has to indicate (using a mouse pointing device) which objects were the targets. A large number of experiments (beginning with studies by Pylyshyn and Storm, 1988) have shown clearly that observers can indeed track up to 5 independently moving identical objects (i.e., objects that are indistinguishable by any property other than their historical continuity with the initially distinct objects). The question to be answered is, how do people do it?

If there had been only one object to track, the answer would be relatively straightforward: Observers could simply track the moving object with their eyes, or perhaps they could track it using attention scanning (such error-driven tracking systems have been common since the development of feedback-control theory and servomechanisms). But how do observers do this task with 4 objects moving along independent random trajectories, interspersed among 4 other randomly moving identical "distractor" objects that must be ignored. One possibility is that observers record and use the locations of each target object and visit them serially. After the initial recording of target locations, they simply go to the location in the list that they have stored and look around for the nearest object, taking that to be the target they are tracking and updating its location code in the list using the following algorithm:

1. While the targets are visually distinct, scan attention to each target and encode its location on a list. Then, when targets begin to move, do steps 2–6.

2. For $n = 1$ to 4, check the nth position in the list and retrieve the location Loc(n) listed there.

3. Scan attention to location Loc(n). Find the closest object to Loc(n).

4. Update the nth position on the list with the actual location of the object found in (3). This becomes the new value of Loc(n).

5. Move attention to the location encoded in the next list position, Loc($n + 1$).

6. Repeat from (2) until elements stop moving.

7. Go to each Loc(n) in turn and report elements located there.

So long as attention moves fast enough from one object to another in relation to the speed of the objects themselves, and so long as targets are sufficiently far from nontargets to prevent frequent mistakes, such a strategy of serial attending and updating a list of locations could explain how observers can track multiple objects. In Pylyshyn and Storm, 1988, however, we were able to show that the motion and dispersion parameters of our original experiments were such that tracking could not have been accomplished using such a serial strategy. The performance of the above algorithm when it is applied to the actual displays used in the Pylyshyn and Storm study results in the performance shown in figure 5.6.

We simulated this serial strategy on the actual trajectories used in the experiments for various attention-scanning speeds (this model assumes

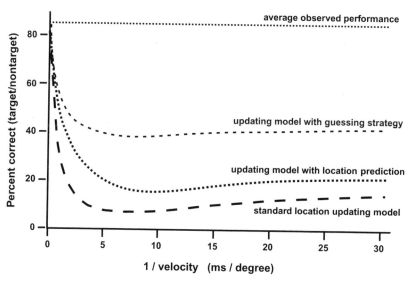

Figure 5.6
Predicted performance of the scanning and location-updating algorithm described earlier, as a function of attention scanning speed, when applied to the actual experimental displays described in Pylyshyn and Storm (1988) shown along with actual observed performance. (Adapted from Pylyshyn and Storm, 1988.)

that to encode location, focal attention must be moved to the object, but it does not assume that either location encoding or disengaging attention require time). The simulation showed that such a serial tracking strategy would very frequently end up switching to tracking nontargets in the course of a trial. Attention-scan speeds have been reported in the range from 4 ms/degree (Posner, 1978) through 8.5 ms/degree (Tsal, 1983), 19 ms/degree (Shulman et al., 1979), 26 ms/degree (Jolicoeur, Ullman, and Mackay, 1983), up to 33.3 ms/degree (Eriksen and Schultz, 1977). So even if we assume the fastest attention-scanning speed ever reported (4 ms/degree, or 250 degrees per second), this strategy could not perform better than about 10 percent correct in tracking the targets (this estimate can be increased to just over 40 percent if we allow for guessing). The observed human tracking performance, by contrast, was about 88 percent correct on average. We have now replicated this result in dozens of different experiments and found that performance in tracking 4 objects in a field of 8 rarely falls below about 85 percent, and for some people it remains over 95 percent. Indeed, many college subjects have no difficulty in tracking five objects.

What this means is that in the multiple-object-tracking studies, observers could not have been keeping track of the targets by using a unique stored description of each object, since at each instant in time the *only* property that is unique to each object is its location. If I am correct in arguing from the nature of the tracking parameters that stored locations cannot be used as the basis for tracking, then all that is left is the object's *individuality*.[10] The individuality of the target objects is initially

10. It has been suggested that one can also think of the *spatiotemporal trajectory* of the object (sometimes referred to as a "space-time worm") as the unique property to which the visual system responds. It is not clear whether this is really different from the proposal I am making since the very notion of a "trajectory" implies that it is a space-time property of a single *individual object*, as opposed to a property defined by time-slices of different objects. In that case responding to a trajectory entails responding to the individuality of an object. The equivalence of these two ways of looking at what the visual system responds to is further supported by the fact that we can represent the display sequence either as a graph in which individual-at-time-t is a node while the correspondences from t to $t + 1$ is an edge, or we can represent it as the dual of the graph, in which a node is a correspondence and an edges is an individual object at a fixed time. Since each graph has a dual, the two may just be notational variants. But individuals, rather than space-time worms, are the natural kinds in our physics, so I prefer to keep to the interpretation I have been giving here.

established by making them distinct (by flashing them). From then on it is historical continuity that determines their identity—where the operative phrase "historical continuity" is defined strictly in terms of the hypothesized primitive mechanism for individuating and tracking: the visual index (or FINST). This mechanism defines a primitive perceptual individuality that persists over time (at least for times as short as 10 seconds and with motion parameters within the range explored in our studies).

The multiple-object-tracking task exemplifies what I mean by "tracking" and by "maintaining the identity" of objects. It also begins to define what a primitive visual object is—it is whatever the early-vision system is capable of tracking in MOT.[11] Tracking, according to this perspective, requires maintaining indexes, and this, in turn requires continually solving the correspondence problem (discussed on pp. 109–112). As I remarked at the end of chapter 4, solving the correspondence problem is tantamount to specifying what constitutes an individual object, from the perspective of early vision. Thus the MOT task can be viewed as operationalizing the primitive notion of "same object"—an object is the *same* if it continues to be bound to the same index despite changes in the object's location and other visual properties. When the early-vision system picks out and keeps track of some cluster of properties, it thereby treats them as an individual object P, rather than as, say, a sequence of time slices of different objects $P_1, P_2, \ldots, P_t$. If the latter were how the visual system parsed the world, then to track an object it would need to re-recognize each of the individual P_ts in some way (say by virtue of their sharing certain properties) so that they might be interpreted as constituting the same individual P. Most reidentifications of familiar things are doubtlessly of this latter kind. To know that the person I saw in a certain movie is the same person whose picture is on my wall and the same person I saw in the store today, I must surely carry out a complex process of describing and comparing descriptions. What I am claiming here is that there are certain primitive cases of identity maintenance that do not require such an apparatus of conceptual descriptions.

11. It is somewhat awkward to keep saying "primitive visual object" to refer to objects as defined by indexing theory or, more particularly, by the tracking task. I have occasionally been tempted to refer to THINGS picked out by FINSTs as FINGs. Now and then I may succumb to this temptation in order to emphasize the mechanism-relativity of this notion of thing or object.

5.3.2   Other properties of visual indexing revealed through MOT
Over the past decade, a large number of additional experiments in our laboratory (McKeever, 1991; Scholl and Pylyshyn, 1999; Sears and Pylyshyn, 2000) and elsewhere (Cavanagh, 1999; He et al., 1997; Ogawa and Yagi, 2002; Slemmer and Johnson, 2002; Suganuma and Yokosawa, 2002; Yantis, 1992) have replicated these multiple-object-tacking results, confirming that people can successfully track several independently moving objects. Some of these studies carefully controlled for guessing strategies and also demonstrated patterns of performance that are qualitatively different from those that would be predicted by any reasonable serial-scanning algorithms we have considered (see Pylyshyn et al., 1994). The results also showed that a zoom-lens model of attention spreading (Eriksen and St. James, 1986) would not account for the data. Performance in detecting changes to elements located inside the convex-hull outline of the set of targets was no better than performance on elements outside this region, as would be expected if the area of attention were simply widened or shaped to conform to an appropriate outline (Sears and Pylyshyn, 2000). Using a different tracking methodology, Intriligator and Cavanagh (1992) also failed to find any evidence of a "spread of attention" to regions between targets in their research.

The sort of "preconceptual" tracking explored in these studies has turned out to have some surprising properties. For example, Scholl and Pylyshyn (1999) showed that tracking can be disrupted by individual objects disappearing for a few hundred milliseconds and then reappearing, whether or not the disappearance and reappearance is abrupt or gradual (e.g., if they shrink into a point and expand from a point). But if the individual objects disappear and reappear in a manner consistent with their going behind an occluding surface (i.e., if they occlude and disocclude at fixed leading contours), tracking is not significantly disrupted—even if the edge of the occluding surface is invisible (i.e., it is a "virtual occluding surface"). This is true even if the occluding surfaces are not global, so that different objects go behind different virtual occluding surfaces. All that is required is that the objects are seen to disappear by having their leading edge accrete as they move behind the occluding surface and then to emerge again as though reappearing at a disoccluding edge (figure 5.7). Viswanathan and Mingolla (1998; 2002) also showed that objects can even occlude one another in their travels, pro-

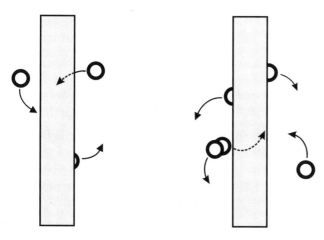

Figure 5.7
Objects can be tracked despite their brief disappearance behind occluding surface and despite self-occlusions when their shapes provide cues (T-junctions) as to which one is in front, as in the case of the rings shown here. (Adapted from Scholl and Pylyshyn, 1999.)

viding there are local cues (e.g., T-junctions) that one is in front of the other. Because of this finding, later versions of multiple-object-tracking experiments have primarily used open circles and have allowed objects free rein in their trajectories—because in this way the trajectories can be made truly independent of one another.

Among the studies we have carried out over the past decade is a set of experiments that explored the question of whether indexes could be assigned voluntarily, or whether only automatic data-driven events could cause indexes to be assigned (Annan and Pylyshyn, 2002). The results were somewhat surprising: they suggested that indexes can be voluntarily assigned based on any visually discriminable property, but only if sufficient time is available. We interpreted this result to mean that although voluntary assignment of indexes is possible, the indexes have to be assigned by serially visiting the objects to be indexed and allowing the assignment to take place (one might say that one can visit objects and "drop off" indexes on the way). If we used straightforward methods of specifying which objects were to be tracked (e.g., numbering them 1 through 8 and telling the subject to track objects numbered from 1 to 4), then, not surprisingly, subjects could do this only if sufficient time was allowed, and they failed if the time available was too brief to allow the numbers to be serially scanned (it is, after all, hardly surprising that the numbers had to be serially read before they could be tracked). But we also introduced a variety of novel procedures for specifying which objects were to be indexed and tracked. Each of these provided information that segregated the set of objects quickly. We then varied the time available to pick one half of the segregated set for tracking. Here is an example of this technique. When 4 of the 8 objects are flashed on and off either very briefly (one on-off cycle of 180 ms) or for a longer time (three on-off cycles totaling 1,020 ms), the flashed objects could be easily tracked in either condition. But when instructed to track the objects that had *not* been flashed, subjects could do so only in the long-flashing condition; they could not track the clearly segregated set if they did not have sufficient time to visit the unflashed objects.

We also explored the question of what sorts of feature clusters qualify as "objects" in our sense. We have shown that not every well-defined cluster of proximal features can be tracked (Scholl, Pylyshyn, and Feldman, 2001). In particular, it appears that certain easily defined *parts* of objects cannot be tracked. Figure 5.8 shows examples where we connected pairs of objects that could easily be tracked. The connections were

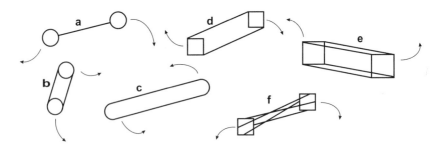

Figure 5.8
Examples of displays in which a target object is paired with a nontarget object by drawing lines indicating connections between them. Objects that had been easy to track by themselves now become difficult when they are shown as parts of other objects, even though they are the same objects and move along the same trajectories. In this set, (c) and (e) are difficult, whereas (a) and (f) are somewhat easier because the parts that have to be tracked are not as integrated into the new objects, despite the fact that (f) involves as many connecting lines between the two squares as does (e). (Adapted from Scholl, Pylyshyn, and Feldman, 2001.)

drawn in various ways, from simple connecting lines to complex connections of various kinds. Some of these lines created perceptually salient and stable new objects, while others created more tenuous new objects. When the connections created salient new objects by merging the original objects, the original objects could not easily be tracked. For example, the endpoints of lines could not be tracked, even though their trajectories were identical to those of dots that were easily tracked. The question of whether the poorer tracking was attributable to the formation of strange elastic objects was addressed recently by Suganuma and Yokosawa (2002), who showed that even if the merged objects were seen as rigid shapes in 3D when viewed stereoscopically, target merging strongly compromised observers' ability to track the individual targets that were merged in this way.

A few of the results we have obtained do seem at first glance to run against the basic assumptions of index theory. One of these will be described to show the sort of methodologies that have been used to investigate this process. We kept finding that as the number of nontarget objects was increased, performance decreased, contrary to the prediction of pure indexing theory (nothing about the nontargets should influence tracking of targets, since tracking is supposed to be determined solely by the indexes that remain attached to individual targets). Chris Sears and I (Sears and Pylyshyn, 2000) reasoned, however, that this decrease in performance might have occurred because as the number of nontargets increased, the chance of mistaking a nontarget for a target and switching to tracking the nontarget would increase. We then devised a method for showing that this was indeed the case. Subjects had to track a number of target figures that moved among a larger set of nontargets. All objects (both targets and nontargets) were shaped like a square 8, and some time during the trial one of the objects changed into either an E or an H. Subjects then had to make a dual response: they had to press one of a pair of buttons indicating that an object had changed into either an E or an H, and they also had to indicate separately whether this change had occurred on a target or a nontarget. As usual, performance on detecting a change on targets was poorer as the number of nontargets increased. But since we had a measure of how often subjects mistook a nontarget for a target, we were able to confirm that the number of switch-over errors increased as the number of nontargets increased, just as we had surmised. Moreover, when we analyzed performance on the objects that observers *said* were targets (whether or not they actually were), performance was *not* affected by changes in the number of nontargets. In other words, if we take into account the increased frequency of erroneously switching to a nearby nontarget, a type of error that went along with there being more nontargets in the display, then tracking was unaffected by the number of nontargets around.

We have also found that when the color or shape of objects changed while they disappeared briefly behind an occluder, not only was tracking unimpaired, but subjects were generally unaware of the changes. When asked, immediately after an object disappeared, what color or shape it had been, subjects' forced-choice responses were at chance. From such studies it appears that objects can be tracked despite the lack of distinctive properties, even when their properties are continuously changing, and despite unpredictable and constantly changing locations. We take the ability to track multiple objects under a wide range of conditions to provide support for the visual-index theory, which hypothesizes a special limited-capacity mechanism for keeping track of individual objects.

The empirical case for the assumptions underlying visual-indexing theory does not rest solely on the multiple-object-tracking procedure. I offer several other experimental demonstrations that support the existence of such a mechanism and the properties we have assumed in table 5.1.

5.3.3 Selecting objects in a search task

Another illustration of some properties of indexes is provided by a series of studies we have performed involving the selection of objects in a visual search task. The search task we used was adapted from one originally introduced by Treisman and Gelade (1980). In the original studies (described briefly on pp. 176–178) Treisman and her colleagues asked subjects to search for a specified (unique) target within an array of nontarget or "distractor" objects. The target in many of these studies (as well as in our variant) was a simple item (such as a short line segment) with several distinctive properties, such as its orientation (/ or \) and color (red or green). Of particular interest was the comparison of two conditions. In one condition, called a single-feature search, the target differed from all distractors in one particular distinguishing property. For example, the target might be the only red object in the display. In another condition, the target differed from the distractors in having a unique combination of two or more different properties. For example, in this condition some distractors had the same color (but different orientation), while others had the same orientation (but different color). The target was defined by the combination of a certain color with a certain orientation (e.g., it was the only green, right-oblique line segment among red right-oblique and green left-oblique segments). This second condition was called a conjunction-feature search, and it proved to be a great deal more difficult. Treisman and her colleagues found that in the single-feature condition, the search slope was very low, that is, the search time increased very little with increasing numbers of distractors. This lead Treisman and Gelade (and many others after them) to refer to the single-feature condition as a "popout," suggesting that the target "pops out" from the set of search objects, rather than having to be serially searched for. In the conjunction-feature condition, by contrast, each item that was added to the array substantially increased the time it took to find the target. This was interpreted as indicating that unique single properties could be detected by a parallel process, whereas pairs of properties had to be searched for serially, item by item. Although the serial-versus-parallel distinction has been subject to a great deal of criticism in recent years, the basic finding that detecting targets that differ from nontargets by a single property shows a different pattern of search than detecting objects that are distinguishable from nontargets by a conjunction of two or more properties remains an important finding, for which various theories have been proposed (see, e.g., Pashler, 1995). From our point of view, the details of the manner in which target items are recognized is not what matters. Rather we are concerned with the way in which the visual system locates items in order to determine their properties. And here we have made use of the interesting difference between searching for single-feature targets and searching for conjunction-feature targets.

In our studies we have used both single-feature and conjunction-feature searches under conditions in which we provided subjects with a way to select a certain subset of items and essentially ignore the items that would ordinarily slow down the search. Visual-indexing theory claims that indexed objects can be accessed directly through the indexes.

Consequently, if a subset of objects was indexed, observers could confine their search to that subset of objects and ignore the rest. The interpretation of these studies in terms of indexes rests on one additional independently verified assumption—that the sudden onset of a primitive object in the visual field elicits indexes. In a series of studies, Jacquie Burkell and I (Burkell and Pylyshyn, 1997) showed that sudden-onset location cues could be used to control searching so that only the precued locations are visited in the course of the search. This is what we would expect if the onset of such cues draws indexes and indexes can be used to determine where to direct focal attention. In these studies (illustrated in figure 5.9) a number of placeholders consisting of Xs (11 in the case illustrated) appeared on the screen and remained there for a period of time (at least one second). Then an additional 3 to 5 placeholders (which

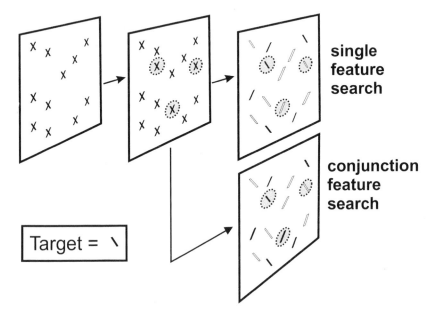

Figure 5.9
Sequence of events in the Burkell and Pylyshyn (1997) subset-selection study. In the first frame the observer sees a set of placeholder Xs for 500 ms. In the second frame, "late onset" placeholders appear for 100 ms, signaling the items that will constitute the search subset. In the last frame all placeholders change to search items, and the subject must try to find the specified target in one of the two conditions. (Adapted from Burkell and Pylyshyn, 1997.)

we refered to as the "late-onset cues") were displayed. After 100 ms one of the segments of each X disappeared and the remaining segment changed color, producing a display of right-oblique and left-oblique lines in either green or red. The entire display had examples of all four combinations of color and orientation, so that the search was technically always a conjunction-search task. The subject's task was to report whether the display contained a prespecified item type (say a right-oblique green line). As expected, the target was detected more rapidly when it had been precued by a late-onset cue, which allowed subjects directly to access those items and ignore the rest. There were, however, two additional findings that are even more relevant to the indexing theory. These depend on whether the precued subset was a single-feature or conjunction-feature search.

As mentioned above, a search of the entire display in these studies would always constitute a conjunction-feature search. However, the subset precued by late-onset cues could be either a single- or conjunction-feature subset. So the critical question is whether the property of the entire display or the property of only the precued *subset* determines the observed search behavior. We found clear evidence that only the property of the subset (whether it constituted a simple-search or conjunction-search task) determined the relation between the number of search items and the reaction time. This provides strong evidence that only the cued subset is being selected as the search set. Notice that the distinction between a single-feature and conjunction-feature search depends on the entire search set, so it must be the case that the entire precued subset is being treated as the search set; the subset effect could not be the result of the items in the subset being visited or in some way processed one by one.

Of particular relevance to the indexing thesis is the additional finding in the Burkell and Pylyshyn (1997) study that when we systematically increased the distance between precued items, there was *no* increase in search time per item, contrary to what one would expect if subset items were being searched for by scanning attention across the display. It seems that the spatial dispersion of the items does not affect the time it takes to examine them, even when the examination appears to be serial (e.g., the time increases linearly as the number of nontargets increases). This is precisely what one would expect if the cued items are indexed and indexes are used to access the items without spatial scanning.

The basic subset result has recently been replicated in a thesis by Elias Cohen using the multiple-object-tracking method to establish indexes, instead of the late-onset method. When all objects in an MOT experiment change into search items and the subject is required to search only among the tracked objects, the same results are found as were found in the Burkell and Pylyshyn experiments. Such studies provide a clear picture of one of the properties of indexes that has not been emphasized in the earlier discussion: indexes provide a *direct access mechanism*, rather like the random-access mechanism found in all modern computers. Once certain elements or primitive visual objects have been indexed, one can make inquiries of them. For each indexed item, one can ask whether it is red or slanted to the right, and so on. Moreover, accessing the items for this purpose does not involve searching the display for a certain property: one can direct an inquiry concerning a certain visual property specifically at a particular item by using the index as one uses a variable or a pointer in a computer-data structure. One can ask "Is item x red?" so long as x is bound to some primitive visual object. Moreover, it appears that one can ask it directly of object x without first searching for an object of a certain type. In other words, one need not search for a target by finding an object having a certain orientation property and then asking whether it has a certain color using a form of question such as, "Is the item that fits the description 'is slanted left and located two-thirds of the way between the fixation cross and the left edge of the screen' colored red?" But this is precisely the sort of process one would have to go through if one could not specify which item one had just found (i.e., one with a particular orientation) except by using a unique description of it.

5.3.4 Inhibition of return

In chapter 4 (pp. 188–189) I described the phenomenon referred to as inhibition of return (IOR), wherein it takes longer for attention to return to an object that had been attended some 500 ms to 900 ms earlier (Klein, 2000). This phenomenon, we saw, was largely object-based: it was not primarily the previously attended location to which attention was slow to return, but the particular previously attended object, which might have moved in the meantime (though location does appear to be relevant as well [Tipper et al., 1994]). But it is also the case that IOR appears to operate simultaneously over several objects, which suggests that it is not the allocation of attention that results in IOR but something more like the indexing of objects. For example, Wright and Richard (1996) showed that as many as four objects can be inhibited at once. Sears (1996) also reported that several loci can be inhibited in an IOR situation and showed that, as in the Burkell et al. findings discussed in the previous section, there was no effect of increasing distance between these loci, which suggests that the effect is both multiple and punctate, just as I argued is the case with visual indexes.

5.3.5 Subitizing

Other studies have shown the power of this framework to account for a large class of empirical phenomena in which simple primitive visual objects are rapidly and preattentively individuated. One of these is the phenomenon called *subitizing* (Jensen, Reese, and Reese, 1950; Kaufman, Lord, Reese, and Volkman, 1949), whereby the numerosity (or cardinality) of sets of fewer than about 4 items can be ascertained rapidly, accurately, and effortlessly.[12] This is a particularly interesting application of indexing theory inasmuch as the determination of the numerosity of a set of items is often taken to be the most elementary signature of what I have been calling *individuation*. In fact, recognizing instances of the same individual is sometimes referred to as recognizing the numerical identity of the two instances (the English words "recognize" and "identity" do not distinguish between the sense in which one

12. Some writers have quarreled with the claim that subitizing and counting involve different processes. For example, Cordes, et al. (2001) have argued that an analysis of error variance shows that the enumeration of both large and small numbers exhibits a constant coefficient of variation (ratio of variance to magnitude), which is a signature of analog-based noise and therefore suggestive of analog processing. I do not make claims here about how the enumeration is carried out (whether by serial counting or by incrementing an analog accumulator) or how the resulting magnitudes are represented. My principal claim—and the one to which the experiments described here are directed—is that a prerequisite for enumeration is a stage of preattentive individuation and access, which is what visual indexes are meant to provide, and which appears be limited to four or five individuals.

might recognize some x as being another instance of a particular individual, as opposed to recognizing x as some known object). It has been known that enumerating sets of 4 or fewer items takes about 60 ms per item (we call this the *subitizing slope*). Above this number the enumeration rate goes up to 100 to 200 ms per item (we call this the *counting slope*).[13] The question of why the slopes should be different has been the subject of speculation, and various alternative explanations have been offered (see the review in Trick and Pylyshyn, 1994b). Subitizing clearly involves both individuating items and enumerating them so as to judge their numerosity. Judging the numerosity of a set of items appears to be a serial process involving visiting each item. But what about the individuation stage? Sagi and Julesz (1984) showed that the shallow subitizing slope of about 60 ms per item is itself not due to the process of individuating items but to the subsequent enumeration process. They demonstrated this by showing that the slope is essentially zero when the task is to judge which of two displays (of size 2 versus 3 or 3 versus 4 items) is more numerous. This is not true outside the subitizing range, where the numerosity of the set does matter a great deal. But if the slope is due to the "counting" process, why is the slope larger for sets of more than 4 items? Our surmise is that in the small (subitizing) sets, the items are individuated preattentively and in parallel by the indexing mechanism. The enumeration can then be achieved without scanning and searching for the items and enumerating them in the process. By hypothesis, the indexes provide a mechanism for direct access to the items (and indeed, it may be possible to enumerate the active indexes themselves). But if there are more than 4 or so items in the display, they cannot all be indexed, so they must be located one at a time and their number determined by some process—perhaps by estimating, or perhaps (as Mandler and Shebo, 1982, have suggested) by segregating the elements into smaller groups and then subitized and adding the results. Thus we

13. The transition between the two parts of the curve was determined by analyzing linear and quadratic components of the pattern of increasing reaction time with increasing number of objects n to be enumerated. Items that are subitized undergo a change at some value of n when the quadratic component of the trend becomes significant. This is taken to be the subitizing point (see Trick and Pylyshyn, 1994b). For sets that are not subitized there is no value of n at which the curve first attains a significant quadratic trend (in most cases the quadratic trend is significant for all $n \geq 3$).

hypothesized that indexes would play the decisive role in enumerating items in the subitizing range. Our analysis of the data yielded strong evidence for this view. The following two findings are particularly relevant.

Subitizing does not occur when preattentive individuation is prevented We have shown that when feature clusters are not automatically individuated and indexed by the early-vision system, no subitizing occurs (Trick and Pylyshyn, 1993; Trick and Pylyshyn, 1994a, 1994b). If, for example, targets are defined by conjunctions of features (which, we have seen, means that to identify them, one has to focus attention on them one at a time), there is no special subitizing slope—the enumeration slope is continuous (and high) throughout the range of numerosities. Similarly, if items to be enumerated are defined by a property known to require focal attention for its detection, then no subitizing is observed. One example of this, discussed in chapter 4, is the enumeration of figures that are arranged concentrically (as opposed to being located side by side). Concentric squares (illustrated in figures 4.5 and 5.10) cannot be subitized, presumably because we cannot individuate them as individual whole figures without tracing their boundaries.

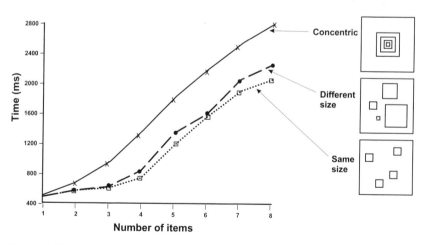

Figure 5.10
A graph of reaction time versus number of items enumerated, for several conditions examined by Trick and Pylshyn (1994b). Concentric squares do not show the characteristic "knee" in the curve that is the signature of subitizing, whereas the same squares placed so they can be automatically individuated do show subitizing. (Adapted from Trick and Pylyshyn, 1994b.)

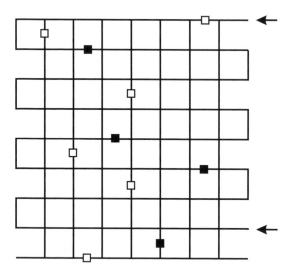

Figure 5.11
An example of a display in which observers had to enumerate either all black dots or all dots lying on the same contour. Only the former can be preattentively individuated and so only they exhibit subitizing. (Adapted from Trick and Pylyshyn, 1993.)

A related condition that we examined is the task of enumerating all items lying on a particular contour (as shown in figure 5.11). This condition does not allow subitizing, since evaluating the property "on the same contour" requires serial scanning (as Jolicoeur, Ullman, and MacKay, 1983, showed). Similarly, subitizing does not occur when items appear gradually (Wright and Richard, 1995), presumably because the gradual appearance of objects does not capture visual indexes.

The spatial layout of a display is unimportant in subitizing We have shown that varying the spatial distribution of objects in a display or even precuing the locations of objects (with either valid or invalid location cues) is relatively unimportant in the subitizing range but critical in the counting ($n > 4$) range (Trick and Pylyshyn, 1994b). These findings are consistent with visual-indexing theory, which claims that the cardinality of the indexed subset can be determined by counting the objects that were indexed, *without* having to spatially scan focal attention over the display (since indexes makes it possible for objects to be accessed directly without search), or even by counting just the number of active indexes. In either case, indexing eliminates the need to search a display for the items to be enumerated and therefore renders location cuing less useful.

These studies show that a preattentive stage of item individuation is critical for subitizing. Such a stage is postulated by the present theory for entirely independent reasons. Simon and Vaishnavi (1996) have argued that this individuation stage is responsible for the limitation in the number of objects that can be subitized. Using an afterimage display, they showed that even when indefinite time is available for counting, the subitizing limit remains. They take this as supporting the contention that it is not the task of counting that is the source of limitation, but the ability to individuate items.[14]

Note that *counting* has been used as a paradigm example of why concepts are needed to pick out individuals. To count things, one must first specify what *sorts of things* are to count as separate and distinct things. So, for example, one cannot say how *many* there are in the room without stipulating conceptual categories by using terms, called *sortals*—such as "furniture," "lamps," "people," and so on—that specify countable things (as opposed, say, to things that are designated by mass nouns like "water," "air," "wind," "talk," or by adjectives like "green" or "big"). How is it possible, then, to count or subitize without the top-down involvement of the conceptual system? If my interpretation of the subitizing studies is correct, it is possible to count active indexes without specifying *what they index*. On the other hand, this does presuppose that one intends to count indexes rather than thoughts or some other mental

14. A question has recently been raised as to whether the limit on the number of objects that could be enumerated from after-images in the Simon and Vaishnavi (1996) study might be due to the eccentricity of the targets being counted. Intriligator (1997) found that "attentional resolution" or the ability to individuate items (which is distinct from the ability to discriminate them) falls off with retinal eccentricity, suggesting that this in itself may account for the Simon and Vaishnavi finding. While this may be true, it can't be the whole story, since allowing eye movements in subitizing does not improve counting accuracy in general, except where it helps to group haphazardly arranged items (Kowler and Steinman, 1977). Moreover, even if the particular numerical limit reached in the Simon and Vaishnavi study resulted from loss of attentional resolution further from the fovea, it still remains true that the limit was indeed due to the *individuation* stage of the process, since attentional resolution is measured in terms of the ability to individuate objects.

particulars. So at that level, sortal concepts *are* involved in counting, just as descriptivist theories suppose. But the conceptual system is not involved earlier in specifying the individuals that elicited indexes. Of course, in cases where one counts something other than primitively indexed objects, we *do* need a concept or sortal to pick out such individuals. For example, in the studies reported in Trick and Pylyshyn, 1994b, there were conditions in which observers were asked to count objects that had certain properties. In those cases, a conceptual selection was presupposed. In fact, it is even presupposed in some of the popout cases, as when one is asked to count Xs in a field of Os or red things in a field of green things. Counting and search may invariably involve a conceptual aspect in a way that tracking may not.

In this section I have presented several types of empirical evidence supporting the view that there are mechanisms in early (preconceptual) vision that pick out individual primitive objects in a way that depends only on the structure of the early vision system and not on what the organism knows or believes. I have also shown that this mechanism (called a *visual index* or *FINST*) is capable of independently picking out several (around 4 or 5) such objects and of keeping track of them when they move around independently in unpredictable ways. There is more that can be said about the properties of this mechanism (and some of this has been presented in various publications, e.g., Pylyshyn, 1998; Pylyshyn et al., 1994). The foregoing provides some of the basic empirically motivated reasons for the postulated visual-indexing mechanism, and thus supports my claims about the relation between mental representations derived from visual perception and the world we perceive. I now turn to the more general issue of why we need such a link.

5.4 Why Do We Need a Special Connection between Vision and the World?

The notion of a visual index, introduced in the last section in the context of certain phenomena of visual attention, has much broader implications beyond clarifying the nature of visual attention and showing the existence of a preattentive stage of item individuation and access. It helps us to understand how visual perception connects with *particular individual things in the world*. This may at first seem like a function already entailed by the very idea of vision. After all, is not vision itself what connects us with the perceived world? Of course this is true, but the usual kinds of theories of world–mind connection are incomplete and inadequate for many purposes. For example, the usual view of vision is that it is a process that constructs a representation of the perceived world. We have already seen that there is some argument about the nature of this representation, and indeed, whether there is a single representation or many. Some feel that the early representation is picturelike, with the picture being laid out spatially, say in the primary visual cortex. Marr's "primal sketch" is, in part, such a representation, though it is augmented with tags that provide symbolic information concerning the depth and orientation of surfaces, as well as information about how certain local features are grouped to form clusters. Others feel that the evidence favors the view that the output of the early-vision system is a symbolic representation that is more languagelike in that it uses a descriptive vocabulary of varying abstractness and, by the time it presents information to the cognitive system, it no longer maps world space onto brain space (or some analogue surrogate) in the representational system. I discussed some of the arguments in chapter 1, and I will have more to say about these issues in chapter 7.

Whatever the ultimate verdict on the nature of visual representation, there remains the question of how the system captures the fact that certain parts of its representation of a scene correspond to certain particular parts of the perceived world. If you take the descriptivist view, you need a way to specify which particular token individual in the world corresponds to a particular symbol or expression in the description. If you take the pictorialist view, you need a way to specify which part of the mental picture corresponds to which part of the world. Even if the mapping were one-one and the mental picture preserved *all* the visible 3D details of the scene, which we know cannot be the case, for both information-theoretic and empirical reasons (see O'Regan, 1992; O'Regan, Deubel, Clark, and Rensink, 2000; Rensink, O'Regan, and Clark, 1997; Simons, 1996), you still need a way to specify that *this* bit of the representation corresponds to *that* bit of the world.[15] Such a mapping of correspondences is essential if the visual process is to make connections among representations of objects in successive glances across saccades and successive elaborations of the representation over time. Such a correspondence matching is also necessary if vision is to make connections with the motor system in order to carry out such actions as moving one's eyes or one's hand to reach and grasp a particular individual (token) object. The motor system cannot individuate objects by virtue of their unique description; it has to have some more direct reference to them. The option of specifying an object by its allocentric coordinates is discussed on pages 179–181, 219–223, and elsewhere.[16]

15. It's not enough to say that this bit of a pictorial representation *looks like* that part of the world, since the latter formulation ("that part of the world") is not available to a visual system that has only pictorial representations (or, for that matter, descriptive representations). The correspondence of part of a picture to part of the world also cannot be carried out by something like template matching since a visual representation is too abstract and ambiguous for that, as Locke noted over 300 years ago. Moreover, templates do not distinguish tokens from types so they do not provide a solution to the problem of matching a particular individual, which has been our main concern.

16. There are at least two ways to deal with the problem of how to command the motor system to carry out some action on a particular visible object, both of which have been adopted by robot designers and neither of which is an empirically valid model of the human visual-motor system. One way relies on error-driven control and requires that the visual system detect both the object and the limb (or whatever is being moved) and then issue a command to move the latter in such a way as to decrease the distance between them (which means that the visual system at least needs to encode relative distances along some monotonic scale that is calibrated against the motor system). But much visual-motor action has a ballistic component which does not use feed back but proceeds automatically once initiated. Also this method cannot account for the multiple-object tracking results described earlier. The other way to deal with the gap between vision and motor control is to include numerical coordinates among the descriptors generated by the visual system. An encoding of proximal location, together with an encoding of the orientation of eyes, head and body in an allocentric (global) frame of reference makes it possible to compute the 3D location of an object in space, calibrated in relation to the organism (or robot). In this way the motor system can be told where to move a limb in terms of world coordinates. However, this option assumes the availability of a complete metrical model of 3D space, which is accessible to the motor system as well as the visual system, and which specifies the location of all relevant objects, including the organism itself. This is an option that we discounted on empirical grounds in chapter 1 and which roboticists have also found to be inadequate (see the discussion in connection with figure 5.13).

What I call a "pure description" view has been the standard form of representation in both artificial intelligence and cognitive science. A pure description is roughly one that uses only a structured arrangement of codes for properties and relations (technically, only predicates and variables bound by quantifiers) in describing a visual scene (for technical details, see note 17, p. 249). Roughly, such representations refer to objects by providing conditions of satisfaction (i.e., description R refers to object O because the description is *satisfied* by O, or is true of O). Such representations might say such things as "There is a unique object that has properties P_1, P_2, P_3, . . ." or "The object that has properties P_i bears the relationship R to the object that has properties P_j," and so on. The important thing is that objects are picked out by definite descriptions. (Sometimes, in computational models, objects may be referred to by *names* such as *Object-5*, as illustrated in figure 5.13. Such names are generally not true proper names, whose reference remains rigidly fixed regardless of context, but only abbreviations for a description.) Pure descriptive representations do not use deictic terms such as "I" or "you" or "now" or "this" or "here," which can be understood (which succeed in *referring*) only in the context in which they are asserted.

Despite the widespread use of descriptive representations, this form of representation will not do in general for a number of reasons. In what follows, I will concentrate primarily on one empirical reason, based on the fact that visual representations must be built up over a series of glances or over a series of what might be called *noticings*, which raises the problem of establishing correspondences between objects at

---

In the absence of such an internalization of the world we are back where we started, because the problem of uniquely picking out individuals reduces to the problem of uniquely picking out particular places in the representation. But even if this way of picking out individuals were possible, it would not eliminate the need for demonstratives or indexes. Even if we have the coordinates of a particular object, there remains the question of whether the object we pick out in this way is a particular individual object we are seeing (i.e., *this* object). We need such a fine grain of individuation because wanting to pick up a particular object is different from wanting to pick up the object at a particular location. Because our intention can include the goal of picking up *that particular thing* we must have a way to represent such an intention. This is why we not only need indexes but have to be able to bind the indexes in two modalities—visual and proprioceptive (a problem on which I speculated in the original expository paper, Pylyshyn, 1989).

different times or in different views. This correspondence problem is one of several reasons for the inadequacy of the "pure description" view. Later I will briefly mention other reasons why the pure-description view will not work, and I will introduce some more general arguments why we need to augment the types of referential terms to include visual indexes, which in many ways work like demonstrative terms such as "this" or "that." This augmentation is needed to meet some important requirements on visual representations, especially when they are used to guide actions.

Consider first the argument from incremental construction of visual representations. It is clear that visual representations are built up over time. There are many reasons for this, some of them empirical and some conceptual. For example, on pages 146–150, I examined some empirical evidence for the articulation of the visual process over time. Also, as we saw in chapter 4, the capacity of the visual system is limited, and this requires allocating attention and consequently leads to a serial component in visual processing. Tsotsos (1988) has argued from a computational, as well as neuroscientific, perspective that the function of serial allocation of attention is to ameliorate the computational complexity of vision. Indeed, Ullman (1984) has made a case that, even if there were no resource limitations in visual information processing, certain visual properties, by their very nature, could only be decided in a serial fashion using what he calls "visual routines."

Another important reason why visual representations must be built up incrementally is the fact that the eye, through which all visual information must initially pass, has a highly limited spatial bound and requires frequent eye movements to build up a percept. In chapter 1 we saw that a superposition explanation of the saccadic integration process runs seriously afoul of the empirical data. Yet anything else raises the question of how information from one glance is integrated with information from a successive glance. Some people have proposed what amounts to a "descriptivist" mechanism for establishing correspondences across glances. For example, Currie, McConkie, and Carlson-Radvansky (2000); Irwin, McConkie, Carlson-Radvansky, and Currie (1994); and McConkie and Currie (1996) have suggested that on each fixation the properties of one significant benchmark (the saccade target) are encoded and on the next fixation those encoded properties are used to locate the benchmark through a fast search. The location of the reidentified benchmark is then used to calibrate the location in space of other items in that fixation. However, this relocation-by-description idea seems implausible for a number of reasons, even if the relocation could be accomplished in the short time available. One reason is that it ought to lead to frequent and significant errors (and failures of visual stability) when the scene is uniformly textured or otherwise free of unique features. Another is that for information from a pair of benchmark objects (in two successive fixations) to calibrate locations of the other items, the observer would have to establish a metrical mapping between real 2D inner displays—a view that we have already seen runs contrary to a great deal of evidence (and which the authors of the benchmark proposal themselves eschew).

The need to build up visual representations incrementally over time brings with it the problem of establishing a correspondence between individuals in successive representations (or glances) of the visual world. Can this correspondence be established within a purely descriptive visual representation? Can we provide a description rich enough to allow correspondences to be established? Sometimes there is a unique description in a certain setting (e.g., "the object in the bottom left of the visual field" or "the only red object in the room"). But a description that uniquely picks out a particular individual would typically have to be changing as the object changes or moves, or else the description would have to include temporal properties (it would have to be tensed or time-stamped), which would mean that it picked out the entire temporal history of the individual (a "space-time worm"). Also, a unique description is often not available to the cognitive system (e.g., allocentric coordinates of objects in a distal scene, or even of their projections on the retina). Even if it were possible to provide a unique description of parts of a scene, based on the immediate proximal input, there would still remain the problem of computing a mapping from this representation to the global representation being constructed. Because objects have a hierarchical part-whole structure, such descriptions are typically complex treelike structures. As a result, the mapping problem is itself generally computationally intractable (it is technically what is known as an NP-complete problem, whose complexity increases exponentially with increasing size of the description). And finally, even if all such technical problems were solved, one would still be left without a critical link that determines which individual in the visual world is the one referred to in a description. That's because a uniquely specifying description is different from a direct causal connection, in ways that I will try to explain later.

In addition to the considerations above, there are a number of empirical reasons to believe that human vision does not work solely in terms of visual descriptions. A critical case arises when a visual representation is constructed incrementally. Suppose that we have a representation of some scene and then we *notice* a new property Q of some object in it (even if we assume no intervening eye movement). To integrate information from the new visual episode with past information, we must incrementally add this newly noticed information to our visual representation. Now we have the following problem: to which object in memory do we attribute the new property Q? When we detect the new property Q, we detect it as the property of *a particular object x*—we do not detect it as occurring on some object that happens to also have property P. In other words, our property detector says something like "Red at object x," and not "Red on object-with-shape-S." But, according to the pure-description view, our memory representation individuates objects only by their properties (by their descriptions). If we are to increment our visual representation by adding to this description, then when we notice that a new property Q holds of a certain object, we need to locate the representation of that object in our evolving visual representation in order to add to it the fact that we now know it has property Q. In other words, we would have to do something like the following. First, we would have to find a unique descriptor of the object in question that does not involve the new property Q. Let's say that this unique descriptor is P. Then we would look for an object in memory that is represented as having property P. Assuming that this retrieves a unique object and that it is the same object that we now noticed to have property Q, we would replace the previous description with the new augmented description that includes both the original property P and the new property Q. This assumes, of course, that the currently unique descriptor P was the one associated with the object in a previous episode, which is in general not true—especially for properties, like location, that change frequently. (If the representation were encoded in predicate logic, we would also have to make sure that property P and property Q are represented as occurring on the same object. The way to specify that two properties hold of the same object is to introduce an identity statement asserting that the object of which P holds and that of which Q holds are the same object.)

If we succeeded in going through this process, we would have augmented our representation of a certain object to include the newly noticed property. Now if a further property R of the same object is detected at some later time, we would have to go through this process all over again: the newly augmented descriptor would have to be inferred from the current properties of the object in question and used to retrieve the object, which would then be augmented (or modified) to include the newly noticed property R, and so on.[17] We can easily show that this could not be the process by which correspondence is established in the incremental computation of a visual representation, or by which the correspondence between object representations at different times is solved, at least in certain situations. For example, in the case of the multiple-object-tracking task, we showed that even if the visual system had an encoding

17. Here is a somewhat more technical way to put what I have been saying. A "pure description" can be understood in relation to descriptive statements in predicate logic in which all variables are bound by quantifiers. Thus an assertion that says an object has property P can be represented as the first-order logic expression $\exists x P(x)$. (Actually, if the description is to specify that P picks out a unique object it would have to be $\exists x[P(x) \land \forall(y)(P(y) \supset (x = y)]$.) This description does not say *which* object has property P. It is up to the visual system to find and pick it out if something further is to be made of it. If we augmented our visual representation by adding clauses to a pure description, for example when we notice that some additional property Q holds of a certain object, we would have to do something like the following. First we would have to find a unique description by which the object in question might have been encoded earlier, say, the complex one given above. Then, on the assumption that the earlier description applies to the object now noticed to have Q, we would conjoin the stored description with the new property Q, resulting in the augmented description $\exists x[P(x) \land \forall(y)(P(y) \supset x = y) \land Q(x)]$. (Inclusion of the equality in this expression would be justified if we found the descriptor $\exists x P(x)$ stored with the object that was noticed to have Q, thus suggesting that it was the same object—so far as the visual system was concerned—and therefore we would state this equality explicitly.) If a further property, R, of the same object is detected at some later time, this new augmented descriptor would have to be retrieved and checked against the current properties of the object newly noticed to have R. If it matches, then the description would be updated again, resulting in the new description $\exists x\{P(x) \land Q(x) \land \forall(y)(P(y) \land Q(y) \supset x = y) \land R(x)\}$. Clearly this is a grotesque way to incrementally construct visual representations, especially since we have no plausible way in general to decide on the description under which the same object had been stored earlier.

of location on the screen for each of the objects being tracked, it could not update locations fast enough (given what we know about the speed of attention scanning) to enable 4 objects to be tracked under the circumstances involved in these experiments (see section 5.2.1, and Pylyshyn and Storm, 1988).

Notice that if we had a direct way to refer to token individuals, as well as a way to tell whether a particular token individual was the one being referred to, we would not run into the problem of locating and updating (momentarily unique) descriptions of objects; we would simply assert that a *particular* object, say the one referred to as x_i, had certain properties, and when we found out it had additional properties, we would add those to the representation of that individual. Of course, in that case we would need to be able to detect that a particular object that just came into view was in fact object x_i and not some other object. This, in general, is a problem that may involve all the faculties of the cognitive system. However, so long as the object remains in view (but see note 20) and so long as the visual architecture has certain properties (such as those I discussed in connection with the theory of visual indexes), a major subset of this problem may be solvable. This is exactly what visual indexes are for. They are there to enable vision to refer to particular token things, as illustrated in figure 5.12.

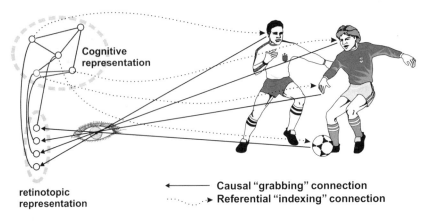

Figure 5.12
Schematic illustration of how visual representations maintain a causal connection to particular token objects in the visual scene.

5.4.1   Essential demonstratives

The problem of updating representations (and of solving the correspondence problem for individual objects over time) is actually much deeper, and indexes or visual demonstratives are needed for more fundamental reasons than this story suggests. Despite my provisional assumption that we might be able to identify token items in a scene by providing a unique description, there is in fact a gap in that story that I glossed over. Think of the visual system as sending messages to the cognitive system and vice versa (a somewhat simplified story that is close enough for our purposes). Suppose that the visual system sends the message "There is an object with properties P and Q in the scene." Now suppose that the cognitive system decides to do something that involves the object in question. If the action is a visual inquiry, it can send the following query to the visual system: "Does the object with properties P and Q also have property R?" But notice that vision and cognition have different sorts of access to the object. Although in principle the visual component has access to *which* object is being referred to (it evaluated the predicates $P(x)$ and $Q(x)$ for a particular x), the cognitive component can refer to the object only by the description provided by vision, so it is only the visual system that can pick out or identify the *particular* object token in question. A consequence of the modularity of vision is that the information flow between vision and cognition is restricted in certain ways—in this case we are assuming that vision did not deliver a direct way of specifying x, such as a proper name of object x. This is why there is a problem about whether objects described in two separate views are the same object. Establishing a correspondence between two descriptions requires making a cross-system judgment: it requires establishing whether an object described as having properties P and Q in one description is the very same object described as having properties P and R in another description. If the visual system could locate objects corresponding to both descriptions in its field of view, it could see whether they were the same, because it could see that there is only one object token despite there being two distinct descriptions. But the cognitive system does not itself enjoy this capability; all it knows (according to the "pure description" view) is that it has two distinct representations. This dilemma leaves the cognitive system unable to refer to particular object tokens, and therefore to take actions toward a particular object token. It cannot, for example, decide to *reach* for a particular object, since, according to the pure-description view, particular object *tokens* are not part of the representational repertoire of the cognitive system (or, for that matter, of the motor system) in the sense that in the descriptive view the cognitive system can't represent a particular individual object *qua individual*, that is, irrespective of its properties. The cognitive and motor systems can only represent facts about *some* object with certain properties, not about a particular object token (understood transparently, i.e., *that* object). Another way to put this is that the visual system and the cognitive system use different vocabularies. Only the visual system can pick out individual objects by their descriptions, and it cannot pass this selection to the motor system using visual descriptors.

We often pick out particular unique individuals when we use linguistic descriptions by using demonstrative terms such as *this* or *that* (or sometimes by giving the individuals distinct names). Note that this way of picking out individuals requires a mechanism over and above the apparatus of pure description. It is not equivalent to individuating objects by their properties, including their locations. Whether or not picking out objects by providing location information (such as their coordinates in some frame of reference) is how our visual system does it is an empirical issue. Some of the evidence I have cited suggests that the human visual system independently detects, and provides access to, what I have called primitive visual objects and then (optionally) encodes some of their properties—including such properties as their color, shape, and location. This does not mean, however, that location plays no role in individuating objects. The theoretical question for us reduces to whether it is possible for visual indexes to point to locations *as such* (i.e., to unfilled places), and that question is not yet settled experimentally, although there is some evidence that the position of an object can persist after the object has disappeared (Krekelberg, 2001), and that at least unitary focal attention may move through the empty space between objects, though perhaps not continuously and not at a voluntarily controlled speed (see note 1 and pp. 340–344).

As a number of philosophers have pointed out (e.g., Perry, 1979), the inadequacy of pure descriptions arises from the fact that a pure description cannot encode certain sorts of beliefs, in particular, beliefs that depend on how and where one is situated in the world (i.e., beliefs that involve deictic references). And it is these beliefs that determine many kinds of actions. A purely descriptive representation does not connect with the world in the right way: there remains a gap between representing the fact that there is something having certain properties and representing the fact that *this very thing* has those properties. Knowing, as a matter of fact, that by extrapolating the pointing stars of the Big Dipper, one can locate the North Star is not the same as knowing that extrapolating from *this* star and *that* star (or from stars named *Merak* and *Dubhe*) will locate the North Star.[18] Only the latter belief will lead you to take certain actions when you are lost. You must at some stage have a representation that connects, in this epistemically direct way, with the token objects on which actions must be based. John Perry gives the following example of how the decision to take a particular course of action can arise from the realization that a particular object in a description and a particular thing one sees are one and the same thing.

18. We could also refer to individuals by using proper names (as I just did) since proper names also refer directly (at least according to certain views). There is a question whether visual indexes are more like demonstratives or more like proper names. The reference of deictic terms such as demonstratives is relativized to the context of utterance. So indexes are like demonstratives insofar as they have a computable reference only in a particular context, i.e., the one in which the referents remain available to perception (although, as we have seen, because of the exigencies of the visual system, this can also include relatively brief periods of time when the objects are actually occluded). On the other hand, we also need indexes to designate objects so that we can determine their correspondence across views. Even if the objects remain continuously in view, if indexes are a type of demonstrative, there is a point when we need to conclude that *this* object is the same as *that* object. Different views are different deictic contexts, so if the index *is viewed as a demonstrative* it initially has a different referent in the two views and the identity of these two referents has to be independently computed. This is the correspondence problem discussed earlier. Names refer to individual objects so they don't have this problem. However, they differ from indexes in that they continue to refer even when the objects are not in view, in fact long after the objects are gone (names are forever). Clearly, visual indexes are not exactly like either demonstratives or names. It's an open question whether it is better to say that indexes refer all the time but their referents are computable only when the objects are in view, or to say that, like demonstratives, what they refer to is relative to the context of utterance. It depends on whether you are more interested in how their semantics turns out or in how they are computed and how they function. (I thank Jerry Fodor and Chris Peacocke for sharing with me their useful—though opposite—views on this question.)

The author of the book *Hiker's Guide to the Desolation Wilderness* stands in the wilderness beside Gilmore Lake, looking at the Mt. Tallac trail as it leaves the lake and climbs the mountain. He desires to leave the wilderness. He believes that the best way out from Gilmore Lake is to follow the Mt. Tallac trail up the mountain. . . . But he doesn't move. He is lost. He is not sure whether he is standing beside Gilmore Lake, looking at Mt. Tallac, or beside Clyde Lake, looking at the Maggie peaks. Then he begins to move along the Mt. Tallac trail. If asked, he would have to explain the crucial change in his beliefs in this way: "I came to believe that *this* is the Mt. Tallac trail and *that* is Gilmore Lake." (Perry, 1979, p. 4)

The point of this example is that to understand and explain the action of the lost author, it is essential to use a direct reference to pick out particulars. This can be done in language using demonstratives, such as "this" and "that." Without a way to *directly* pick out the referent of a descriptive term and to link the perceived object token to its cognitive representation, we would not be able to explain the person's actions. The same applies to incrementally creating visual descriptions of the sort I have been discussing. Unless at some point one can think the equivalent of "*This* has property *P*," one cannot refer to a particular object token in a way that will allow it to be bound to the arguments of a visual predicate or to serve as the basis for action (e.g., to point toward or grasp the token object in question). But what I have called a "pure description" does not allow us to do that.

What all this means is that the cognitive representation of a visual scene must contain something more than descriptive information in order that it may refer to individual visual objects. What is needed is a device for ensuring that we can find correspondences between parts of an evolving visual representation and token visual objects—as we could if we could label individual objects in the world. What we need is what natural language provides in part when it uses names (or labels) that uniquely pick out particular individuals, or when it embraces demonstratives, terms like "this" or "that." With such a mechanism we can refer to particular individuals, and in so doing, we can elaborate descriptions while ensuring that we continue to describe the *same thing*. And we can also keep track of a particular individual object, as the same object, even while it changes its properties and moves in an unpredictable way. This latter requirement should now make it clear that the function we need is precisely what was postulated in the theory of visual indexes.

According to the theory, visual indexes realize the equivalent of a direct reference, much like a demonstrative, within the visual system.

Apart from being able to refer to particular individual objects as such, another advantage of having a mechanism like a visual index is that it makes it possible to use a particular efficient strategy (which Ballard et al., 1997, have dubbed a "deictic strategy") in dealing with the visual world. In the deictic strategy people encode only those aspects of the visual scene that are relevant to a particular task, and they rely on a deictic reference mechanism for getting back to encode more as the need arises. We saw earlier that the rich panorama of perceptual detail that we feel we have access to in vision is not only illusory, but also unnecessary, since the world we are observing is there before us to examine and reexamine as we need. There is considerable evidence (some of it sketched in chapter 1) to suggest that the visual system makes use of this fact by not encoding a rich and informationally dense panorama. Rather, it records those aspects that are relevant to some task at hand, whether solving a problem or merely pursuing some theme for its own intrinsic interest.

Take, for example, the study by Ballard et al. (1997). They showed that when subjects carry out a task of reproducing a pattern of colored blocks by using a supply of additional blocks provided for the task, they appear to memorize very little of the target pattern on each glance, relying instead on their ability to move their eyes back to reexamine the source pattern. They appear to encode only something like the relative position or color of one or two blocks—far less than they could recall in short-term memory. Instead of memorizing the pattern, they keep glancing back at it, picking up bits of information each time. Such a deictic strategy is a useful one if making an eye movement is less costly by some measure than encoding and recalling several items of information. Such a strategy is feasible, however, only if there is some easy way to keep track of *where* (in the sense of "at which object") the relevant information is, without actually recording the details of what the information is at that object. This, in turn, implies a mechanism like a visual index. In fact, it suggests that we have several such indexes (around 4 or 5), just as do the multiple-object-tracking experiments discussed earlier. What would not make sense is to recall where the relevant visual information was by storing a unique description of the object in question. That would nullify the point of the deictic strategy. Since there is already considerable evidence for the existence of multiple indexes in the visual system, the deictic strategy makes a great deal of sense.

5.4.2 Situated vision for robots

In the field of artificial intelligence and robotics there has been a growing interest in the use of strategies such as the deictic strategy discussed by Ballard et al. Some of this interest developed among investigators interested in showing that cognition is "situated"—a term used to emphasize the role played by environmental information in cognitive activity (some proponents of the "situated" camp even maintain that no representations of any sort are needed to guide robots [Brooks, 1991], a thesis I believe is demonstrably false even though it contains an important insight). The basic idea that the real environment provides an important basis for thinking and planning has been widely explored. For example, Simon (1975) describes a variety of strategies for solving the "Towers of Hanoi" problem, one of which, often adopted by people solving this problem, relies on the visible positions of disks on pegs for keeping track of the current state of problem solving, instead of relying on memory.[19] The same is true of more mundane problems like addition or subtraction.

19. The Towers of Hanoi problem is attributed to Edouard Lucas, who in 1883 published it in a four-volume work on mathematical recreations under the name of M. Claus (an anagram of Lucas). But the problem has also been associated with an ancient legend. Douglas Hofstadter's *Metamagical Themes* column in *Scientific American* (March 1983, pp. 16–22) describes the legend colorfully as follows:

In the great temple of Brahma in Benares, on a brass plate under the dome that marks the center of the world, there are 64 disks of pure gold that the priests carry one at a time between these diamond needles according to Brahma's immutable law: No disk may be placed on a smaller disk. In the beginning of the world all 64 disks formed the Tower of Brahma on one needle. . . . When the last disk is finally in place, once again forming the Tower of Brahma but on a different needle, then will come the end of the world and all will turn to dust.

The problem has fascinated mathematicians and computer scientists and is frequently used as a class exercise to illustrate recursive programming. Various versions of this problem have been used to study human problem solving, where a typical starting configuration has only five or so disks located on an initial peg. The tricky part is to move the disks from the first peg to the third peg, using the second peg for temporary storage, without at any time placing a larger disk on top of a smaller one.

VanLehn and Ball (1991) show that in solving simple arithmetic problems, subjects do much of their planning and keeping track of their subgoals by relying on the numerical display itself. Van Lehn and Ball claim that accounts of human problem solving overemphasize planning and plan-following to the exclusion of what they call the externalized or situated nature of memory, and especially of goal memory. They claim that much of human behavior is "situated" rather than "planned," where the latter refers primarily to formal "planning systems" that were developed in the field of artificial intelligence in the 1970s, systems that generated completely specified plans in advance of their execution as series of steps to be carried out to achieve some goal (see, e.g., Georgeff, 1987). This idea of formal plan-generation has come under criticism in a number of quarters as relying too little on information in the environment. Alternative approaches such as "reactive planning" have been proposed (Kabanza, Barbeau, and St-Denis, 1997) and have led to the study of what is referred to as "situated actions" (Suchman, 1987). These ideas are very much in the spirit of the visual-index theory inasmuch as indexing is a mechanism by which representations in memory can be integrated with information in the visual environment (as I argued in Pylyshyn, 2001b).

There has been considerable interest in the idea that a better way to describe the world for a robot might be in deictic terms, that is, in terms that make essential reference to such contextual concepts as "myself," "here," "now," "this," "that," and so on, whose referents are indeterminate outside of the specific occasion of their use. Although artificial intelligence researchers rarely talk in these terms (for a notable exception, see Lespérance and Levesque, 1995), the spirit of this approach can be seen in what is sometimes called "situated vision" or "situated planning." The reasons for favoring such an approach are related to the reasons I have explored for needing visual indexes, and to reasons philosophers have given for needing "essential demonstratives" (discussed in the previous section). The alternative to the use of deictic terms is to describe the world in user-independent or allocentric frames of reference, which is not useful for performing actions on objects in this world, or navigating through it, since a global frame of reference is rarely available to a robot, and if it were it would become obsolete very quickly as either the robot or the objects in the environment (including people and other robots) changed locations.

As I pointed our earlier in this section, a purely descriptive representation is connected to the world by semantic relations: objects in the
world either satisfy or fail to satisfy the description. Consequently, the
only way that a robot can tell whether some particular thing in the world
corresponds to an item in its representation is by checking whether the
description is satisfied by that part of the visual scene. Since, as we saw
earlier, an indefinite number of things in the world could, in principle,
satisfy a particular description, this is always an ambiguous connection.
Moreover, the matching process itself can be computationally intractable
(matching descriptions is in general an exponentially complex, or what
is technically known as an "NP-complete" problem). Even in a benign
world where everything remained in place except the robot, and in which
the robot's position in a global frame of reference was always known,
operating successfully in such a world would depend entirely on keeping
the global model in precise correspondence with the world at all times.
That's because the robot would in fact be making all decisions based on
its global model and only indirectly on the perceived world. If the relevant part of the world was dynamic and the robot had to rely on visual
perception to find its way around, then the problem of updating its model
would become extremely complex. One solution to this dilemma is to
provide the equivalent of deictic references or indexes to certain objects,
locations, or properties in the scene and to allow the robot to reason
using deictic terms, as suggested by Lespérance and Levesque (1995).

The different forms of representation that a robot could have are illustrated in figure 5.13. A representation such as the one labeled (2) is inherently better for a mobile robot than the descriptive model labeled (1).
The literal alternative labeled (3) is either a version of (1) or is the totally
impractical proposal that the robot have a small version of the room in
its memory. (I will return to that class of proposals when I discuss mental
imagery and mental models in chapters 6 to 8.) The pointers in the representation labeled (2) might be implemented in various ways that need
not concern us here, since they need not have any psychological import.
But just in case the reader is wondering whether something miraculous
is being proposed, consider that an obvious implementation might be to
use direction of gaze as the main pointer and to provide a way for the
robot to direct its gaze to where the other pointers indicate, thus making
use of direction of gaze to realize several pointers. In any case there are
many technical ways of providing a functional equivalent of having

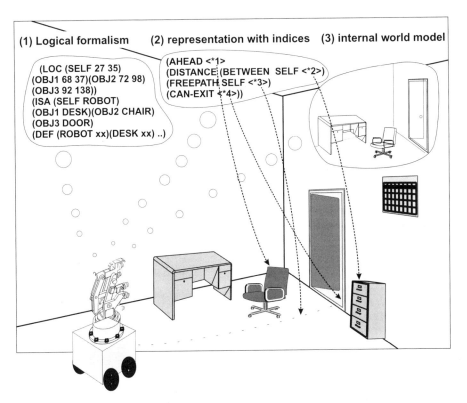

Figure 5.13
Illustration of several possible ways for a robot to represent a room. The middle form, which uses indexical pointers like the FINST visual indexes discussed in the text, is not only more efficient, but is also necessary for the robot to navigate without first identifying objects and encoding their locations in an allocentric coordinate system. (From Pylyshyn, 2000.)

several pointers. Any technique that allows either the direction of gaze or a locus of visual attention to be moved to a particular object without first having to retrieve a description of that object's properties would provide the basis for a functional pointer. (Appendix 5.A provides a partial network implementation of retinotopic-based pointers.)

5.5 Indexes and the Development of the Object Concept in Infants

The idea of a visual index has also been used to explain interesting find-ings concerning the development of the *object* concept and of numeros-ity (or, as some people call it, "arithmetic" ability [Wynn, 1998]) in infants between the ages of about 6 and 12 months (Leslie, Xu, Tremoulet, and Scholl, 1998). Interestingly, in that age range, infants appear to be sensitive to the numerosity of sets of objects, although in the earlier end of the range (under ten months) they do not seem to keep track of individuals by their properties, but rather by something like their individuality. Evidence presented by Spelke, Gutheil, and Van de Walle (1995); Wynn (1992); and Xu and Carey (1996), as well as more recent evidence by Tremoulet, Leslie, and Hall (2001), suggests that at the age of only a few months, infants respond to the numerosity of items that disappear behind a screen; they do so by showing a "surprise" reaction (measured in terms of increased looking time) to a display of fewer (or more) items than they earlier had seen being placed behind the screen.

A typical experiment is one reported by Wynn (1992) and illustrated in figure 5.14. A five-month-old infant is shown a single doll on a stage. A screen is then raised to cover part of the stage, obscuring the doll. With the screen still covering the doll, a hand appears from the side of the

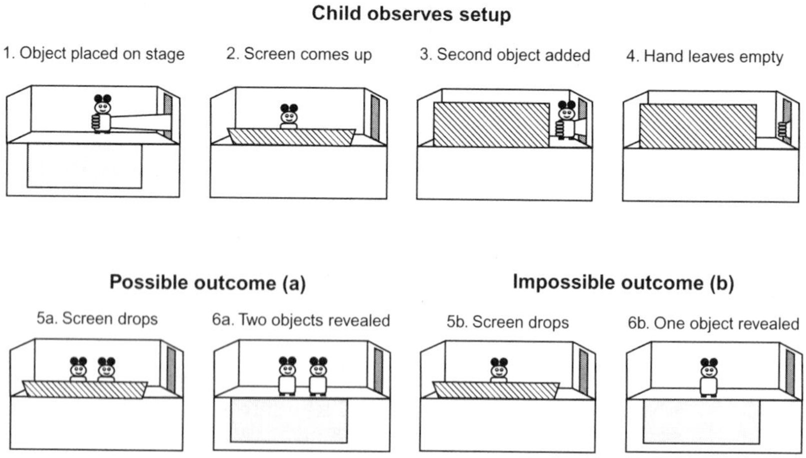

Child observes setup

1. Object placed on stage	2. Screen comes up	3. Second object added	4. Hand leaves empty

Possible outcome (a)

5a. Screen drops	6a. Two objects revealed

Impossible outcome (b)

5b. Screen drops	6b. One object revealed

Figure 5.14
Illustration of a study by Karen Wynn. An infant sees a doll being placed behind a screen. A hand then delivers a second doll behind the same screen and leaves empty. The screen then comes down and the infant sees one of two outcomes. The one labeled "impossible outcome," in which only one doll is seen, leads to longer looking times than the one labeled "possible outcome." Wynn (1992) interpreted this and related findings as revealing a primitive arithmetic ability in infants as young as five months of age. (Adapted from Wynn, 1992.)

stage holding a second doll, moves briefly behind the screen, and returns empty. The screen is then lowered revealing either one or two dolls. Wynn found that infants looked longer at the "impossible" condition in which there is only one doll ("looking time" is known to be related to violations of the infants' expectations). Similar evidence for numerical sensitivity occurs when the number of objects decreases. Suppose the stage initially contains two dolls that are then obscured by the screen. If an empty hand moves from the side to behind the screen and returns holding one doll, then when the screen is lowered, infants look longer at the stage when there are two dolls there (the impossible condition).

Simon, Hespos, and Rochat (1995) extended Wynn's study by adding a condition in which the numerosity of the resulting stage contents was correct but the *type* of doll was different. Infants in this study showed no looking time differences when the identity of objects was violated, only when numerosity was violated. These basic results were confirmed by Xu and Carey (1996), who also showed that it mattered whether the objects were seen simultaneously or one at a time before they were placed behind a screen. Xu and Carey used two objects that differed greatly in their appearance (and which could be clearly distinguished by the infants) and placed them behind a screen, one from each side. In one condition, infants saw the two objects simultaneously before they were both moved behind the screen. In the other condition, they saw one being placed behind the screen, and then, once the first object was hidden, the other was brought out and placed behind the screen (the objects appeared from each side of the stage). Then, as in the other experiments, the screen was removed and infants' looking time was measured. Xu and Carey found that for younger infants (10 months of age) looking time was sensitive to numerosity (i.e., as revealed by their looking time to one versus two objects) *only* when they earlier had seen the two objects simultaneously, one on each side of the screen. When they had seen only one of the two objects at a time, as they were about to be placed behind the screen, they showed no preference for resulting numerosity when the screen was removed. In contrast, older (12-month-old) infants were sensitive to numerosity regardless of whether they had seen the objects simultaneously or serially. This suggests that the younger infants could not individuate objects by their visual properties, but only by their being in discrete locations.

More recently, Tremoulet et al. (2001) further clarified the Xu and Carey finding concerning the distinction between simultaneous and serial viewing of objects. They used two objects that could vary in color (red or green) and in shape (triangle or circle). Like Xu and Carey, they showed that 12-month-old infants could individuate objects (i.e., determine that two objects were distinct) by using differences in either shape or color. This was demonstrated by the fact that the infants showed sensitivity to the numerosity of the displays when the objects that differed in color or shape were placed on the stage one at a time. The Tremoulet, Leslie, and Hall studies also asked whether the infants could recognize if the shapes and colors of the objects in the display were the same as those shown earlier (before they were hidden by the screen). They found that 10-month-old infants did *not* show surprise when the final display contained a different colored object, although they did show surprise when the final display contained an object of a different shape. The design of the relevant studies is illustrated in figure 5.15 (which illustrates results from several studies).

What is of special interest to us is that this study suggests a distinction between the process of individuation and the process of recognition. It shows that properties that allow for individuation may be different from the properties that allow for recognition. The 10-month-olds in the Xu and Carey study were capable of individuating objects according to location (they were shown side by side), but they failed to correctly anticipate numerosity when they were required to individuate objects according to their visual properties (when they were shown one at a time). In the Tremoulet et al. study, 12-month-old infants could individuate objects by both color and shape, as demonstrated by the fact that they showed a sensitivity to the number of objects when the evidence for their numerosity was attributable solely to the different visual properties (being shown a red object and then a green object was evidence that there were two distinct objects and led the infants to expect two objects in the final display). Despite being able to individuate objects on the basis of color and shape and use this information to determine how many there were, 10-month-old infants could not recognize when a display failed to contain the right pair of colors. In other words, they could not use color to re-recognize an object as *the same one* they had seen before. In terms of the indexing theory, this suggests that the assignment of *different*

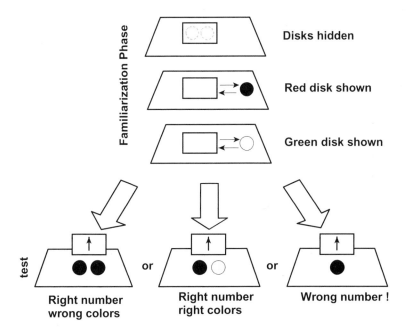

Figure 5.15
This figure illustrates the experimental condition in which objects are shown sequentially to ten-month-old infants. Infants always show increased looking times when the wrong number of objects appear in the test phase, but they show no difference in looking times when the colors are different from those they saw in the familiarization trials. This result appears to show that infants at age ten months are sensitive to the numerosity of the objects but they do not encode objects' colors. Yet it was the fact that the objects' colors were different that specified that there were two distinct objects. It appears that the properties used for individuating need not be the same properties that are used for recognition. (The actual single-object condition, presented here for completeness, was not part of the same experiment but was carried out separately by familiarizing infants to a single object and testing them with the same two-object outcomes as shown here. Infant looking times were longer for outcomes with unexpected number of objects but not for outcomes with unexpected colors.) (The figure is based on descriptions in Leslie et al., 1998 and Tremoulet et al., 2001.)

indexes might make use of such distinguishing properties as differences in location and perhaps also differences in other properties, yet these properties might not be involved in what I have called identity maintenance. I have suggested that primitive identity maintenance is a direct result of a primitive tracking capacity built into the early-vision system and as such may involve quite different properties than those that "grab" indexes. Indeed, as we saw earlier, under certain conditions (i.e., when objects can be visited serially) any distinguishable property can be used to allocate indexes, yet changing objects' properties does not affect tracking performance.

Leslie et al. (1998) explained the above findings by appealing to the theoretical construct of an "object index," a construct derived from visual-index theory described in this chapter. Their analysis differs in a number of ways from the one presented here (as they acknowledge). The differences lie not so much in differences between their notion of an object index and my notion of a visual index, but in their failure to draw a distinction between conceptual and perceptual mechanisms in the process of individuation. As pointed out on numerous occasions in earlier discussion, *conceptual* individuation and re-recognition of objects is the general rule in dealing with individuation and objecthood. I have gone to some length to distinguish the traditional full-blooded sense of individuation from primitive perceptual individuation by positing the notion of a *primitive visual object* as distinct from the notion of physical object. Whether or not infants have the full concept of physical object at an early age is an empirical question, though they clearly do develop such a notion. Indeed, by about 10 months of age they appear to have the full notion of a sortal as a concept that characterizes certain kind of things in the world (e.g., dogs, cats, people, tables, toys) (see, e.g., Xu, 1997).

Perhaps the most surprising in the series of studies of babies' sensitivity to numerosity are experiments that appear to show that when babies (age 8 months) have an opportunity to witness objects being taken apart and put back together, they treat them as collections as opposed to individuals; and they do not keep track of the numerosity of collections in the sorts of experiments described above (i.e., they do not show sensitivity to the numerosity of collections [Chiang and Wynn, 2000]), even though they are perfectly capable of tracking certain visual clusters, such as moving groups of lines (Wynn, Bloom, and Chiang, 2002). Nor do infants appear to keep track of the numerosity of piles of substances, as opposed to individual objects. If instead of seeing objects being placed behind a screen (as in figures 5.14 and 5.15) they see individual piles (e.g., of sand) being poured, they also do not treat them as individuals in numerosity experiments such as those just discussed (Huntley-Fenner, Carey, and Salimando, 2002). Since piles of sand and rigid objects in the shape of piles of sand are visually identical (as are objects seen to be put together from parts, compared with the same objects without a history of being taken apart and put together) it seems that whether or not certain entities invoke numerosity judgments depends on their immediately prior history. To explain numerosity effects in terms of indexes, the immediate history of an object may have to be taken into account. There is some suggestive evidence that objects cannot be tracked in MOT if they appear to "pour" or slither from place to place, the way a Slinky toy might move, so it may be the mode of movement that makes the difference in these studies (van Marle and Scholl, in press). This will not explain all the infant results just mentioned, but it does suggest that certain temporal properties enter into determining whether elements can be tracked. Visual-index theory does not prohibit temporal properties, or any other properties, from influencing what can or cannot be tracked. But since the tracking process is hypothesized to be nonconceptual, how objects are interpreted (what they are seen *as*) should not affect whether they are tracked. At the present time there does not appear to be good reason to reject this hypothesis.

5.5.1 Do the numerosity data suggest that infants have the concept of an object?

In the above discussion I have focused on a primitive sense of individuation and tracking for two reasons. One is that psychophysical evidence suggests that there is a preconceptual stage of individuation and tracking, whose character does not depend on what is known about the properties of the object being tracked. The other is that the full-blooded sense of individuation and tracking, a sense that does require appeal to a variety of conceptual (encoded) properties, must rest on some more basic mechanisms of the perceptual architecture that individuates objects in a more primitive sense and allows their properties to be detected and encoded. Keeping track of objects by appealing to their properties, although essential to full individuation, cannot be the whole story since at some point there must be a basic primitive "thing" or "perceptual object" (or what I will call a "FING" to emphasize its relation to FINSTs) to which conceptual properties are ascribed. At some level, the nature of the visual system must dictate what sorts of things are trackable and countable, which, in turn, places constraints on how the world is parsed and on the things that can be conceptualized. The demarcation of things provided by our conceptual system, that is, by sortal properties, cannot extend to arbitrary cuts through the physical-temporal continuum. Rather, it must capitalize on the equivalence-classes given by our visual architecture, operating over properties of the visible world. These arise from such things as the way the visual system solves the correspondence problem. According to the view presented here, this solution begins with the mechanism of the visual index, which parses the visible world in a way that can be accessed by cognition, and thus interpreted and described by our system of concepts.

The above story commits us to the claim that the FINGs picked out by visual indexes are not conceptualized and therefore are not based on the concept of an object or on what philosophers call sortals (or sortal concepts). But many people have suggested that the infant numerosity literature sketched earlier shows that infants have the concept of an object early in life (Carey and Xu, 2001; Xu, 1997; Xu and Carey, 1996). Visual-index theory takes no position on the question of whether infants have the concept of an object or whether they just keep track of FINGs, except that, as just noted, no sortal-based tracking can occur without some preconceptual parsing of the world. This sort of parsing need not pick out the same sets of things as are referred to by the term "object," but it does pick out *some* set of observer-dependent or sensorium-dependent properties. In fact, there is reason to believe that it picks out some rather odd disjunctions of physical properties, since we can track a wide range of individual FINGs, while at the same time we fail to track some perfectly well defined clusters of visual features (as we saw on p. 230).

As to the infant results sketched above, it is not clear whether they entail that at a certain age (around 6 months) babies possess the sortal "physical object," which may be a relatively impoverished concept, or that they merely track primitive FINGs, which have no independent characterization other than that provided by the structure of the early-vision system. There are reasons for thinking it may be the latter. Some sortal concepts (e.g., that of "Spelke-Objects," defined after Spelke, 1990, as "bounded, coherent, three-dimensional objects that move as a whole") no doubt develop early, but it is not clear that the infant data require the assumption of such a concept. The issue is, of course, whether or not infants have the *concept* of an object, or whether they have a perceptual system that enables them to track something (a "proto-object") that is partially coextensive with the adult notion of an object. It may well be that no object concept is needed to track something that disappears behind a screen, for the same reason that no concept is needed in the multiple-object-tracking studies described earlier. But what about the case where the object disappears behind the screen, remains there for 10 seconds or more, and then reappears when the screen is removed (either by itself or with another object)? Is the infant's lack of surprise a result of its visual system maintaining an index directed at the occluded object during the entire time, or does the infant re-recognize the reappearance as the same sortal (i.e., *object*) as in the earlier disappearance? The data are inconclusive: at present either option remains possible.

Although we cannot answer this question with the available data, it is important to understand exactly what is at stake and perhaps what would count as evidence one way or the other. Consider what we know about the early-vision system (the autonomous visual system described in chapters 2 and 3). It is a complex system that does much more than transduce the optical inputs. As we saw, it can compute visual representations in ways that seem quite intelligent. It appears to take into account conflicting possible interpretations and comes up with a "solution" that often appears remarkably "intelligent." The operating principles used by the visual system seem to be based on a variety of built-in assumptions, often called "natural constraints," that typically apply in our kind of world. These are not rational principles such as those the cognitive system uses to draw inferences. Since the visual system is encapsulated it cannot make use of relevant knowledge other than what is wired into the visual system itself. In addition, even though the processes in early vision are generally based on local cues, they exhibit many global effects (e.g., the global cohesion effects found in the apparent motion of multiple elements discussed on pp. 109–111 and 190–191). In the same "natural constraint" spirit, we have seen that indexing and tracking one or more primitive objects can go on even when the objects disappear from view (Scholl and Pylyshyn, 1999; Yantis, 1995). It is not known whether indexing can be sustained if the occlusion duration is 10 or 20 seconds or more as it is in the baby experiments (although some low-level visual persistence phenomena have been reported for periods as long as 5 minutes [Ishai and Sagi, 1995]). The point is that nothing in principle prevents early vision from carrying out the sorts of functions that are exhibited in the infant studies, such as keeping track of objects that are hidden by a screen or that go out of sight in other ways.[20] Given the often surprising nature of early vision it would seem premature to conclude that these sorts of phenomena have to involve the conceptual system.

5.6   Possible Implementations of the FINST Indexing Mechanism

I have tried to show that one needs a nonconceptual binding mechanism to connect mental particulars, such as tokens of symbols, to primitive

20. One might wonder what exactly the index points to when the object is temporarily out of view. But then one might equally wonder what an index points to when the object is distributed over some region of the display (as in the studies by Rock and Gutman, 1981), or when it is a more general kind of object (as in the case of the Blaser et al. studies discussed on pp. 192–193), or even when the motion is illusory, and so on. It seems that the indexing system can individuate and track FINGs that are not highly localized in either space or time and can track them even though they may be absent at particular moments in time and at particular places. Such results suggest that punctate time and space may be an inappropriate way of characterizing indexing and tracking and that the term "pointing" may itself be misleading. Larger chunks of space-time my be involved, such as happens in predictive tracking using an adaptive filter (e.g., a Kalman filter). Perhaps we should take seriously (at least as a first approximation) the principle enunciated earlier, that indexes pick out *primitive visual objects* (or FINGs) without regard for such properties as their location, extent, or duration. There is no need to be entrapped by the idea that because we view an index as a pointer it must literally point to an exact geometrical *point* in time or space. It may simply point to a FING, as defined by the architecture of early vision, the properties of which are to be discovered by empirical inquiry and which may not correspond to a simple physical description except in special circumstances. This is, after all, what happens with other ways of referring, such as using a proper name or a deictic reference (e.g., a demonstrative such as *that*).

visual objects or FINGs. But how is this possible? It almost sounds as though I am hypothesizing something like an elastic band that connects symbols with things. In a functional sense this is useful way to look at the FINST mechanism. As illustrated in figures 5.4 and 5.12, an index corresponds to two sorts of links or relations: on the one hand, it corresponds to a *causal chain* that goes from visual objects to certain tokens in the representation of the scene being built (perhaps an *object file*), and on the other hand, it is also a *referential relationship* that enables the visual system to refer to those particular FINGs. The second of these functions is possible because the first one exists and has the right properties. Mental symbols refer to certain objects because those objects caused an (initially empty) object file to be created.

A primitive object or FING is both an object of thought and the starting point of a causal chain. This situation is no different from the one that obtains in perception generally. When we perceive, our percept is of something in the world—what Gibson called a *distal* stimulus. We do not perceive retinal stimulation or the action of rods and cones; we perceive *things in the world*. But a theory of perception must deal with the fact that this perception of a distal object is accomplished by a whole chain of causal connections mediating between the distal scene and the organism's sensors. Such a theory must include a description of processes operating over a *proximal* stimulus—or the stimulus actually impinging on the sense organs or transducers, even though we do not *perceive* the proximal stimulus.

It is this proximal aspect of the causal chain that I now address. We must ask how a visual mechanism might implement the functions summarized in table 5.1. These include at least the following functions: (a) the appearance of primitive visual objects in the field of view causes the individuation of some of these objects; (b) a subset of the individuated elements causes the activation of a small number of indexes, a unique one for each object up to a limit of about 4 or 5 indexes; (c) so long as the objects' motion is constrained in certain ways (some of which were discussed earlier in section 5.3.2, but many of which remain to be discovered), these indexes continue to be maintained so that each index keeps being associated with the same primitive visual object; and (d) once an index is activated it becomes possible to interrogate each unique object to determine its properties or combination of properties—so the link has a downward as well as an upward connection. I begin by viewing these requirements in a purely functional manner and describe an easily constructible black box that approximately achieves these functions.

Consider first the question of how indexes might be evoked by the appearance of a small number of visual objects in a scene in such a way that it is then possible to probe each individual object (putting off for now the question of how tracking occurs). It turns out that this function can be accomplished fairly easily by any of a number of possible mechanisms, one of which I sketch for purely expository purposes. For simplicity I provide a simple functional description of what the mechanism does. Readers who are interested in how one could implement such a function in a network can see some of the details briefly spelled out in appendix 5.A at the end of this chapter. Those who are not interested in the question of how a mechanism might implement an index may skip the rest of this section altogether. The only value of the discussion that follows is that it may clarify what is being claimed about indexes and may serve to demystify it by fleshing it out in the form of a particularly simple black box function.

Here is the picture of what the simple mechanism does. Think of the mechanism as consisting of boxes such as shown in figure 5.16, in which an array of detectors provides the inputs (see note 22 on my use of the term "array"). These will need to be more than just luminance detectors; they will be preprocessed inputs, perhaps as in Wolfe's activation map (Wolfe, Cave, and Franzel, 1989) or Treisman's feature maps (Treisman and Gelade, 1980). The middle box detects the n most active of the input lines (I have set $n = 4$ for illustrative purposes). When it has done this it lights up n of the lights shown on the box. For this illustration, assume that the first light corresponds to the most active input line (whichever that might be), the second light corresponds to the second most active line, and so on. Beside each light is a button. These buttons allow a signal to be sent back to the source of the input lines as follows: when you press the first of these buttons it sends a signal to the input element that activated the corresponding detector and caused the first light to come on. Pressing the second button sends a signal to the element that caused the second light to come on, and so on. Notice that whoever (or whatever) presses the button does not know *where* the signal from the button will go, only that it will go to whatever caused the corre-

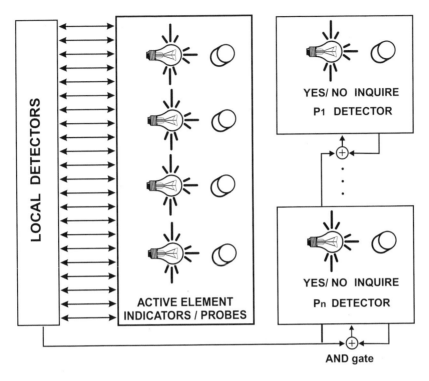

Figure 5.16
Sketch of a possible "black box" implementation of a FINST mechanism (see text for explanation).

sponding light to come on (this ensures that two buttons do not send a signal to the same detector). The function just described can be implemented as a winner-take-all circuit, which I describe in appendix 5.A (it is based on a design of a network for attention-scanning proposed by Koch and Ullman, 1985).

The function just described is the heart of the indexing system, for it provides a way to "probe" particular elements in the input without knowing what or where they are, only that they have activated an index (represented here functionally as the active-element indicator light). This, in turn, provides a way to ask about certain detectable properties of any of the activated elements. To do that we need a set of global sensors for properties $P_1, P_2, \ldots, P_m$, each of which is connected to every element in the input (in other words, there is a detector for each property $P_1, P_2,$

P_3 and so on at each site in the input array; for example, each site has a detector for red, green, blue, luminance, nth order derivatives of luminance in various directions, and so on). We now arrange things so that a property detector for P_i will fire only if the (unique) element being probed by the system just described has property P_i. Here's how it's done. We have a number of YES/NO P DETECTOR indicators and P INQUIRY buttons, one for each distinct property P_i, as well as a bit of simple logical circuitry.[21] The idea is simple: a P DETECTOR fires only if it gets two or more inputs. One of these comes from an input element that has property P_i and the other comes from what we call the probe, which originates with the buttons on the central ACTIVE ELEMENT box. If (and only if) the item being probed has the property being inquired at the P DETECTOR button, the light on the corresponding P DETECTOR indicator will be illuminated. Thus the procedure for using this black box requires two hands: if you want to know whether a particular element—one that was salient enough to cause light X_i to come on—has property P_i, you press the button beside light X_i and also press the button marked "P INQUIRY" for property P_i. The P-DETECTOR indicator will then light up if the element associated with light X_i has property P_i. This protracted description is presented to make only one point: it is easy to make a circuit that tells you whether an active detector element has a particular property, *even if you don't know anything about the active element in question* (e.g., where it is located).

This gives us what we want of our indexing mechanism: a way to inquire directly about particular properties of certain salient items without first having to locate the items. It even allows one, for example, to ask whether a particular salient object has both property P_i and property P_k. Just press both the P-INQUIRY buttons while pressing a button

21. I have arbitrarily made the P-detectors active inquiry systems, rather than passive transponders. If they were passive, then *all* property indicators for properties of the probed element would light up, so as soon as a button in the middle box was pressed, all properties of the element in question would be indicated. It seems more plausible that indexes are used to inquire about particular properties of indexed objects rather than all properties of the probed object at once, since there may be a very large number of potential properties. Nonetheless the choice between these two schemes is an empirical matter and not a matter of principle.

on the main box corresponding to an active element: if the P_i and P_k indicators both light up, it means that there is an individual element that has both property P_i and property P_k. Notice that, contrary to the assumption of most theories of visual search (see section 4.4.2), a conjunction of properties is detected in this system without first retrieving the location of one of the conjuncts. When a light is illuminated on the main "active element" box it tells us only that *some* element is bound to an index. When n lights are illuminated it tells us that n distinct primitive objects are bound to distinct indexes. Beyond that the illumination of a light does not tell us *anything* more about that object (even the ordinal position of lights in the middle box, which I spoke of as marking activation ranking, is not required and is invoked here only as a way to keep the objects distinct). In particular, the box provides no information about the location of the objects that caused the lights to come on. Certainly the circuits inside the box must make the connections to the appropriate locations, but this information is unavailable to the outside. In this way the box comes close to providing the function of indexing a number of primitive objects in the input matrix so as to allow the indexed objects to serve as arguments to visual predicates.

The alert reader will notice that as it stands this box does not quite meet all our functional requirements. That's because what is being selected and inquired of in this case is a particular (stationary) element of the proximal stimulus. It is not an object in the world, inasmuch as the system does not, for example, keep addressing the same distal cause of activation as the proximal projection of the latter moves around in the array. But this can be changed so that functionally the system in figure 5.16 behaves roughly as required by the indexing theory—it will keep addressing (interrogating) a moving item in the input matrix as long as that item moves in a trajectory that meets certain constraints. It is not technically difficult to arrange matters so that the particular input element that is probed by a particular button changes appropriately to correspond with continuous movements of the pattern of stimulation in the input. It is simply a matter of providing some mechanism, operating over local neighborhoods of the input, that ensures that the same connection between cells and lights/buttons is maintained when adjacent cells become activated/deactivated (i.e., when the activation maxima move continually over the spatial matrix).[22] When property-inquiries are carried out in such a system, they would then typically detect properties associated with the same moving object. When two properties are detected in association with the same index (i.e., the same light), these will be joint properties of the same moving object. The function of the box shown in figure 5.16 therefore mirrors the properties required of indexes, including automatic selection of primitive visual objects, and object-based or "sticky" indexes that are transparent to object location.

In appendix 5.A I discuss a possible implementation of such a mechanism, using a connectionist or "neural net" architecture, that enhances neighboring elements in the input and increases the chances that they will become associated with the same indicator light and thus will be the target of the same probe inquiries. This provides a rough tracking mechanism for continuous smooth motion. Many mechanisms can be imagined that could track continuously moving patterns of local excitation maxima, including a parallel predictive mechanism based on techniques such as Kalman Filters (e.g., Lee and Simon, 1993) or parallel mechanisms that compute apparent motion over brief disappearance of the objects (such as those proposed for apparent motion by Dawson and Pylyshyn, 1988). The only neurologically motivated constraint that we impose on such a mechanism is that it should operate on the basis of *local information support*. This means that any predictive tracking should be based on spatially local information. Beyond that, the tracking mechanism can take into account any property of the movement of the activation pattern and in principle can even track objects that disappear behind an occluding surface in certain ways or that take part in

22. When I refer to a "map" or a "array" in the present context I make only weak claims about its spatial character. For example, distances in the array need not map onto some monotonic function of distances in the world. The only spatial properties that such a map needs to have is (a) the detectors have to be spatially local (i.e., they have to have limited receptive fields) and (b) there must be connections between individual detectors and the detectors of neighboring sites. This is assumed here only because the notion of "neighborhood" plays a role in the suggested mechanism for favoring continuity of motion. The actual units in the mechanism illustrated in figure 5.16 do not themselves have to be situated in a 2D spatial array, and indeed the operation of the mechanism illustrated here is indifferent to the input being spatially scrambled, as long as immediate-neighbor connections are preserved.

apparent motion. Sometimes surprisingly global patterns can be computed in this way. For example, the mechanism for computing apparent motion discussed on pages 109–110 operates on the basis of strictly local information and yet predicts global effects of apparent motion (such as the preference for coherent group motion).

The network shown in appendix 5.A illustrates a possible implementation of this mechanism. This implementation is not in itself of particular interest except as an existence proof that the function being assumed is realizable in a simple network based on local computations (such as would be expected in the nervous system) and that such functions as enabling selective probing of moving objects can be accomplished without first *locating* the objects in question, at least in the sense of encoding their coordinates.

Appendix 5.A Sketch of a Partial Network-Implementation of the FINST Indexing Mechanism

The function described in section 5.6 can be implemented in a network of simple elements. Such networks are sometimes referred to as artificial neural networks (ANNs), but I do not make any such neural claim. What is important about this network, from our perspective, is that it illustrates how a simple mechanism can realize the function described earlier (and therefore can approximately realize some of the properties of the FINST indexing mechanism) while operating with the kind of input that is natural for the visual system, at least to a first approximation. The network I have in mind uses a slightly modified version of what is known as a fully connected winner-take-all (WTA) network. When provided with an array of inputs that vary in their activation level (i.e., that have different magnitudes of inputs), the WTA network settles into a state in which the unit with the most highly active input retains its value while the activity level of all the others is reduced to zero. This is, in fact, a maximum-finding circuit. Since we usually don't want the values of the actual inputs to be changed, we think of these units as copying their values into a duplicate array that we call a buffer array. So far the picture is like that shown in figure 5.17. An array of input units activates an array of buffer units. Each of the buffer units feeds into a unit of a WTA network. The network eventually settles into a state where all the buffer

inputs buffer   WTA Network

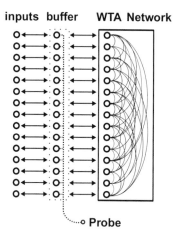

·······o **Probe**

Figure 5.17
A winner-take-all (WTA) "maximum-finding" network, the first step to a possible mechanism for implementing FINST visual indexes in a network architecture. WTA is a completely interconnected network in which each unit inhibits
all the others (from Pylyshyn, 2000). See the text for an explanation.

units have value zero except the one that received the largest input from
its corresponding input unit.[23] When this happens, the network signals
its success by generating an output (in some versions it might generate
such an output only if the maximum input value exceeds some
threshold).

Because we now have a buffer in which every unit but one is turned
off, a simple bit of logical circuitry allows us to send a signal (call it the
"probe signal") to the input unit corresponding to the selection. (This is
easily accomplished by summing the probe signal with the activity level
of each buffer unit, using an AND gate, so that it succeeds in reaching

23. The simplified version of the network described here—in which each unit is
connected to every other unit—is unsatisfactory for a number of reasons (e.g.,
it is not guaranteed to converge, the number of connections grows exponentially
with the number of units, etc.). There are various ways to implement such a
network that overcome these problems, one of which is described by Koch and
Ullman (1985). In addition, it may be desirable for a number of reasons to
arrange the connectivity to emphasize closer units, for example by having the
density of connections fall off as the distance between units increases. This helps
the smooth-tracking problem by preventing indexes from "jumping" to remote
but more active inputs.

the only input unit whose corresponding buffer unit is currently on.) Thus the probe signal only reaches the buffer unit that had the maximum value at the outset.

Another AND gate (or summation and threshold unit) accomplishes the property of "interrogation." The details can be filled in many ways, but for the sake of the present example, let's assume that at every input site there is a detector for each property P (e.g., for a property such as "red"), which sends its output to the appropriate indicator box shown on the right in figure 5.16. This detector fires and sends a signal to its indicator box *only if* (a) the receptive field of that input unit has property P and (b) a probe signal arrives at that input unit. In other words, the property is detected on a particular input element only if that element has been probed by a signal from the middle box in figure 5.16. In this way the output of each detector and the signal from the inquiry button are summed (through an AND gate, shown in figure 5.16). If we wanted to know whether the *object selected by the probe* in the middle box had a particular property P, we would send a signal to one side of an AND circuit associated with the P detector and the detector would send a signal to the other side (as shown in the figure). If both were nonnull, the indicator in that particular box would light up.

The point of this exercise is to show that once you have figured out what properties of objects are treated as salient (and cause the WTA network to converge), it is easy to think of ways to use such a network to allow a signal to be sent to the input that is selected in this way, and thereby to test the selected input for specified properties. It is important to notice that this elementary circuit allows an element to be interrogated without any information about it other than that it was the most active (i.e., salient) unit. In particular, it provides a way to test for properties associated with a unit *without knowing where that unit is*. No part of the system contains the coordinates (or any other location information) of the unit whose associated properties are being tested.

This particular network does not track a moving object, nor is it able to select several objects at one time. Neither of these limitations is insurmountable. For example, it is easy to augment the network so that it can follow a moving signal—in fact, one possible technique was described by Koch and Ullman (1985). The likelihood that a particular input will be selected by the WTA network depends on the magnitude of its activation signal—the source of which I have left completely unspecified (although it can easily assimilate the assumptions in such theories of attention as Wolfe's guided search model [Wolfe et al., 1989]). Consequently, anything that increases the input that a particular buffer unit receives will tend to make it a more likely candidate for selection. One possible source of this increase, suggested by Koch and Ullman (1985), is activation from spatially nearby units. It is easy enough to arrange for each selected unit to pass activation to its immediate neighbors. The consequence of this type of connection is to give the region surrounding a selected object an increased probability of being subsequently selected. What this means is that if an object moves smoothly across the display it will keep enhancing its immediate neighborhood, leading to continuous tracking. This is a very crude means of causing a certain type of tracking behavior. It is like tracking the bump when a cat is moving around under a blanket. Other locally based activation mechanisms are also possible. For example, on pages 109–110 we discussed a proposal that Michael Dawson and I offered (Dawson and Pylyshyn, 1988) for modeling apparent motion, based on summation of labeled information from neighboring units. The resulting network displays apparently global properties—such as increasing the likelihood of apparent motion occurring in a manner consistent with the natural constraint of coherence of matter—even though it is based entirely on local information from neighboring regions. Similarly, in Pylyshyn and Eagleson (1994), we proposed a network that performs statistical extrapolation (based on Kalman filters) using only spatially local information. The point here is that tracking is compatible with a locality constraint on index assignment. And tracking does not require that certain visual properties first be identified in order for a correspondence to be established (as we saw earlier in section 5.1).

The alert reader might notice that these activation-spreading mechanisms only increase the likelihood that a neighboring element is selected next. This still leaves open the question of whether this element is the *same* one as was selected earlier, and if so what makes it the same one. As far as the mechanism I have described is concerned, a *different* index might be assigned to the nearby element as a result of the spreading activation. But for the network to keep tracking the same token moving element, the element has to keep being attached to the same index. How does one ensure that nearby elements keep the same index? Within the context of the network model of indexing, this too can be viewed as a technical (as well as empirical) problem rather than a matter of principle. Both the multiple-object-tracking and the same-index-tracking problem might be solved by the same design principle. For example, if buffer units were randomly connected to other buffer units so that the probability of a connection between a pair of units is greater the closer the units are to one another, then we might prevent indexes from jumping to more distant units that have higher immediate activation. This would favor spatial-temporal continuity in assigning particular indexes.

As it stands, the network is also incapable of selecting multiple objects, as required by indexing theory. If we had several networks such as the one discussed above they would converge on the same object, so the problem that needs to be solved is how to keep the different objects distinct—or how to prevent distinct visual objects from capturing the same *index*. But once again alternative ways to solve this problem are available. For example, Acton (1993) developed a multiple-object-tracking version of the network by using time-based marking. The most highly activated object captures the first index and then enters a refractory period while the second most active object captures the next index. The indexes are synchronized to a clock, which provides an easy but not very satisfying solution to the index separation problem (since it requires a clock to pulse the network). Also, varying the density of connections as a function of distance, as suggested earlier, could prevent two distant active units from grabbing the same index. Other mechanisms include capitalizing on a process known as inhibition of return, wherein an activated or attended object inhibits reactivation for a period of time (as in the well-known refractory period between nerve firings). Although these particular solutions may or may not be appropriate as a general solution, they do point out that alternative implementations are easily found and show the in principle realizability of the indexing proposal.

6

Seeing with the Mind's Eye: Part 1, The Puzzle of Mental Imagery

6.1 What Is the Puzzle about Mental Imagery?

In earlier chapters I discussed various connections among the world, the visual system, and the central cognitive system that is responsible for reasoning, inference, decision making and other rational processes. In the course of this analysis we have found much that is counterintuitive about how the mind is organized and how it connects with and represents the world. Yet nowhere does our intuition go astray more than when we consider what happens when we recall a past event by imagining it or when we reason by imagining a situation unfold before our "mind's eye." Our introspection is very persuasive here, and it tells us quite unequivocally that when we imagine something we are in some important sense *seeing* it and that when we solve a problem by imagining a situation unfold in our "mind's eye" we have but to pay attention and notice what happens. No intervention on the part of reasoning appears to be involved in much of this process.

Imagine a baseball being hit into the air, and notice the trajectory it follows. Although few of us could calculate the shape of this trajectory, none of us has any difficulty imagining the roughly parabolic shape traced out by the ball. Indeed, we can often predict with considerable accuracy where the ball will land (certainly a properly situated professional fielder can). It is often the case that we can predict the dynamics of physical processes that are beyond our ability to solve analytically. In fact, they may be beyond anyone's ability to solve analytically. Consider the behavior of a coin that has been spun on its edge. As it topples, it rolls around faster and faster until, with a final shudder, it lies still. The physics of this coin, which accelerates as it loses energy, has only recently been mathematically analyzed (Moffatt, 2000). Yet many people can imagine the behavior in question when asked to visualize the situation. Why? Is it because something in their imaging mechanism inherently obeys the relevant laws? Or is it perhaps because, under the right circumstances, they recall having seen a dropped coin behave this way? The intuition that the behavior of one's image is automatic is very strong. There seems to be something involuntary and intuitive about how the action unfolds in one's image. The impression that it is properties of the image, rather than any involvement of reasoning, that is responsible for the action one passively observes with the mind's eye, is very strong. Can this possibly be true?

Imagine that you climb a ladder and drop a ball from a ten-foot height. Observe it in your mind's eye as it falls to the ground. Now do the same but imagine that you drop it from a five-foot height. Does it not take longer to fall to the ground from a height of ten feet than from a height of, say, five feet? How much longer? You could measure the time it took for the ball to drop in your imagined scenario and get an exact answer, which would surely confirm that it takes longer to drop from a greater height. You could even plot the time as a function of distance and perhaps even as a function of imagined weight (and you would probably find, as Ian Howard did, that the time was proportional both to the height and to the weight—unlike what would happen if you actually dropped a real ball).[1] Now imagine that you are riding a bicycle along a level road, pedaling as hard as you can. Then imagine you have come to a hill. Does not the bicycle slow down without your having to think about it? What about when you come to the downhill side of the hill? You can even imagine that you have stopped pedaling completely, and you will probably find that the bicycle in your imagination continues to speed down the hill.

1. In a series of unpublished studies, Ian Howard of York University showed that people's naive physics, as measured by their predictions of falling objects, conformed to Aristotelian rather than Newtonian or Galilean principles. Howard dropped metal rings of various sizes behind an opaque screen and asked subjects to catch them by poking a rod through one of several carefully located holes in a screen. The measured times showed that subjects assumed a constant velocity, rather than the correct constant acceleration, and that the assumed velocity increased with the weight of the ring, contrary to Galilean principles (i.e., that objects fall with constant acceleration rather than constant velocity, and that the acceleration is independent of mass).

The illusion of the autonomy of the imagined scene is even more persuasive in the case of purely visual or geometrical properties. Imagine a very small mouse in the far corner of the room. Can you "see" whether it has whiskers? Now imagine that you are very close to it (perhaps it is in your hand). Isn't it much easier now to see whether it has whiskers? Close your eyes and imagine you are looking at the bottom left corner of the wall in front of you. Now imagine that you shift your gaze to the upper right corner. Did your gaze move through the intermediate points as you shifted from one corner to the other? Did you notice any of the things on the wall as you shifted your gaze? Do you think it would have taken you longer to shift your gaze if the region you were imagining had been smaller (say, confined to just a picture on the wall)? Or imagine a rectangle, and imagine drawing the diagonal from the top left corner to the bottom right corner. Now imagine drawing another line, this time from the bottom left corner to the middle of the right-hand side. Does this second line cross the first one you drew? And if so, does it cross it below or above its midpoint? Did you have to do any geometrical analysis to answer that question, or did you just "read it off" your image? Imagine an upper case letter D. Imagine it rotated counterclockwise by 90 degrees. Now imagine the letter J attached to it from below. What is the shape of the resulting combined figure? It seems as though you can do this entirely in your mind's eye and "notice" that the combination of the two figures "looks like" an umbrella without thinking about it. Such examples seem to show that mental imagery has a "life of its own" and unfolds without your rational intervention. They also seem to show that imagery makes use of the process of *visual* recognition. But does it? Notwithstanding one's strong intuitions about all these examples, there is much more to what your mental image does and what it "looks like" than meets the eye—even the "mind's eye." As we saw in chapter 1, the more familiar and vivid our experience of our inner life is, the less we can trust our impressions to provide the basis for a scientific theory of the underlying causes. I will return to more examples of this later.

Opposing the intuition that your image has an autonomous existence and unfolds according to its own laws and principles is the obvious fact that it is *you* alone who controls your image (of course the same might be said for other forms of conscious thought, such as inner dialogue, which are subject to the same erroneous intuitions, as we will see in chapter 8). Perhaps, as Humphrey (1951) once put it, the assumption that the image is responsible for what happens in your imagining puts the cart before the horse. It is more likely that the image unfolds as it does because you, the image creator, *made* it do so. For example, does it not seem plausible that the way things unfold in your image is actually guided by what you know would happen in real life? You can imagine things being pretty much any size, color, or shape you choose, and you can imagine them moving any way you want. You can, if you wish, imagine a baseball sailing off into the sky or following some bizarre path, including getting from one place to another without going through intervening points, as easily as you can imagine it following a more typical baseball trajectory. You can imagine all sorts of impossible things happening—and cartoon animators frequently do, to everyone's amusement. The wily coyote chasing the roadrunner runs into what turns out to be a picture of the road or sails off the edge of the cliff but does not fall until he sees that there is no support under him. Or the roadrunner sees the coyote approaching and suddenly appears behind his back. We can easily imagine the laws of physics being violated. In fact, unless we have learned certain Newtonian principles of physics we do not even correctly imagine what happens in certain real situations—such as in the earlier example of the time course of an object falling to earth (as mentioned in note 1).

If we can imagine anything we like, why then do we imagine the things we do in certain circumstances? Do we imagine things happening a certain way merely because we *know* that this is how they would happen? What if we couldn't predict what would happen without going through the process of imaging them; would this mean that images contain different kinds of "knowledge" than other forms of representations? And what exactly would that mean? Would it mean that imagery involves the use of *different* sorts of reasoning mechanisms? It may feel as though we can imagine pretty well anything we like, but is that so? Are there events, properties, or situations that we cannot imagine, and if so, why not? We can imagine the laws of physics being violated, but can we imagine the axioms of geometry being violated? Try imagining a four-dimensional block, or how a cube looks when seen from all sides at once, or what it would look like to travel through a non-Euclidean space (in which, for example, one side of a triangle was longer than the sum of the lengths of the other two sides). Before concluding that such examples illustrate the intrinsic geometry of images, however, consider whether your inability to imagine these things might not be due to your not *knowing*, in a purely factual way, how these things might look. The answer is by no means obvious. For example, do you know where various edges, shadows, and other contours would fall in a four-dimensional or non-Euclidean space? If you don't know how something would look, then how could you possibly have an image of it? Having an image of something *means* imagining how it looks. It has even been suggested (Goldenberg and Artner, 1991) that certain deficits in imagery ability that result from brain damage are a consequence of a deficiency in the patient's knowledge about the appearance of objects. At the minimum we are not entitled to conclude that images have the sort of inherent geometrical properties that we associate with pictures.

We also need to keep in mind that despite our intuitions about such examples, there is reason to be skeptical about what our subjective experience reveals about the nature of the mental image (both its content and its form). After all, when we look at an actual scene, we have the unmistakable subjective impression that we are examining a detailed panoramic view; yet as we saw in chapter 1, there is now considerable evidence that we encode and store very little in a visual scene unless we explicitly attend to the items in question, which we do only if our attention or our gaze is attracted to it (Henderson and Hollingworth, 1999). The natural implication of our phenomenology appears to be quite wrong in this case, even though the phenomenology itself is not to blame; things appear to us the way they appear—it's how we interpret this appearance that is in error. The information we have about a scene is not in the form of a global picture, for reasons discussed in chapter 1 (e.g., because nonretinal information appears to be much more abstract and conceptual than retinal information, because information from successive glances cannot be superimposed, because we fail to notice major changes in sequentially presented pictures, and so on). It is thus reasonable to expect that our subjective experience of mental imagery would be an equally poor guide to the form and content of the information in our mental images.

What needs to be kept in mind is that the content of our mental images, both the explicit information it contains and the dynamics of how that changes, is the joint consequence of (a) what we intend our mental image to show, (b) what we know about how things in the world look and how they tend to unfold in time, and (c) the way our mind (or perhaps only the part of it that specializes in mental imagery) constrains us (there are some other possible extrinsic reasons as well; see pp. 325–327). Discovering the boundary between the two major determiners of image content (in particular, between what we *know* or *intend* and the constraints imposed by the mechanisms or the particular form of representation used—in other words, by the way our brain is structured) is the central problem in the study of mental imagery. Both the impression that we can imagine whatever we please and the impression that our images have a life of their own are illusions. Our task as scientists is to try to steer our way between the Charybdis of total plasticity and the Scylla of autonomous unfolding. This task is no different from the one faced by cognitive scientists in every area of cognition, since what we can and do think is similarly a joint consequence of the plasticity of thought (we believe we can think any thought there is to think) and the constraints imposed on them (on what we can represent, conceptualize, or infer) by the nature of mind. The latter constraints arise from what is known as *cognitive architecture*, and I will have more to say about this concept later. In the case of a particular cognitive activity accompanied by vivid experiences, such as the experience of seeing an image in our mind's eye or experiencing ourselves thinking in sentences of our language, the temptation to reify the experiential content into a theory of the form of our representations seems nearly inescapable, leading to the ubiquitous view that the mind has two distinct modes of thought: linguistic and imagistic (or pictorial). In fact, these two ways of experiencing our thoughts neither exhaust the ways in which we can think nor provide a useful characterization of what thinking consists of—but more on this in the chapter 8. It is precisely the power of introspection, on the one hand, to provide a window into what we are thinking *about* and, on the other hand, to mislead us into believing that we can see the *form* in which our thoughts are encoded and the nature of the thinking process itself, that creates difficulty in coming to an understanding of the nature of perception and thought. It is the main reason why there is a ubiquitous problem of grasping what a scientific theory of reasoning with mental images might be like.

The view to which we are tempted by introspection is the view discussed earlier in chapter 1 (it is what Dan Dennett has called the "Cartesian Theater" view of the mind in Dennett, 1991). It is the view that when we think using mental images we are actually creating a picture in our mind, and when we reason in words we create sentences in our mind. In both cases there is the concomitant assumption that someone (or something) perceives these pictures or sentences. Henceforth I will refer to such views (at least as applied to the visual modality) as the "picture theory" of mental imagery. This is sometimes contrasted with an alternative that posits symbol structures, of the sort that are used in artificial intelligence or other computational models. As we will see in chapter 8, there are very good reasons for believing that thought takes place not in natural language or images, but in what has sometimes been called the "language of thought" (LOT) or *lingua mentis* (Fodor, 1975). For present purposes I will not be concerned with the LOT theory of the mental structures that underlie the experience of mental imagery. Rather I will be concerned to show that the intuitively appealing *picture theory* of mental imagery is implausible on a number of grounds. Part of the argument will be that the phenomena and experimental findings that are cited in support of this theory in fact have no bearing on the format of mental representations used, only on their content. Thus they do not provide evidence favoring one format (e.g., a picturelike format) over some other possible format (e.g., a languagelike format as posited by MOT). Consequently they provide no evidence for the view that the form of representation involved when we have the experience of "seeing a mental image" is different from the form of representation involved when we have some other experience, or no experience at all. The view that thoughts have the same underlying form (though usually with different contents insofar as they are about different things) regardless of how they are experienced I will call the *null hypothesis*.

But why should we shun the intuitively appealing view in favor of something so counterintuitive? In chapter 1 I alluded to some of the reasons why, in the case of visual perception, the intuitive view is inadequate and incapable of accounting for the empirical facts. Before elaborating on this argument and extending it to cover the case of mental imagery, let us stand back and try to get a broader picture of the problem of mental imagery that needs explaining. Before doing so, however, I want to clarify one point that is often misunderstood. Contrary to what many critics have assumed, I do not claim that images do not really exist or are merely "epiphenomenal" (Shepard, 1978b). The notion of something being an epiphenomenon is itself misleading. Usually what people mean when they accuse me of making this claim is that they do not agree with my view (as Block, 1981, has correctly pointed out). There can be no question of whether the experience of imagery exists, nor is there even much disagreement about its phenomenal character. The scientific problem is the explanation of the causal events that underlie this phenomenal experience. In cognitive science, these causal events typically take the form of information-processing operations performed on representations (the reason they take this form is explored in detail elsewhere [Pylyshyn, 1984a]). The explanation of what underlies this process need not, and in general will not, appeal to how they are experienced—to the fact that they appear to us to be like pictures of a scene we are viewing. This is much like saying that the way physical objects look to us is not part of our theory of how they take part in physical and chemical reactions. For that we need a different theory, a theory of their underlying causal structure, which always adverts to invisible things and invisible properties and forces.

Of course, the phenomenology is also interesting, and one may be able to tell a fascinating story about how things appear. In fact, Shepard (1978a) has done a remarkable job of illustrating many of his hypnagogic (near-sleep), entoptic (externally caused, though not by light), and dream images. These are fascinating accounts, but it is not clear how they should be taken within a causal theory. In commenting on a paper of mine, Dalla Barba, Rosenthal, and Visetti (2002) remark that phenomenology was never intended to provide a causal explanation. What it does is provide an account of how things are experienced, and in so doing it may show how some experiences are like others—it may provide a taxonomy of how things appear. On the basis of their (and other writers') phenomenal experience of mental imagery and of perception, Dalla Barba et al. conclude that images are pictorial but that they also differ significantly from the experience of vision. Whether phenomenally based taxonomies can be accommodated in an information-processing theory, or whether they can help to decide among alternative theories, is at present an open question (both in the study of mental imagery and in the study of vision).

The most important idea that must guide us in trying to understand the nature of mental imagery is the question of which properties and mechanisms are *intrinsic* or *constitutive* of having and using mental images, and which arise because of what we believe, intend, or otherwise attribute to *that which we are imagining*. The central question we need to ask is which aspects of "visual" or imaginal (or imagistic) thinking occur because of the special nature of the imagery system, rather than because of the nature of thinking in general, together with our tacit knowledge of the situation being imagined, how this knowledge is organized, and how we interpret the imagining task. We also need to ask whether what is special about imaginal thinking might simply be the fact that mental imagery is associated with certain contents or subject matter, such as the appearances of the things we are thinking about, and not on the way the information is encoded or on any special mechanisms used in processing it. Notice that it *could* be the case that when we think about spatial layouts, or about the appearance of objects (e.g., their shapes and colors) or other visual properties that tend to elicit the experience of mental imagery, we find that certain psychophysical phenomena are observed because we are then thinking about concrete visible properties rather than abstract properties. This would be no different from finding that certain properties (like differences in reaction times to different words or the ability of different secondary tasks to interfere with thinking) are observed when we think about economics or music or sports. It is plausible that when you are solving problems in economics your performance is degraded by secondary tasks involving economic concepts, in the same way that thinking about spatial topics is disrupted by tasks that themselves involve spatial concepts. Differences attributable to the *topic* of thinking are clearly not what those who postulate a separate image system have in mind. If what goes on during episodes of thinking with images is just the sort of thing that goes on when imagery is not being used, then the postulation of a special image system would be redundant and gratuitous, *regardless of whether we have a worked-out theory of any kind of reasoning*.

A number of important distinctions have to be made before evidence from hundreds of experiments dealing with mental imagery can be properly interpreted. As I suggested above, one serious possibility is that in experiments that ask subjects to solve a problem or answer a question by using their mental image, the subject may interpret the request as one of saying what would happen if he or she were to *see* the corresponding imagined event taking place. But this deflationary explanation requires that we distinguish between (1) explicit and tacit knowledge, (2) patterns of reasoning that arise from habit or preference and patterns that arise because of the nature of the fixed mechanisms involved, and (3) patterns that are intrinsic to reasoning with images and patterns that would arise no matter what form of reasoning was being used. Even if we do find that there are properties intrinsic to reasoning with images, we must still ask whether these arise because certain imagery-specific forms of representation or processing are being deployed or, as is generally claimed, because imagery involves applying specifically *visual* mechanisms to perceive an inner picturelike (depictive) pattern.

6.2   Content, Form, and Substance of Representations

One thing that everyone agrees on is that mental images are *representations*: they encode information about the world. In this and subsequent chapters we will be concerned with visual images that primarily, though not exclusively, encode information about the visible world. When we speak of a representation, there are at last three levels of analysis at which we can theorize (for a detailed discussion of these "levels" see Pylyshyn, 1984a).[2] At the *first* level we can ask about the representation's content, or what the representation *represents*—what it is *about*. The thing represented need not even exist (e.g., we can represent unicorns with no difficulty), and even if it does exist, the content of the representation is different from the thing in the world being represented. That's because the content of the representation consists not only in some particular thing in the world, but also the interpretation or the concept under which it is represented or what it is represented *as*. If we repre-

2. Newell (1980b) refers to these levels as the knowledge level, the symbol level, and the physical level, respectively. He also mentions additional levels that are important in actual digital computers (e.g., the register transfer level). There may, in fact, be reason to include other levels in the case of mental processes (e.g., an abstract neurological level that accounts for additional generalizations) but as far as I am aware none has been proposed so far. (Hebb's 1949 cell assemblies and other such aggregates do not constitute a different level since they do not conform to different principles than do cells themselves.)

sent a certain physical thing as Dr. Jekyll, the representation has a different content than if we represent the very same physical thing as Mr. Hyde. If we represent a certain point of light as the planet Venus, the representation has a different content than if we represent it as the morning star or as the evening star, even though all these representations refer to the very same physical body. The difference in how it is represented (or what it is represented as) has real consequences for potential behavior; how a person represents something will affect how he or she interacts with the world. A great deal has been said about the notion of content in philosophy, but for our purposes we only need to acknowledge that there is more to being a representation than having a certain form.[3] For many purposes we also need to talk about the content of the representation, and we need to distinguish between properties of the representation's form and properties of the representation's content.

At the *second* level of analysis, we can inquire about the *form* of the representation, the system of codes by which mental states can represent aspects of the world. These codes need not be discrete symbols, but they do have to embody some principles by which they combine and by virtue of which they are able to represent novel things—they need to form a productive system (see Fodor and Pylyshyn, 1988). In the case of language, these principles are referred to as the *syntax* of the language. Differences in representational content (in what the linguistic objects represent) arise from corresponding differences in the *form* of the representation, which means the particular terms (codes) that are used and the way they are syntactically structured. I will devote considerable attention in this and the next chapter to the question, What is the *form* of mental images? It is at this level that we can raise such questions as whether mental images use a system of encoding different from that of other forms of thought. The formal or symbol level divides into two kinds of questions: (a) What are the (relatively) fixed computational resources that make up the processes and determine the form that representations may take, and how are they organized (e.g., are they

3. This quick sketch does not do justice to this complex subject. For example, the content of a representation also includes certain logical components (given by logical constants like AND, OR, and NOT) as well as quantifiers (SOME, ALL, EVERY, EXISTS), modalities (MUST, CAN, SHOULD), and propositional attitudes (BELIEVES, KNOWS, FEARS, HOPES).

encapsulated, like early vision, or can they communicate freely among themselves)? (b) What is the structure of representations underlying images (e.g., are they two-dimensional displays, as some have claimed?) and what are the particular processes that underlie reasoning with mental images (e.g., are they visual)?

The *third* level of analysis of mental representations is concerned with how representations are realized in biological tissue. In chapter 7 I will consider evidence at this third level of analysis. We will see that the distinction between the information-processing level and the biological or physical level often gets blurred because both are concerned with the question, *How is the function realized?* These two levels often use the same terminology. For example, they may refer to the "size" of mental images, where a systematic ambiguity is retained between some formal property of images that may be responsible for certain observed experimental phenomena and a literal physical property of its instantiation in brain tissue. We can ask how some process is carried out or how something works in at least two senses or at two different levels of abstraction. One level considers functional or computational mechanisms in information-processing terms, whereas the other focuses on brain mechanisms described in neuroanatomical terms. Unfortunately, knowledge of neural mechanisms is not sufficiently advanced to allow this level of analysis to elucidate the computations or algorithms involved,[4] so typically the most that we get from this level is a general *taxonomy of functions* derived from brain damage and neural imaging data. The other level at which we can address the question of how something is done in the brain is by asking what basic operations and formal properties the brain makes available. This question really belongs to the second (formal) level, though it is often confused with the biological level.

One of the discoveries of the last forty or so years of information-processing psychology is that it is possible to ask the question, *How is it done?* without requiring an answer in terms of biology or physics. To ask how it is done in this more abstract sense is to ask how it is realized

4. Indeed, Randy Gallistel (1994) has pointed out that theorizing about how the brain may carry out certain basic functions is currently stuck in a psychology that was discredited decades ago—a psychology that takes association to be the basic operation, rather than the manipulation of symbols (including real-valued magnitudes processed in a register architecture).

by information-processing resources (basic operations, forms of encoding, types of memory, and so on) that constitute what is known as the *cognitive architecture*. To characterize the cognitive architecture is to provide a more abstract description of the way the brain or computer functions in relation to its capacity to process representations. It is a level of description that captures the essential aspect of information processing abstracted from the sorts of details that differ from occasion to occasion and from person to person.

This notion of cognitive architecture is absolutely central to theorizing about cognitive processes. Elsewhere I have written extensively on the topic of cognitive architecture (Pylyshyn, 1984a, 1991a, 1996). For present purposes I wish to emphasize that the distinction between cognitive architecture and knowledge-based processes arises because these two levels involve different types of explanatory principles, which are often confused in discussions about mental imagery. For example, we have already seen how mental images are often discussed as having a certain form or having certain special properties (e.g., size, distance), when what is meant is that the *content* of those images (or the things referred to or depicted in the images) have these properties. The property of being larger or smaller or being farther or closer are among such properties. There is clearly a difference between claiming that you have an image of something big (or red or heavy or slow, etc.) and claiming that the image itself is big (or red or heavy or slow, etc.).

Although there is general agreement that we need all three levels of description when we discuss systems of representation, these levels have not always been kept distinct. In particular, when one claims that images have certain properties it is important to be clear as to the level at which our claims apply. In chapter 7 we will see that this is especially true when we consider claims such as that images *have* or *preserve* metrical or spatial properties of the world they represent.

6.3   What Is Responsible for the Pattern of Results Obtained in Imagery Studies?

6.3.1   Cognitive architecture or tacit knowledge
The distinction between effects attributable to the intrinsic nature of mental mechanisms and those attributable to more transitory states, such

as people's beliefs, utilities, preferences, habits, or interpretation of the task at hand, is central not only to understanding the nature of mental imagery but to understanding mental processes in general. The former sorts of effects (those attributable to the intrinsic nature of mechanisms) invoke propertie of the cognitive architecture (Fodor and Pylyshyn, 1988; Newell, 1990; Pylyshyn, 1980, 1984a, 1991a, 1996)—one of the most important ideas in cognitive science. Cognitive architecture refers to the set of properties of mind that are fixed with respect to certain kinds of influences. In particular, cognitive architecture is, by definition, not directly altered by changes in knowledge, goals, utilities, or any other representations (e.g., fears, hopes, fantasies, etc.). In other words, when you form an interpretation of a certain task, find out new things about a situation you are thinking about, draw inferences from what you know, or weigh the options and make a decision, your cognitive architecture does not change. Of course, if as a result of your beliefs you decide to take drugs or to change your diet or even to repeat some act over and over, this can result in changes to your cognitive architecture, but such changes are not a direct result of the changes in your cognitive state. A detailed technical exposition of the distinction between effects attributable to knowledge or other cognitive states and those attributable to the nature of cognitive architecture are beyond the scope of this book (although this distinction is the subject of extensive discussion in Pylyshyn, 1984a, chapter 7). This informal characterization and the following example will have to do for present purposes.

To make this point in a more concrete way, I invented a somewhat frivolous but revealing example, involving a mystery box of unknown construction whose pattern of behavior has been assiduously recorded (Pylyshyn, 1984a). This box is known to emit long and short pulses with a reliable recurring pattern. The pattern (illustrated in figure 6.1) can be described as follows: pairs of short pulses usually precede single short pulses, except when a pair of long-short pulses occurs first. In this case the observed regularity, though completely regular when the box is in its "ecological niche," is due not to the nature of the box (to how it is constructed) but to an entirely extrinsic reason. This distinction between two sorts of "reasons" for the observed pattern (intrinsic or extrinsic) is analogous to the architecture versus tacit knowledge distinction and is crucial

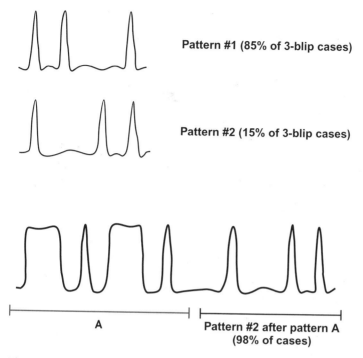

Figure 6.1
Pattern of blips recorded from a box in its typical mode of operation (its "ecological niche"). The question we ask is: Why does it exhibit this pattern of behavior rather than some other? What does this behavior tell us about how it works?

to understanding why the box works the way it does, as well as to why certain patterns of cognition occur.

The reason why this particular pattern of behavior occurs in this case can be appreciated only if we know that the pulses are codes, and the pattern is due to a pattern in *what they represent*, namely, English words spelled out in International Morse Code. The observed pattern does not reflect how the box is wired or its *architecture*; it is due entirely to a pattern in the way English words are spelled (the principle being that generally *i* comes before *e* except after *c*). Similarly, I have argued that many of the patterns observed in mental image research reflect a principle that subjects believe holds in the imagined world, and not a principle of their mental architecture. The patterns arise from the fact that subjects know what would happen if they were to see certain things unfold before their eyes, and so they make the same thing happen in their imagined simulation. The reason that the behavior of both the mystery code box and the cognitive system do not reveal properties of its intrinsic nature (its *architecture*) is that both are capable of quite different regularities if the world they were representing behaved differently. They would not have to change their nature (their "wiring" or their causal structure) in order to change their behavior. The way the behavior can be altered provides the key to how you can tell what is responsible for the observed regularity. This is the basis for the methodological criterion I called "cognitive penetrability" (to be described on pp. 321–325).

Clearly, it is important to distinguish between architectural and knowledge-based explanations in understanding mental imagery. I noted earlier that to understand what goes on in mental imagery it is essential to distinguish the case where (a) people are merely making the mental representation underlying their phenomenal image (whatever that turns out to correspond to in the theory) have the contents that they independently believe would be seen or would occur in certain situations, from the case where (b) it is the very fact of putting their thoughts in the particular form of representation corresponding to a mental image—and thus being constrained by the properties of this form of representation— that is responsible for the outcome. In case (b), the claim is that properties intrinsic to images, to their form or their particular realization in the brain, result in thoughts unfolding the way they do. In other words, in this second case we are claiming that the observed properties of the image-based thoughts are a direct consequence of properties of the special cognitive architecture used in mental imagery. In case (a), where people simply make their image do what they believe would happen if they were seeing the event happen, the properties of the image representation are irrelevant to explaining the way the thoughts unfold: nothing is gained by postulating that an image representation has certain properties, since these properties figure in no explanation and in no way constrain the outcome. Thus, saying that an image is like a picture may reflect the phenomenology of imagery, but if case (a) were the correct analysis of what is going on, the pictorial format would be theoretically irrelevant to explaining the outcome of thinking with images. Thus the phenomenology-based theory of the representation underlying a mental image would be doing no work because the real explanation would lie elsewhere, for example, in what people decided to put into their phenomenal image or what they made it do.

To see that the distinction between knowledge-based and architecture-based accounts of why things work the way they do makes a difference to our understanding of how imagery works, try to imagine a situation whose physical principles are unknown to you. For example, imagine that you have a jar filled with sugar and a jar filled with water. Imagine, in your mind's eye, that the water is slowly poured into the jar of sugar, as shown in figure 6.2. Does the water in the sugar-filled jar begin to overflow, and if so, at what point in the pouring does it do so? In this case it seems clear that what will happen in your imagination will depend on what you know (or believe) would happen in the world if you observed such an experiment being performed. Clearly, your imagination does not embody the subtle principles by which solids dissolve in liquids, which involves understanding how molecules of certain solids can take up the spaces between molecules of the liquid. What happens in your imagination is just exactly what you *think* would happen (perhaps based on what you once saw happen), nothing more. If you believe that it is up to your image to determine what will happen and that it is the properties of your imagery system that generates the result, you would be letting your phenomenal experience cloud your judgment. To see that properties of your image system do not determine how your image behaves, try making your image do something different just by willing it to.

Take another example, one that does not involve such an obscure principle of physics. Ask yourself what color you see if you look at a white

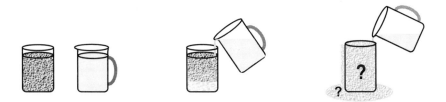

Figure 6.2
What happens when you pour a beaker of water slowly into a beaker already full of sugar? Does the water in the sugar-beaker overflow before the water-beaker has been emptied?

wall through a yellow filter and then gradually superimpose a blue filter over the yellow filter. The way that many of us would go about solving this problem, if we did not know the answer as a memorized fact, is to "imagine" a yellow filter and a blue filter being superimposed. We generally use the "imagine" strategy when we want to solve a problem about how certain things would look. Try this out on yourself. Imagine looking at a white wall through a blue filter and a yellow filter and then bring them into overlapping positions, as illustrated (without the benefit of color) in figure 6.3. What color do you "see" in your mind's eye in the overlap region? More important, why do you see *that* color in your mind's eye rather than some other color? Some people (e.g., Kosslyn, 1981) have argued that the color you see follows from a property of the imagery "medium," from the intrinsic character of the color encoding and display mechanism deployed in imagery, just as the parallel case of visual color mixing arises from the intrinsic character of the color receptors in the eye, together with the character of light that is transmitted through colored filters. But since there can be no doubt that you can make the color of the overlap portion of the filters in your mental image be *any* color you wish, it can't be that the image format or the architecture involved in representing colors is responsible. What else can it

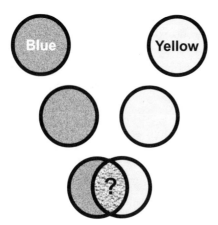

Figure 6.3
Imagine that the two disks shown here are blue and yellow filters or beams of light. Close your eyes and imagine that the disks are moved closer until they overlap. What color do you see in your mental image where the two disks overlap? Why do you see *that* color rather than some other color?

be? This is where the notion of *tacit knowledge* plays an important role in cognitive science (Fodor, 1968; see also pp. 321–325).[5] It seems clear in this case that the color you "see" depends on your tacit knowledge either of principles of color mixing or of these particular color combinations (having seen something like them in the past). In fact, people who do not know about *subtractive* color mixing generally get the above example wrong; mixing yellow light with blue light in the right proportions produces white light, but overlapping yellow and blue filters leads to green light being transmitted.

When asked to do this exercise, some people simply report that they see no color at the intersection, or a washed-out indefinite color. Still others claim that they "see" a color different from the one they report when asked to answer without imagining the filter scenario (as reported in Kosslyn, 1981). Cases such as the latter have made people skeptical of the tacit knowledge explanation. There are indeed many cases where people report a different result when using mental imagery than when they are asked merely to answer the question without using their image. Appeal to tacit (inexplicit) knowledge may be crucial, but that does not mean one can solicit the relevant tacit knowledge by merely asking a subject. It is a general property of reasoning that the way a question is put and the reasoning sequence used to get to the answer can affect the outcome. As I will suggest on pages 313–316, knowledge can be organized in many different ways and it can also be accessed in many different ways—or not accessed at all if it seems like more work than it is worth.

To illustrate this point, consider the following analogue of the color-mixing task. Imagine your third-grade teacher writing the following on a blackboard: "759 + 356 = _____?" Now, as quickly as you can, without stopping to think about it, imagine that the teacher continues writing on the board. What number can you "see" the teacher write in the blank? Now ask yourself why you saw *that* number rather than some other number being written in the blank. People will imagine different things in this case depending on whether they believe that they are

5. Outside of epistemology, people typically do not distinguish between "belief" and "knowledge," so that it may turn out that some "knowledge" might be false or at any rate not justified. I use the term "knowledge" simply because it has been in general use in psychology and in artificial intelligence and the distinction between belief and knowledge is immaterial in the present context.

supposed to work it out or whether in the interest of speed they should guess or merely say whatever comes to mind. Each of these is a *different task*. Even without a theory of what is special about visual imagery, we know that the task of saying what something would look like can be (though it needn't be) a different task from the task of solving a certain intellectual puzzle about colors, as you can see if you consider the difference between the various ways you might go about filling the blank in the arithmetic example. The difference can be like the difference between free-associating to a word and giving its definition. The task of imagining something unfolding in your "mind's eye" is a special task: it's the task of simulating as many aspects of the visual situation as possible, as many aspects as you can—not because you are being led on by the experimenter and not because of some special property of mental imagery, but *because this is what it means to "imagine X happening."*

In most of the cases studied in imagery research, it would be odd if the results did not come out the way picture theories would predict, and if they did, the obvious explanation is that subjects either did not know how things work in reality or else they misunderstood the instructions to "imagine x." For example, if you were asked to construct a vivid and detailed auditory image of a competent performance of the "Minute Waltz," played on a piano in front of you, the failure of the imagined event to take approximately one minute would simply confirm that you had not carried out the task properly (or at all). Taking roughly one minute is inherent in a real performance and thus it is natural to assume it to be indicative of a good imagined re-creation or simulation of such a performance. To realistically imagine a musical performance of a piece *means* to imagine (i.e., think of) each token note being played in the right order and at the right loudness and duration, whether or not it entails that certain sensory qualities are "perceived" by the "mind's ear." In other words, regardless of what else you believe goes on when you imagine hearing the piano piece being played, one thing that the task requires is reproducing a sequence of mental states or thoughts corresponding to "hearing" the sequence of notes in the right order and at roughly the right durations. Thus, in this case, the form of representation involved does not determine the observed outcome (i.e., the time taken) because the outcome is attributable to some of the person's tacit knowledge about the "Minute Waltz."

Finally, let me emphasize again what kind of tacit knowledge is relevant to this discussion, because there has been serious misunderstanding on this question. The only knowledge that is relevant is knowledge of *what things would look like* in certain situations, in particular in situations like the ones in which subjects in mental imagery experiments are to imagine themselves. Thus it is not a criticism of this type of explanation to point out, as Farah (1988, pp. 314–315) does, that people are unlikely to know how their visual system or the visual brain works. That's not the tacit knowledge that is relevant. Nor is it merely the tacit knowledge of what results the experimenter expects (sometimes referred to as "experimenter demand effects") as many have assumed (Finke and Kurtzman, 1981b). Of course, the latter is highly relevant as well and may even explain some of the findings in imagery studies (as suggested by Banks, 1981; Intons-Peterson, 1983; Intons-Peterson and White, 1981; Mitchell and Richman, 1980; Reed, Hock, and Lockhead, 1983; Richman, Mitchell, and Reznick, 1979), but it is not what I mean by the tacit knowledge explanation. All I mean is that subjects in studies where they are asked to "imagine X" use their knowledge of what "seeing X" would be like to simulate as many aspects of the corresponding visual event as they can. Doing this successfully, of course, depends on having certain psychophysical skills, such as the ability to generate time intervals proportional to certain computed magnitudes (Fraisse, 1963), or to compute the time-to-contact of moving objects (as we will see, p. 340).

6.3.2 Problem solving by "mental simulation": Some additional examples

The idea that what happens in certain kinds of problem solving can be viewed as *simulation* has had a recent history in connection not only with mental imagery (Currie, 1995) but also with other sorts of problems in cognitive science (Klein and Crandall, 1995). Take, for example, the question of how we manage (rather successfully) to predict other people's behavior in everyday life. One proposal, referred to as the "off-line simulation" view (so-called because the simulation is not getting its inputs directly from the things being simulated), argues that we do not need to assume that people have a tacit theory of how other people's minds work to anticipate what they will do or how they will feel in various situations. Instead all we need is to put ourselves in their position and ask what *we* would do. This way of putting it still leaves open the question of whether the latter predictions come from a special behavior-generating mechanism in our brain (our cognitive architecture) or from a tacit theory, and the difference is hotly debated in the case of social cognition (some of the arguments are reviewed in Nichols et al., 1996). These two alternatives differ only if the mechanism being appealed to is different from our general reasoning capacity. This in turn means that to be a true alternative to what some have called a theory-theory explanation, the simulation explanation must appeal to an encapsulated or modular architectural system. If it requires general reasoning, which is able to access any relevant knowledge, then the two options are indistinguishable.

Granted that the "simulation mode" of reasoning is used in many kinds of problem solving, two questions remain: (1) Why should this mode be used at all, as opposed to some more direct way of solving the problem, and (2) When it is used, what does the real work of solving the problem—a special part of our mental architecture that deals with a special form of image representation, or a general reasoning system that draws inferences from tacit knowledge? I have already suggested one major reason why subjects might use the simulation mode in imagery studies: the task of imagining something invites it, since the task of "imagining X" is properly understood as the task of pretending that you are looking at situation X unfolding and you report the sequence of events that you would see (in the right order and in roughly correct relative times). Even without instructions from an experimenter, the simulation mode is often natural because of the nature of the task. For example, if it is a task that you would normally carry out by making a series of actions and observing what happens, you might be tempted to imagine doing the same thing. Imagery is most often used for tasks that ask what would happen in a certain counterfactual (what if . . . ?) situation involving perceivable spatiotemporal events.

In what follows I will sketch a number of extremely influential experimental results and compare explanations given in terms of inherent properties of the image (the architecture of the image system) and those given in terms of the simulation-from-tacit-knowledge explanation (and other considerations as well) that need not assume any particular form of representation.

Scanning mental images   Probably the most cited result in the entire repertoire of research motivated by the picture theory is the image-scanning phenomenon. Not only has this experimental paradigm been used dozens of times, but various arguments about the metrical or spatial nature of mental images, as well as arguments about such properties of the mind's eye as its "visual angle," rest on this phenomenon. Indeed, it has been referred to as a "window on the mind" (Denis and Kosslyn, 1999).

The image-scanning result is the following: it takes longer to "see" a feature in a mental image the further away it is from an object in the image on which one has been focusing. So for example, if you are asked to imagine a dog and inspect its nose and then to look at its tail, it will take you longer to "see" the tail than if you were asked to first inspect its hind legs and then to look at its tail. Here is an actual experiment, perhaps the most cited result in all the imagery research literature (first reported by Kosslyn 1973). Subjects were asked to memorize a map such as the one in figure 6.4. They were then asked to imagine the map and to focus their attention on one landmark on it, say, the "church." In a typical experiment (there are many variants of this basic study), the experimenter says the name of a second landmark in the image (say, "beach" or "tree"), whereupon subjects must examine their image and press a button as soon as they can "see" the second-named place in their image. What Kosslyn (and many others since) found is that the further away the second place is (on the actual map) from the place on which subjects are initially focused, the longer it takes to "see" the second place in their "mind's eye." From this result most researchers have concluded that *greater distances on the imagined map are represented by greater distances in some (mental) space*. In other words, they concluded that mental images *have* spatial properties, that is, they have spatial magnitudes or distances. This is a strong conclusion about cognitive architecture. It says, in effect, that the symbolic code idea I discussed earlier does not apply to mental images. In a symbolic encoding two places can be represented as a certain distance away in many ways, for example it can

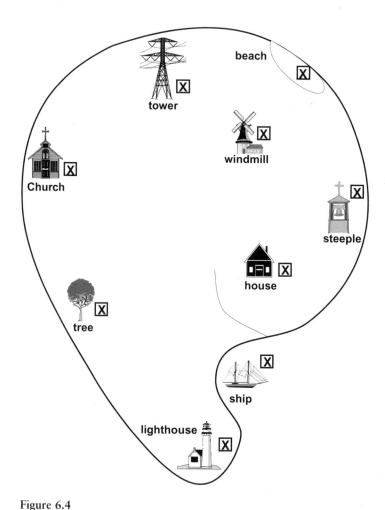

Figure 6.4
Example of a map, such as that used by Kosslyn (1973) and others, that is memorized and then imagined in order to study mental scanning. Subjects are asked
to fix their attention on one landmark in their image and then to glance up at
another named landmark and report (by pressing a button) when they can see
it in their "mind's eye." The reaction time to report "seeing" the second landmark in their image is measured and is found to be a linear function of the distance between the two landmarks in the original map. The question raised in the
text is: Why does this linear relation hold and what does it tell us about the form
of the mental representation of the map?

be done the way it is done in language; by saying the places are *n* units from one another. But the representation of larger distances is not itself in any sense larger. The question then is: Is this conclusion about architecture warranted in the case of mental images? Does the difference in time in this case reveal a property of the architecture or a property of what is represented? This exactly parallels the situation in the color-mixing example I discussed earlier where I asked whether a particular regularity revealed a property of the architecture or a property of what people know or believe—a property of the represented situation of which they have tacit knowledge. To answer this question we need to determine whether the pattern of increasing scanning time arises from a fixed capacity of the image-representation or image-processing system, or whether the time it takes can be changed by changing the beliefs that subjects hold about how things are in the world or about what they are supposed to do in this experiment. In other words, we need to ask whether the empirical regularity is cognitively penetrable.

This is a question to be settled in the usual way, by careful analyses and experiments. But even before we do the experiment there is reason to suspect that the time-course of scanning is not a property of the cognitive architecture. Do the following test on yourself. Imagine that there are lights at each of the places on your mental image of the map in figure 6.4. Imagine that a light goes on at, say, the beach. Now imagine that this light goes off and instantly another light comes on at the lighthouse. Did you need to scan your attention across the image to see this happen—to see the light come on at the lighthouse? Liam Bannon and I repeated the scanning experiment (see the description in Pylyshyn, 1981b) by showing subjects a real map mounted on a display board, with lights at the target locations, as I just described. We allowed the subjects to turn lights on and off. Whenever a light was turned on at one location it was simultaneously extinguished at another location. Then we asked subjects to imagine the map and to indicate (by pressing a button) when they could "see" the second illuminated place in their image. The time it took to press the button was recorded and its correlation to the distances between illuminated places on the map was computed. We found that there was no relation between distance on the imagined map and time. You might think: of course there was no increase in time with increasing distance; subjects were not asked to imagine scanning that distance! But that's just the point: you can imagine scanning over the imagined map if you want to, or you can imagine just hopping from place to place on the imaginary map. If you imagine scanning, you can imagine scanning fast or slow, at a constant speed or at some variable speed, or scanning part way and then turning back or circling around. You can, in fact, do whatever you please since it is *your* image and *your* imagining.[6] At least you can do these things to the extent that you know what it would be like if you were to see them and so long as you are able to generate the relevant measurements, such as the time you estimate it would take to get from point to point.

My proposal regarding the scanning experiment and many other such experiments involving mental images is that the task of imagining invites observers to pretend (in whatever way they can) that they are looking at some situation and then to use whatever knowledge they have and whatever problem-solving technique seems to them most relevant, to generate the appropriate sequence of mental states (notice I do not say that they generate the answer they believe is wanted, but that they generate some sequence of mental states). The criticism of the scanning studies is not that the investigators have failed to control for something and have allowed an artifact to contaminate the results. It is that a proper understanding of the task requires that subjects try to do certain things; that is what is meant by a "task demand." Other investigators have confirmed the relevance of task demands (Intons-Peterson, 1983; Intons-Peterson and White, 1981; Mitchell and Richman, 1980; Reed et al., 1983; Richman et al., 1979). Yet when these criticisms are discussed in the literature, they are often understood as the criticism that the results are obtained by the experimenter leading the subject, or by subjects' complying with the experimenter's expectations. This may often be true, but the deeper point is that subjects are mostly just doing the task, as they

6. When we first carried out these studies we were (quite rightly, in my view) criticized on the grounds that it was obvious that you did not have to scan your image if you did not want to, and if you did you could do so according to whatever temporal pattern you chose. It still seems to me that the studies we did (including the one described below) only demonstrate the obvious. That being the case one might well wonder what the fuss is about over the scanning phenomenon (as well as the image size phenomenon describe below); why dozens of studies have been done on it and why it is interpreted as showing *anything* about the nature of mind, as opposed to choices that subjects make.

understand it, that is pretending that they are looking at a map and seeing places on it (or seeing some sequence of events occur).

Notice that whether or not you choose to simulate a certain temporal pattern of events in the course of answering a question may depend in part on whether simulating that particular pattern seems to be relevant to the task. It is not difficult to set up an experimental situation in which simulating the actual scanning from place to place does not appear to be so obviously relevant to solving a particular problem. For example, we ran the following experiment that also required retrieving information from an imagined map by focusing attention on various locations on the map (Pylyshyn, 1981b). Subjects were asked to memorize the same map as I described above and to refer to their image of the map in solving the problem. Rather than imagining looking at one place on the map and then looking for a second named place and indicating when they could "see" it (as in the original studies by Kosslyn et al., 1978), the task was instead to indicate the direction (in terms of a clock face) from the second named place to the previously focused place (for example, using the map in figure 6.4, they might be asked to focus on the tower and then to indicate what direction the tower is from the tree; the correct answer being "at 1 o'clock"). This direction-judgment task requires that the subject make a judgment from the perspective of the second place, so if anything requires using the image and focusing at the second place on the imagined map this is certainly a good candidate. Yet in this experiment, the question of how you get from focusing on the first place to focusing on the second place on the map was less prominent than it was in the task to "examine the map and indicate when you can see *X*," especially when that request was presented right after the subject had been asked to focus on another place on the map. The second task required that subjects concentrate on the relative directions between two places once both places had been retrieved, rather than on how they got from one place to the next or on how far away the two places were on the map. In this case we found that the distance between places had no effect on the time taken to answer the question. Thus it seems that the effect of distance on reaction time is cognitively penetrable.

People have sometimes suggested that one can accommodate the finding that the "scanning effect" is cognitively penetrable by noting that the observed behavior depends both on the form of the image and on the particular processes that use it, so that the differences in the process in this case might account for the different result one gets in different contexts. This is true; but then what explanatory work is being done by the alleged spatial property of the image? Whenever we appeal to the nature of the process, then the hypothesized properties of the image play no role. The claim has to be that under specified conditions the metrical properties of images is exhibited. But the specified conditions mustn't be defined circularly. The claim that we get the scanning effect only when subjects imagine that they are scanning their attention from place to place and not when they are hopping from place to place may well be true, but then is there anything that the image format restricts them from imagining? The answer is surely that people can imagine whatever they wish. What, then, does claiming that images are spatial commit one to? So long as the assumption that there is a spatial representation that "preserves metrical distance" does not constrain possible behavior, it plays no role in the explanation; it remains theoretically irrelevant.[7]

Not only can observers move their attention from one imagined object to another without scanning continuously through the space between them, but we have reason to believe that they actually *cannot* move their attention continuously, as though smoothly tracking an imagined movement. In interviews after the study, many subjects said that they did not feel they moved or scanned their attention *smoothly* through intermediate locations. They claimed that they did not notice (or "see") objects at intermediate locations in their mental image in the course of their scanning, unless the objects were relevant to the task. This led us to wonder whether it was even possible to continuously scan an image as required by Kosslyn's display-scanning model. The model claims that in getting from *A* to *B* in a mental image you must trace a path that takes you through all intermediate points (within the resolution of the image), just

7. Kosslyn insists that the medium does provide constraints. According to Kosslyn, "The subjects apparently can control some aspects of processing, such as speed of scanning, but not others; in particular, they could not eliminate the effects of distance on the time to shift attention across an imaged object" (1994, p. 11). But this is flatly contradicted by our data, as well as one's personal experience of being able to hop around on one's image. In fact, Kosslyn's earlier model (Kosslyn et al., 1979) had a jump operation specifically to acknowledge that flexibility.

as a moving spot or a smooth eye movement would visit such places in the corresponding case of a real map. Without this assumption there is no reason to predict that the time it takes to scan a certain distance should be proportional to the distance. But both introspection and objective studies suggest that we are unable to actually *move* an imagined point through a smooth set of invisible places along a mental scan path. In fact, Jonathan Cohen and I (Pylyshyn and Cohen, 1999) carried out a number of experiments that show that observers are poor at judging where an imagined moving object is located at various times during its imagined passage through a region where there are no visible elements (e.g., in the dark). This suggests that the imagined object does not actually *pass through* a sequence of locations, a suggestion that I will defend later in this chapter (p. 340).

Given that the times for mental scanning are actually computed, as opposed to observed in the course of scanning a mental image, one might well wonder why people bother to imagine a point of focus being scanned (even if not continuously) across their image? In the case of scanning while looking at a scene, the answer is clear; the physics of the eye and the architecture of attention scanning requires that the point of focus pass through intervening locations. But why should people persist on using this method when scanning entirely in their imagination where the laws of physics and the principles of spatial attention scanning do not apply (since there is no real space)? Assuming that people actually do use the mental scanning strategy in their imagination, a possible reason, already alluded to earlier, is that when using the simulation mode to imagine solving a problem, people may carry over strategies that they use in real situations, where the strategy is clearly the appropriate one. Inasmuch as they are being asked to imagine that they are seeing something, it makes sense to imagine what would have happened in the visual case.

Consider the example presented by Pinker, Choate, and Finke (1984), in which people claim they "extrapolate" an arrow, whose location and direction is not seen but retrieved from memory, to determine whether the arrow points at a particular dot in a recalled image. In this task, Pinker et al. found an effect of distance on response time (although interpreting this result is not unproblematic given that the response times involved are much longer than reported mental scanning times; see

Pylyshyn, 2002). But extrapolating a line from the arrow is clearly the right strategy *if you have ruler and a rigid surface*, since in that case you would be able to see whether the extrapolated line would intersect the dot. It may also be the right strategy to use if you can see the arrow and the dots, since that judgment can make use of some of our precise psychophysical skills, such as judging whether several visual elements are collinear or whether two line segments are aligned, as they are in the case of vernier acuity measurement. It may even be the right strategy to use when a perceived arrow is superimposed on a perceived screen and subjects have to judge whether the arrow points to dots that had been on the screen shortly before (as was the case in the earlier experiment by Finke and Pinker, 1982), since in that situation subjects can use their ability to visually index features in the display (even a uniform screen), and their high-capacity visual short-term memory. But in the purely imagined case (where both the arrow and the dot must be recalled from memory), the problem for the theorist is not to explain why that strategy was used (it was probably used because it was the appropriate thing to do in the situation being imagined and the subject was simulating what would happen in a perceived situation), but rather to explain how such a strategy could possibly work without a real display. Unless you believe in a literal picture theory (in which case you have a lot of other problems, as we will see in the next chapter), drawing a mental line in mental space cannot solve the problem, because mental lines do not actually *have* the property that when they are extrapolated they intersect appropriately situated mental objects. In imagining the line being drawn you don't actually draw anything, all you do is *imagine that* (i.e., think the thought that) the line is initially short and gets progressively longer. And you don't need a special form of representation to do that. All you need is a representational system capable of representing (not of *having*) various lengths and distances. But if there is no physical line on a physical surface, of course, no perceptual judgments can be based on such thoughts (which may account for the strong allure of the literal picture theory). Therefore, the judgments are being made by some other means, which, as usual in such cases, is not available to introspection. This question is closely related to the general question of where the spatial character of mental images comes from. I will take up that question in the next chapter (especially in section 7.3).

The "size" of mental images   Here is another example of a widely cited result that might well be attributed to the use of tacit knowledge to simulate the imagined event. Consider the finding that it takes more time to report some visual detail of an imagined object when the object is imagined to be small compared to when it is imagined to be large (e.g., it takes longer to report that a mouse has whiskers if the mouse is imagined as tiny than if it is imagined as huge; see Kosslyn, 1980, chap. 9). This seems a clear candidate for being the result of an implied requirement of the imagery task. For if you are asked to imagine something small then you are likely to imagine it as having fewer visible details than if you are asked to imagine it looming large directly in front of you, *whatever* form of representation that involves. One reason you might do this is that when you actually *see* a small object (or an object that is far away) you can make out fewer of its details owing to the limited resolution of your eye. If you are to accurately simulate the visual experience of seeing an object, then in the case of a small object you have to take additional steps to make the details available (e.g., imagine bringing the object closer or zooming in on it). But what does it mean to make your image "larger"? Such a notion is obviously meaningful only if the image *has* a real size or scale. If the image is encoded as a symbol structure, then size has no literal meaning. You can *think of* something as larger or smaller, but that does not make some *thing* in your brain larger or smaller. On the other hand, *which details are represented* in your imagination does have a literal meaning: you can put more or less detail into your working memory or your active representation. So if this is what the task demands when the mouse is imagined as "large" then the result is predictable without any notion of real scale applying to the image.

The obvious test of this proposal is to apply the criterion of cognitive penetrability. Are there instructions that can counteract the effect of the "image size" manipulation, making details easier to report in small images than in large ones and vice versa? Can you imagine a small but high-resolution or very detailed view of an object, in contrast to a large but low-resolution view or a view that for some reason lacks details? Surely you can, though I know of no one who has bothered to carry out an experiment such as asking subjects to report details from a large blurry image versus a small clear one. There is a good reason to forgo such an experiment. Consider what it would mean if such an experiment were done and showed that it takes longer to report details in a large blurry object than in a small clear one? Would this show that it is the presence of visible details rather than size that is the relevant determiner of response time? Surely we expect that examining a blurry object will lead to difficulty in reporting its fine-grained properties. To see that there is a semantic issue involved here, think about what it would mean if, instead, people were *faster* in reporting details from a blurry mental image than from a clear one or if it was faster to report details from a small image than from a large image. The strangeness of such a possibility should alert us to the fact that what is wrong lies in what it *means* to have a small versus a large mental image, or a blurry versus a clear image. Such results would be incompatible with what happens in *seeing*. If one failed to see fine details in a large object there would have to be a reason for it, such as that you were seeing it through a fog or out of focus or on a noisy TV, and so on. As long as examining a visual image *means* simulating what it is like to see something, this must necessarily be the case.

Given the rather obvious reason for the parallels between vision and imagery in such cases one might even wonder how studies of mental image inspection could fail to show that it parallels the case of seeing, assuming that observers know more or less what it would be like to see the object that is being imagined. This applies to any property of seeing of which observers have some tacit knowledge or recollection. For example, it applies to the finding that the acuity map of mental images appears to roughly duplicate the acuity map of vision (Finke and Kosslyn, 1980). As noted earlier, observers do not need to have articulated scientific knowledge of visual acuity; all they need is to remember roughly how far into the periphery of their visual field things can be before they cease to be discriminable, and it is not surprising that this is duplicated in imagery, especially when subjects are asked to turn their head (with eyes closed) and pretend to be looking at objects in their visual periphery. This methodology also illustrates the well-known phenomenon that recall is better when the recollection takes place in an environment similar to the one that obtained in the situation being recalled.

The case of image size is a classical example of the common confusion (referred to in philosophy as the "intentional fallacy") between properties of the represented world and properties of the representation, or the vehicle through which the mind represents the world. It is the error of attributing to the representation properties that hold of what is represented. It can also be seen as the failure to keep clear the distinction between the semantic or knowledge level and the syntactic or symbol level in psychological explanations. This failure (to which we will return in section 7.2.1) is well illustrated in the cartoon by the science cartoonist Sydney Harris (fig. 6.5).

Mental "paper folding"   The examples discussed so far suggest that many of the mental imagery findings may be a result of subjects' simulating what they think would happen if they were witnessing the imagined event taking place. But why should people go through the trouble of simulating a situation if they already know (albeit tacitly) what the answer is? Several reasons were considered earlier (pp. 301–302)

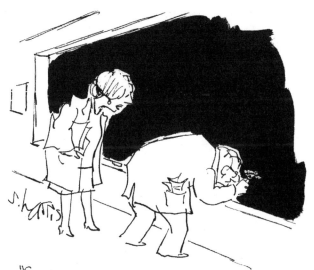

"SURE, WE'RE DEALING WITH TINY PARTICLES, BUT YOUR FORMULA IS JUST A SYMBOLIC REPRESENTATION."

Figure 6.5
The point of this cartoon is self-explanatory: We must not confuse properties of what is represented with intrinsic properties of representations themselves. (S. Harris, from *American Scientist*, 66, p. 647; reprinted with the artist's permission.)

including the implied task demands. But there is another important reason we have not yet discussed, related to how the relevant tacit knowledge is organized. Consider the question: What is the fourth (or *n*th) letter after "M" in the alphabet? To answer that question, people normally have to go through the alphabetical sequence (and it takes them longer the larger the value of *n*). (This works even if the question is "Is R *before* M in the alphabet?"—the time it takes depends on how far apart the two letters are in the alphabet).

A somewhat more complex example, which may well also involve the same principle, applies to a paper-folding task studied by Shepard and Feng (1972). In their experiment, subjects are asked to mentally fold pieces of paper shown in a drawing (examples of which are shown in figure 6.6), and to report whether the arrows marked on the paper would touch one another. Try this yourself. You will find, as they did, that the more folds it would require to actually fold the paper to check whether the arrows coincide, the longer the task takes when done using imagery. Shepard and Feng (1972) took this to indicate that working with images parallels working with real objects. Elsewhere, Shepard and Chipman (1970) call this principle "second-order isomorphism" and claim that it

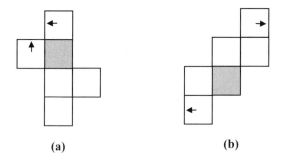

(a)   (b)

Figure 6.6
Two of the figures used by Shepard and Feng (1972) to study the mental operations involved in "mental folding." The task is to imagine the outlined shape as paper templates and to imagine folding the paper (using the dark shaded square as the base) until you can judge whether the arrows in the templates will coincide. The time it takes to solve this task in your mind increases with the number of folds that would be required actually to fold such a paper template. (Adapted from Shepard and Feng, 1972.) Again, the question is: What does this tell us about how the paper template is represented and how the task is carried out, and why it is carried out in that way rather than in some other way?

is a general property of mental images (though I have argued that such a principle may be true of any empirically adequate functional model, regardless of the form of representation used; see Pylyshyn, 1984a, p. 203).

The question we need to ask about this task is the same as the question we asked in the case of the color-mixing task: what is responsible for the relation between time taken to answer the question and the number of folds it would take to fold the corresponding real piece of paper? This time the answer is not simply that it depends on tacit knowledge, because in this case it is not just the content of the tacit knowledge that makes the difference. Possessing the relevant tacit knowledge would explain why it was possible for subjects to imagine folding the paper at all. As in the earlier examples, if you are asked to imagine folding a sheet of paper then you are required (on pain of failing to follow the instructions) to imagine each individual step of the folding. But in the present case one would presumably get the same result even if one did not ask the subject to imagine folding the paper. Yet it is still hard to see how you could answer this question without imagining going through the sequence of folds. Why should this be so? A plausible explanation, which does not appeal to properties of a special imagery system, is that the observed time difference has to do with how knowledge of the effect of folding is organized—just as in the alphabet example. What we know by rote about the effects of paper folding is just this: *we know what happens when we make one fold.* Consequently, to determine what would happen in a task that (in the real world) would require four folds, we have to apply our one-fold-at-a-time knowledge four times.

Recall the parallel case with letters: to name the fourth letter after M we have to apply the "next letter" rote knowledge four times. In both the alphabet case and the paper-folding case subjects could presumably memorize the results of macro-operations. They could commit to memory such facts as which letter of the alphabet occurred two (or *n*) letters after a given letter; or, in the case of the paper-folding task, they could memorize such facts as what results from double folds of different types. If that were how knowledge is organized, the results discussed above would most likely no longer hold. The important point, once again, is that the experimental result may tell us what sequence people go through in solving a problem (that's the "second-order isomorphism" phenomenon), but it tells us nothing about *why* people must go through that sequence rather than some other. It also does not tell us about how the states of the problem are represented and whether one needs to appeal to any special properties of image representations to explain the results. In this case it tells us only what knowledge the person has and how it is organized.

The role played by the structure of knowledge is ubiquitous and may account for another common observation about the use of mental imagery in recall. We know that some things are easier to recall than others and that it is easier to recall some things when the recall is preceded by the recall of other things. Knowledge is linked in various intricate ways. To recall what you did on a certain day it helps first to recall what season it was, what day of the week it was, where you were at the time, and so on. Sheingold and Tenney (1982), Squire and Slater (1975), and others have shown that one's recall of distant events is far better than one generally believes because once the process of retrieval begins it provides clues for subsequent recollections. The reason for bringing up this fact about recall is that such sequential dependencies are often cited as evidence for the special nature of imagery (Bower, 1976; Paivio, 1971). Thus, for example, to determine how many windows are there in your home, you probably need to imagine each room in turn and look around to see where the windows are, counting them as you go. To recall whether someone you know has a beard (or glasses or red hair) you may have to first recall an image of that person. Apart from the phenomenology of recalling an appearance, what is going on is absolutely general to every form of memory retrieval. Memory access is not well understood, but at least it is known that it has sequential dependencies and other sorts of access paths and that these paths are often dependant on spatial arrangements (which is why the "method of loci" works well as a mnemonic device).

Mental rotation   One of the earliest and most cited results in the research on the manipulation of mental images is the "mental rotation" finding. Shepard and Metzler (1971) showed subjects pairs of drawings of three-dimensional figures, such as those illustrated in figure 6.7, and asked them to judge whether the two objects depicted in the drawings were identical except for orientation. Half the cases were mirror-images

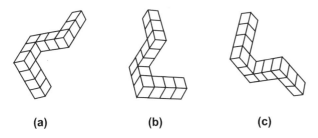

(a)   **(b)**   **(c)**

Figure 6.7
Examples similar to those used by Shepard and Metzler (1971) to show "mental rotation." The time it takes to decide whether two figures are identical except for rotation, as in the pair (a, b), or are 3D mirror images (called "enantiomorphs"), as in the pair (a, c), increases linearly as the angle between them increases, no matter whether the rotation is in the plane or in depth. What does this tell us about how the shapes are represented and what operations we are required to perform on them to solve the problem? (Adapted from Shepard and Metzler, 1971. Copyright 1971, American Association for the Advancement of Science.)

of one another (or the 3D equivalent, called "enantiomorphs") and therefore could not be brought into correspondence by a rotation. Shepard and Metzler found that the time it took to make the judgment is a linear function of the angular displacement between the pair of objects depicted (except when the angle is over 180 degrees, when, in some cases, the time it took was proportional to the angular distance remaining—i.e., to the angle measured counterclockwise).

This result has been universally interpreted as showing that images are "rotated" continuously and at constant speed in the mind and that this is, in fact, the means by which the comparison is made: we rotate one of the pair of figures until the two are sufficiently in alignment that it is possible to see whether they are the same or different. The phenomenology of the Shepard and Metzler task is clearly that we rotate the figure in making the comparison. I question neither the phenomenology, nor the description that what goes on in this task is "mental rotation." But there is some question about what these results tell us about the nature of mental images. The important question is not whether we can or do imagine rotating a figure, but what it means to say that the image is rotated—what exactly is rotated—and whether we solve the problem *by means of* mental rotation. For mental rotation to be the mechanism by which the solution is arrived at, its utility would have to depend on some intrinsic property of images. For example, it might be the case that during mental rotation the figure moves *as a rigid form* through a continuum of angles, thus capitalizing on an intrinsic property of the image format that maintains the form in a rigid manner. Also relevant to this explanation is the question of whether we are *required* to apply this particular transformation in order to compare two shapes in different orientations. Not surprisingly, it turns out to be important that the mismatches be ones in which the figures have the same features but are enantiomorphic images; otherwise, observers simply look for distinguishing features and no mental rotation ensues (Hochberg and Gellman, 1977). There are two points to be made about this mental rotation phenomenon.

First, contrary to the general assumption, the figural "rotation" could not be a holistic process that operates on an entire figure, changing its orientation continuously while rigidly retaining its shape. In the original 3D rotation study (Shepard and Metzler, 1971), the two comparison figures were displayed at the same time. A record of eye movements made while doing this task reveals that observers look back and forth many times between the two figures, checking for distinct features (Just and Carpenter, 1976). This point was also made using simpler 2D figures, where it was found that observers concentrate on significant milestone features when carrying out the task (Hochberg and Gellman, 1977), and that when such milestone features are present, no "rotation" is found. In studies reported in Pylyshyn, 1979b, I showed that what counts as the "rate of rotation" (the rate of change of reaction time as a function of the angle of mismatch) depends both on the complexity of the figure and on the complexity of the postrotation comparison task (I used a task in which observers had to indicate whether or not a misoriented test figure was embedded in the original figure, as shown in figure 6.8). The fact that the apparent the "rate of rotation" depends on such organizational factors shows that whatever is going on in this case does not appear to consist merely in "rotating" a shape in a rigid manner until it is in rough correspondence with the reference figure.

Second, even if the process of making the comparison in some sense involves the "rotation" of a represented shape, this tells us nothing about the form of the representation and does not support the view that the

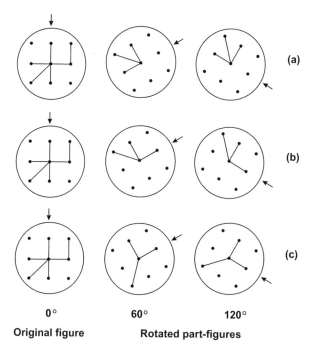

0°   **60°**   **120°**

Original figure   **Rotated part-figures**

Figure 6.8
Figures used in Pylyshyn (1979b) to show that mental rotation is not a holistic process. The task was to indicate whether the figures in the second and third columns are *parts of* the figure in the first column. The part-figures varied in how "good" a subpart they were (as reported by Palmer, 1977) and in the angle through which they would have to be rotated to fit into the whole figure. Row (a) shows a "good" subpart, row (b) shows a "poor" subpart, and row (c) shows a figure that is not a subpart of the original figure. Results showed a "rotation" effect (larger angles took longer) but the "rate of rotation" depended on how good a subpart the probe figure was. (From Pylyshyn, 1979b.)

representation is pictorial. The notion that a representation maintains its shape because of the inherent rigidity of the image while it is rotated cannot be literally what happens, notwithstanding the phenomenology. Since the *representation* is not literally being rotated—neither the brain cells that encode the figure nor any other form of encoding is being moved in a circular motion—the closest to a "rotation" that might be happening is that a representation of a figure is being processed in such a way as to produce a representation of a figure at a slightly different orientation, and then this process is iterated. There are undoubtedly good reasons, based on computational resource considerations, why the process might proceed by iterating over successive small angles (thus causing the comparison time to increase with the angular disparity between the figures) rather than attempt the comparison in one step. For example, small rotations, at least in 3D, result in small relative displacements of component parts of the form and decrease the likelihood of a new aspect coming into view.[8] As a result, incremental rotation might require less working memory to ensure the maintenance of the relative location and connectivity of parts of the figure, using a constraint propagation method such as is commonly used in computer vision systems (and discussed on pp. 99–106). Recognition of constraints on working memory led Marr and Nishihara to hypothesize what they called a SPASAR mechanism for rotating simple vertices formed by pairs of lines and obtaining their projection onto a new reference frame (see Marr and Nishihara, 1976; a slightly different version that left out the details of the SPASAR mechanism was later published in Marr and Nishihara, 1978). This was an interesting idea that entailed a limited analog operation on a small feature of a representation. Yet the Marr and Nishihara proposal did not postulate a pictorial representation, nor did it assume that a rigid configuration was maintained by an image in the course of its "rotation." It hypothesized a particular operation on parts of a structured representation (which might be viewed as an analog operation) that was responsive to a computational complexity issue.

In the context in which two differently oriented figures are being compared for whether they are identical or mirror images, the linear relation

---

8. An *aspect* is a topological structure of the edges, junctions, cusps, and other discontinuities, of a single viewpoint of an object. As the point of view changes, a small amount an aspect is likely to remain the same, constituting a set of stable vantage points. With larger changes new discontinuities come into view, resulting in sudden changes in aspect called *events*. The graph of discrete aspects and their interconnections is termed a graph of the *visual potential* (sometimes called an aspect graph) of an object and has been used in computer vision for characterizing a shape by its potential aspects (Koenderink, 1990). Going from one aspect to a very different one in the course of recognizing a complex object is computationally costly; consequently, in recognizings figures from two different vantage points, it makes sense to move gradually through the aspect graph, traversing adjacent aspects one at a time. This suggests that one should compare pairs of misaligned shapes by a gradual aspect-by-aspect change in point of view, resulting in a discrete sequence that may appear as a "rotation."

between angle and time seems to be robust and does not appear to be cognitively penetrable. It is thus not a candidate for a straightforward tacit knowledge explanation (as I tried to make clear in Pylyshyn, 1979b). Rather, the most likely explanation is one that appeals to the computational requirements of the task and to general architectural (e.g., working memory) constraints. It therefore applies regardless of the form of the representation. Nothing follows from the increase in time with angle concerning either the form of the representation of the figures or the inherent properties of a representational medium, which ensures the maintenance of the shape of an object through different orientations. Nor does the empirical finding suggest that the representation must be manipulated as a whole and must pass smoothly through intermediate angles. The problem of accounting for the linear relation of the angle between figures and the time to make the comparison is not resolved by talk of image "rotation." After all, we still need to say what, if anything, is rotated in mental rotation experiments. An "image rotation" story can be explanatory only if we are willing to attribute causality to the phenomenal experience, which few people are willing to do once it is pointed out that this is what the account entails.

6.3.3   A note concerning cognitive penetrability and the appeal to tacit knowledge

How can you tell whether certain patterns of observations made while a subject is solving a problem tell us about the nature of the architecture of the imagery system or about the person's tacit knowledge and the way it is organized? One diagnostic I have advocated, and discussed at length in Pylyshyn, 1984a, is to test for the cognitive penetrability of the observed pattern. Because many of my criticisms of particular conclusions that have been drawn from imagery research have been based on this criterion, the criterion has been criticized by picture-theorists. And because so much of this criticism has been based on misunderstandings of the role that this criterion plays, I will devote some space to a discussion of this issue.

If the reason for a particular pattern of observations (say, the pattern of reaction times for variants of the task) is that people are simulating a situation based on their tacit knowledge of what it would look like, then if we alter the knowledge or the assumptions about the task, say, by varying the instructions so as to change people's beliefs about the task situation, the observations may change accordingly in a way that is rationally connected with the new beliefs. This is the basis of the criterion of cognitive penetrability. For example, if we instruct a person on the principles of color mixing, we would expect the answer to the imaginal color-mixing question discussed earlier to change appropriately. Similarly, if you ask people to tell you when they see certain details in an image after they have been focusing on a certain place, then depending on subjects' beliefs, the time it takes may be altered. For example, if subjects do not believe that they have to scan the image to see the details, or if they believe that in the visual situation a light will come on immediately after the second place is named, then there may not be a linear relation between distance in the image and reaction time (as I showed experimentally; see pp. 305–307). But, as is the case with all methodological criteria, cognitive penetrability cannot be applied blindly. Even when some behavior depends on tacit knowledge, the behavior cannot always be appropriately altered with instructions, and you certainly can't discover what tacit knowledge subjects have merely by asking them. This is a point that has been made forcibly in connection with tacit knowledge of grammar and of social conventions, which also typically cannot be articulated by members of a linguistic or social group, even though violations are easily detected.

In using the cognitive penetrability criterion, it is important to recognize that the fact that an imagery-related pattern of observation is cognitively impenetrable does not mean that the pattern arises from properties of the mental image or of image-manipulating mechanisms. Many behaviors that are clearly dependent on specific knowledge are immune from cognitive influence (e.g., phobias and obsessive behaviors). In general, when people are shown that some belief they hold is false, they do not immediately change it; beliefs are generally resistant to change, so being impenetrable by relevant information is not sufficient for concluding that some regularity arises not from tacit knowledge but rather from a property of the architecture of the image system. Moreover, as I noted earlier, not every aspect of patterns observed in mental imagery experiments is due to tacit knowledge, and therefore not all aspects of these patterns need be cognitively penetrable. Consider the following example, in which the cognitive impenetrability of some part of a pattern of observation has been taken as evidence against the tacit knowledge explanation of the entire pattern. In a series of experiments on mental scanning, Finke and Pinker (1982) found that the time required to judge that an arrow points to a memory image of a dot increases the further away the dot is from the arrow. Nonetheless, Finke and Pinker argued that this case of mental scanning could not have been due to tacit knowledge (contra my claim, discussed on pp. 303–310). The reason they gave was that although subjects correctly predicted that judgments would take more time when the dots were further away, they failed to predict that the time would actually be longer for the shortest distance used in the study. Of course, neither could the authors—and the reason is that the aberrant short-distance time was most likely due to some entirely different mechanism (perhaps the effect of "attentional crowding" in the original visual display) from that which caused the monotonic increase of time with distance, a mechanism not known to either the subjects or the experimenters.

A major reason why one sometimes observes phenomena in imagery studies that are not attributable to knowledge is precisely the reason recognized by Finke and Freyd (1989): most observed phenomena have more than one cause. Even when tacit knowledge is the main determiner of the observed pattern, other factors also contribute. Because of this, cognitive impenetrability has to be used to examine specific proposed mechanisms, not entire experimental results. Moreover, cognitive penetrability is a *sufficient but not necessary condition* for attributing a pattern to the tacit knowledge held by subjects in these experiments. If a particular pattern is penetrable by changing beliefs, we can conclude that it is due to tacit knowledge; but if it is not penetrable, it may or may not be due to tacit knowledge, and it may or may not be attributable to some property of the imagery architecture.

Another example of the mistaken inference from cognitive impenetrability to assumed properties of the imagery system concerns what has been called "representational momentum." It was shown that when subjects observe a moving object and are asked to recall its final position from memory, they tend to misremember it as being displaced forward. Freyd and Finke (1984) attributed this effect to a property of the imagery system (i.e., to the nature of the imagery architecture). However, Ranney (1989) suggested that the phenomenon may actually be due to tacit knowledge. Yet it seems that at least some aspects of the phenomenon are not cognitively penetrable (Finke and Freyd, 1989). Does this mean that representational momentum must then be a property of the imagery architecture, as Freyd and Finke assumed? What needs to be recognized, in this and other such cases, is that there may be many other explanations besides tacit knowledge and imagery architecture. In this particular case there is good reason to think that part of the phenomenon is actually visual and takes place during perception of the moving object, rather than in its representation in memory. There is evidence that the perception of the location of moving objects precedes the actual location of such objects (Nijhawan, 1994). Eye movement studies also show that gaze precedes the current location of moving objects in an anticipatory fashion (Kowler, 1989, 1990). Thus, even though the general phenomenon in question (the forms of visualized motion) may be attributable to tacit knowledge, the fact that in these studies the moving stimuli are presented visually may result in the phenomenon also being modulated by the visual system operating on the perceived scene. The general point in both these examples is that even genuine cases of failure of cognitive penetrability do not mean that the phenomena in question reveal properties of the architecture of the imagery system.

A final point that needs emphasizing is that no criterion can be applied blindly to the interpretation of empirical results without making collateral assumptions. No cognitive mechanism (nor, for that manner, any physical law) can be observed directly. Even something as clearly a part of the architecture as a "red" detector, may or may not be deployed in a particular situation, depending on the observer's beliefs and goals. A red detector can be used to find a red car in a parking lot, yet the overall task of looking for the car is clearly cognitively penetrable (it matters what color you believed the car was and where you believe you left it). To distinguish the functioning of the detector from the functioning of the cognitive system in which it is embedded, we need to set up the appropriate control conditions and we also need to make some (independently motivated) assumptions about how the task is carried out. As I have repeatedly said (e.g., Pylyshyn, 1978), observed behavior is a function of the *representation-process* pair, and one cannot be observed without the other. But that does not mean (as Anderson, 1978, has concluded) that we cannot in principle decide the nature of either the process or the structure of the representation. As I argued in my reply to Anderson (Pylyshyn, 1979c), the situation here is no different from the one that applies in any science, where theory is always underconstrained by data. The history of information-processing psychology (as well as in other sciences) has shown that the problem of deciding between alternative theories is not principled, but only practical (at least outside of quantum mechanics). Cognitive penetrability is not a panacea, but a tool, much like reaction time or fMRI, to be used in carefully controlled experiments. Although one can always argue about individual cases, the cases of cognitive penetration that I have cited here and elsewhere (Pylyshyn, 1981b, 1984a) seem to me clear cases that show that particular hypotheses about the constraints imposed by the mental imagery mechanism are not tenable.

6.3.4   Summary of some possible reasons for observed patterns of imagery findings

As I mentioned throughout this section, there is more than one reason why particular systematic patterns of observations are found in studies of mental imagery, other than inherent properties of the imagery system (i.e., the architecture of mental imagery). Here is a summary of some of the reasons discussed in this section concerning why imagery experiments may produce the pattern of observations they do.

(1) First and foremost, the pattern may be due to the *use of tacit knowledge to simulate aspects of real-world events, as they would appear if we were to see them unfold*, including the stages through which such events would proceed and their relative durations. Subjects may cause the observed results to come out in certain ways because they know how things in the world work and because they interpret the task as that of simulating how things would look to them if they were actually to happen in the world. We call the body of knowledge and beliefs that are brought to bear in this simulation *tacit knowledge*—"tacit" because people may not be able to articulate what they know, as is generally the case with knowledge of naive physics, of the conventions of social interactions, of the structure of one's language, and of what motivates and guides other people's behavior. Although such knowledge must be inferred indirectly by observing its consequences on behavior, it must also meet the criteria of being knowledge: it must enter into inferential

processes (so that its effect depends on what else observers know and what their utilities and goals are) and have generalized effects beyond a narrow domain.

(2) The pattern may be due not only to the content of tacit knowledge, but also to *how this knowledge is organized*. It is commonplace in psychology to find that to solve a problem people may be forced to go through a sequence of steps dictated by the way their knowledge is organized. A simple example of this that I gave earlier is the task of saying what the *n*th letter is after a given letter in the alphabet. The time it takes to carry out this task depends on the fact that our knowledge of the alphabet happens to be organized in the form of a list to be accessed in sequence (presumably because it was learned that way). Similarly, the pattern we observe may arise from the fact that in using imagery certain access paths to relevant knowledge may be easier to use or more salient. It is also a commonplace finding in studies of reasoning that rewording a problem in a different but logically equivalent way may result in it being either much easier or much more difficult to solve (Hayes and Simon, 1976; Kotovsky, Hayes, and Simon, 1985). A prime candidate for this sort of explanation is the phenomenon concerning mental paper-folding, discussed on pp. 313–316.

(3) The pattern may be the result of a *habitual way of solving certain kinds of problems* or of more frequent patterns of solution. This is the basis for the widely studied phenomenon known in the problem-solving literature as "mechanization," an example of which is the Luchins water jug experiment (Luchins, 1942). In this example subjects are shown a series of problems concerning measuring out a specified amount of liquid using containers of certain sizes. After successfully solving a series of problems using a certain combination of containers, subjects were unable to solve a new (even simpler) problem requiring a different combination of containers. Another is the so-called functional fixedness phenomenon studied by Anderson and Johnson (1966), in which people get stuck with one view of the function of an object (say, viewing a matchbox as a container) and then have a great difficulty solving a problem that is easily solved by viewing the object in a different way (say, as a potential shelf). This sort of effect is also common with tasks involving imagery, where we tend to use a particular, often habitual way of imagining a situation— particularly when we have a habitual way of solving a problem in reality when we can actually carry out certain actions and watch the solution emerge (as in the case discussed earlier of determining whether a line can be extrapolated to intersect a visible object).

(4) The pattern may be due to the nature of the task itself. As Ullman (1984) has argued, some tasks logically *require* a serial process for their

solution. Depending on what basic operators we have at our disposal, it could turn out that the stages through which a solution process passes and the time it takes may be essentially determined by task requirements. Newell and Simon (1972) have also argued that what happens in certain segments of problem solving (as it shows up, for example, in what they call a "problem behavior graph") reveals little about subjects' strategies, because in those episodes subjects' choices are dictated primarily by the demands of the task. That is, subjects are doing what must be done to solve the problem or the obvious thing that any rational person would do in that state of the problem solving process.

(5) The pattern may also be due to general computational complexity constraints that result in trading off increased time for less complex operations, as hypothesized for mental rotation by the SPASAR theory (Marr and Nishihara, 1976), or as hypothesized by Tsotsos (1988) in connection with the question of why certain operations are carried out sequentially rather than in parallel. A candidate for this sort of explanation is the mental rotation phenomenon, discussed on pages 316–321.

It is also possible that when we carry out experiments on mental imagery we will find effects that are due not to one of the above reasons alone, but to a combination of reasons. A phenomenon may have multiple causes; it may be due to the interaction between the tacit knowledge used in the mental simulation and also certain properties of the cognitive architecture involved in reasoning. The architectural properties may be general ones (e.g., limitations of the short-term memory in which image representations are stored during processing) or ones that are specific to creating and manipulating visual mental images. What we need to do is determine whether tacit knowledge will explain the effect, since if it can we are left with the "null hypothesis." If it cannot, then we need to look for other effects, including interactions.

Having laid out some of the issues, as well as some alternative explanations of certain well-known empirical observations associated with the study of mental imagery phenomena, I now turn to a more detailed examination of some of the theoretical views concerning what makes mental imagery a special form of cognitive activity—views that have now become as close as anything can get to being received wisdom within psychology and parts of philosophy of mind.

6.4   Some Alleged Properties of Images

6.4.1   Depiction and mandatory properties of representations

It has been frequently suggested that images differ from symbolic forms of representation (such as those sometimes referred to as "language of thought") in that images stand in a special relationship to what they represent, a relationship often referred to as *depicting*. One way of putting this is to say that to depict some state of affairs, a representation needs to correspond to the spatial arrangement it represents the same way a picture does. One of the few people who have tried to be explicit about what this means is Stephen Kosslyn, so I quote from him at some length.[9]

A depictive representation is a type of picture, which specifies the locations and values of configurations of points in a space. For example, a drawing of a ball on a box would be a depictive representation. The space in which the points appear need not be physical, such as on this page, but can be like an array in a computer, which specifies spatial relations purely functionally. That is, the physical locations in the computer of each point in an array are not themselves arranged in an array; it is only by virtue of how this information is "read" and processed that it comes to function as if it were arranged into an array (with some points being close, some far, some falling along a diagonal, and so on). In a depictive representation, each part of an object is represented by a pattern of points, and the spatial relations among these patterns in the functional space correspond to the spatial relations among the parts themselves. Depictive representations convey meaning via their resemblance to an object, with parts of the representation corresponding to parts of the object. . . . When a depictive representation is used, not only is the shape of the represented parts immediately available to appropriate processes, but so is the shape of the empty space. . . . Moreover, one cannot represent a shape in a depictive representation without also specifying a size and orientation. . . . (Kosslyn, 1994, p. 5)

This quotation introduces a number of issues that need to be examined closely. One idea we can put aside is the claim that depictive representations convey meaning through their resemblance to the objects they depict. This relies on the extremely problematic notion of resem-

9. I don't mean to pick on Stephen Kosslyn, who, along with Allan Paivio and Roger Shepard, has done a great deal to promote the scientific study of mental imagery. I focus on Kosslyn's work here because he has provided what is currently the most developed theory of mental imagery and has been particularly explicit about his assumptions, and also because his work has been extremely influential in shaping psychologists' views about the nature of mental imagery. In that respect his theory can be taken as the received view in much of the field.

blance, which has been known to be inadequate as a basis for meaning (certainly since Wittgenstein, 1953). Resemblance is neither necessary nor sufficient for something to have a particular reference: images may resemble what they do not refer to or what they depict (e.g., an image of John's twin brother does not depict John) and they may depict what they do not resemble (an image of John taken through a distorting lens depicts John in the sense that it is an image of John, even though it does not resemble him).

Despite such obvious problems, the notion of resemblance keeps surfacing in discussions of mental imagery, in a way that reveals how deeply the conscious experience of mental imagery contaminates conceivable theories of mental imagery. For example, Finke (1989) begins with the observation, "People often wonder why mental images resemble the things they depict." But the statement that images resemble things they depict is just another way of saying that the conscious experience of mental imagery is similar to the conscious experience one would have if one were to see the thing one was imagining. Consider what it would be like if images did not "resemble the things they depict." It would be absurd if, in imagining a chair, one had an experience that was like that of seeing a dog. Presumably this is because (a) what it means to have a mental image of a chair is that you are having an experience like that of seeing a chair, and (b) what your image looks like, what conscious content it has, is something on which you are the final authority. You may be deceived about lots of things concerning your mental image. You may be, and typically are, deceived about what sort of thing your image is (i.e., what form and substance underlie it), but surely you cannot be deceived about what your mental image looks like, or what it resembles. That is not an empirical fact about imagery, it's just a claim about what the phrase "mental image" means.

What gives representations a role in thought is the fact that it is possible for processes in the organism to obtain relevant information from them and to make inferences from them, thereby making explicit some otherwise implicit information. There might be a weak sense of "resemblance" wherein a representation can be used to provide information about the appearance of an object or to allow such information to be made explicit when it was only implicit (for more on the question of how *real* visible images allow one to draw certain kinds of inferences, see section 8.3). But in this sense, every representation of perceptible properties (including a description of how something looks) could be said to "resemble" its referent. Any stronger sense of resemblance inevitably imports an intelligent and knowledgeable agent for whom the representation "looks like" what it represents (i.e., what it would look like if it were perceived visually). This agent is the means by which one eliminates the inherently many-to-many relation between an image and its meaning that Wittgenstein and others talked about. As Wittgenstein reminded us, an image of a man walking upstairs is exactly the same as the image of a man walking downstairs backward. An intelligent agent could select one of these interpretations over the other, but he or she would do so on the basis of reasoning from other (nonimage) considerations.

In contrast to the problematic criterion of resemblance, the proposal that images are decomposed into "parts," with the relations between parts in some way reflecting the structure of the corresponding parts of the world, does deserve closer scrutiny. It is closely related to a criterion discussed by Sloman (1971), although he suggested this as characteristic of analog representations. Fodor and I referred to this sort of part-whole structure as the compositional character of representations and claimed that it is a requirement on any form of representation adequate to explain the representational capacity of intelligent organisms and to explain the capacity for thought and inference (Fodor and Pylyshyn, 1988). Thus, if images are to serve as vehicles of thought, they too must be compositional in this sense. And if they are compositional then they have what might be called interchangeable parts, much as lexical items in a calculus do. This, however, makes them more languagelike (as in the "language of thought" proposal of Fodor, 1975) than pictorial and says little about the alleged depictive nature of images since it applies equally to any form of representation. Indeed, it is doubtful that images are compositional in the required sense, even if they do have parts.

Another proposal in the Kosslyn quotation above is that in depictive representations it is mandatory that certain aspects be made explicit. For example, according to Kosslyn, if you choose to represent a particular object you cannot fail to represent its shape, orientation, and size. This claim too has some truth, although the questions of which aspects are mandatory, why they are mandatory, and what this tells you about the form of the representation remain open. It is in fact a general property of representations that some aspects tend to be encoded (or at least assigned as a default) wherever other aspects are. Sometimes that is true by definition of that form of representation or by virtue of the logical entailments of certain facts that are represented. So, for example, you can't represent a token of a spoken or written sentence without making a commitment as to how many words it has, you can't have a representation containing four individual objects without implicitly representing the fact that there are at least four of them, and so on. Of course, the converse is not true; the sentence "there are four plates on the table" does not contain four distinct representations of individual plates. Also the tendency to represent certain clusters of properties sometimes may be just a matter of habit or of convention or a reflection of the frequent co-occurrence of the properties in the world: when you represent someone as riding a bicycle you may also represent him as moving the pedals (even though you need not), when you represent someone as running you might also represent her as moving quickly, and so on, none of which is mandatory even if they are all plausibly true. It may also be that certain patterns are frequent (if not mandatory) in visual images simply because they are frequent in the world being represented.

So the question is, when you represent some object in the form of an image is it mandatory that you represent its shape and size, and if so, why? What about its color and shading? Must you represent the background against which you are viewing it, the direction of lighting, and the shadows it casts? Must you represent it as observed from a particular point of view? What about its stereoscopic properties; do you represent the changing parallax of its parts as you imagine moving in relation to it? Could you choose to represent any or none of these things? Is there something special about the encoding of shape, orientation, and size of an object? We know that retinal size and retinal location can be factored away from the representation of an object (in fact it is hard to demonstrate that these are even encoded into long-term memory), but can the shape and orientation of an object also be factored away? Studies in rapid search suggest that we can identify the presence of a shape without identifying its location and we can identify both color and shape but miscombine them to form "conjunction illusions" (Treisman and Schmidt, 1982). In fact, these studies appear to show that in representing shape, abstract properties such as having a "closed contour" may be factored apart from other properties of shape and miscombined. These studies do not tell us which properties must be contained in an imaginal representation, but they do suggest that in the process of visual encoding, properties such as shape, color, location, and even closure can be factored apart from one another (i.e., they are represented as separate codes). In chapter 4 (and in Pylyshyn, 2001b) I suggested that very early in the visual process, all such properties (shape, color, location) are factored from (and are initially secondary to) the individuality of visual objects. What Kosslyn may have had in mind in the earlier quotation is that when you ask someone to imagine an object, say, the letter "B," the person will make a commitment to such things as whether it is in upper or lower case. It does seem that you can't imagine a "B" without imagining either the upper case letter "B" or a lower case letter "b." But is this not another case of an implicit task requirement? Are you not being asked to describe what you see when you see a *printed token of a particular letter*? Were you actually to see a token of a printed letter you would have to see either a lower or an upper case letter, but not both and not neither. If someone claimed to have an image of a B that was noncommittal with respect to its case, what would you conclude? You might be tempted to say that the person did not have a visual image at all, but only some idea of the letter.

Yet most of our representations are noncommittal in many ways (see chapter 1 for examples). In particular, they can be noncommittal in ways that no picture can be noncommittal. Shall we then not call them images? Is an image generated in response to the letter-imaging example mentioned above not an image if it is noncommittal with respect to its color or font or whether it is bold or italic? Such questions show the futility of assuming that mental images are like pictures. As the graphic artist M. C. Escher once put it, "A mental image is something completely different from a visual image, and however much one exerts oneself, one can never manage to capture the fullness of that perfection which hovers in the mind and which one thinks of, quite falsely, as something that is 'seen'" (1960, p. 7).

One of the most important claims of the Kosslyn proposal, as expressed in the quotation on page 328, is the idea that although images are inherently spatial, the space in question need not be physical but may be "functional." Both parts of this proposal (that images are spatial and that the relevant space might be a functional one) have been extremely influential and have led to new lines of research, some of which have involved neural imaging. The claim that images are spatial and the new lines of research that focus on this claim will be discussed in detail in chapter 7. For the present I will take up the question of whether there is any evidence to support the claim that images are the sorts of things that can be examined visually, as is clearly implied by the notion of "depiction" as a mode of representation.

6.5 Mental Imagery and Visual Perception

Perhaps the most actively pursued question in contemporary imagery research has been the question of whether mental imagery uses the visual system. Intuitively the idea that imagery involves vision is extremely appealing for a number of reasons, not the least of which is the fact that the experience of mental imagery is very like the experience of seeing. Indeed, there have been (disputed) claims that when real perception is faint because of impoverished stimuli, vision and imagery can be indistinguishable (Perky, 1910a). I will return to the similarity of the experience of vision and imagery later (pp. 350–357) when I raise the question of what significance ought to be attached to this experiential evidence. In this section I look at some of the psychophysical evidence for the involvement of vision in imagery. In chapter 7 I will consider a new and, to many investigators, much more persuasive class of evidence for the involvement of vision in mental imagery, evidence that derives from neuroscience (especially neuroimaging studies and clinical reports of brain-damaged patients).

In examining the question of whether (and in what way) vision may be involved in mental imagery, it is important to make a clear distinction between the visual system and the cognitive system, since cognition clearly is involved in some stage of both mental imagery and what we generally call visual perception. To see how intimately imagery involves the visual system we must first provide some criteria for when we are observing the operation of the visual system, as opposed to the system that includes reasoning and cognition in general. This is why we need to identify a narrower technical sense of "visual system," as I attempted to do in chapters 2 and 3 (and in Pylyshyn, 1999) where I used the term "early vision" to designate the modular part of vision that is unique to that modality. In investigating the involvement of the visual system in mental imagery we must also distinguish between effects attributable to the operation of a special visual architecture and effects attributable to the fact that in visual imagery we are concerned with different subject matter. For example, in visual imagery, we are typically concerned with visual (optical, geometrical) properties of some scene (actual or hypothetical). The "null hypothesis" strategy I introduced in section 6.1 (i.e., that in the absence of evidence to the contrary we shall assume that all thoughts use the same format) says that we need to ask whether a system that does not have a special *form* of encoding or a special architecture might nonetheless exhibit the observed characteristics when it reasoned about visual properties. We might, after all, expect that certain distinct characteristics might be exhibited when we reason about some special subject matter, such as emotions, feelings, interpersonal relations, or mathematics, or perhaps when we reason about such psychologically distinct categories as animate versus inanimate things (e.g., there is reason to think that such subject matters may even involve different parts of the brain; see Dehaene, 1995; Samson, Pillon, and De Wilde, 1998). What this means is that we have to insist that certain distinctions be honored when asking whether imagery involves the visual system. In what follows I will examine a number of lines of evidence that have persuaded people that mental imagery involves the visual system, while keeping in mind the need for a finer technical distinction between the narrow sense of "visual system" and the rest of the cognitive mind.

Many of the experiments described earlier (including the image-scanning experiments and the studies involving projecting images onto visual stimuli) have been interpreted as suggesting that mental images are inspected by the visual system. I have already discussed the finding that it takes longer to judge the presence of a small feature in a small image than in a large one. There is also a well-documented relation between the relative size of a pair of imagined objects and the time it takes to judge which one is larger. For example, when we make certain judgments by examining a visual image we find the same psychometric function as we get when we do the task visually: it takes longer to judge from an image whether a toaster is larger than a person's head than to judge whether a toaster is larger than a horse. That this relation is the same as when real objects are being viewed has suggested to some people that the same visual mechanisms are being used in both cases. Although this phenomenon received a great deal of attention in early work on mental imagery, it soon became clear that it had nothing to do with the putative *visual* aspect of mental images since the effect occurs with any comparison of magnitudes, including judgments of such abstract properties as the relative cost or attractiveness of different objects, or the relative magnitude of numbers (it is faster to judge that 374 is larger than 12 than that 21 is larger than 19). This more general phenomenon is called the "symbolic distance effect" (Friedman, 1978) and has been used to argue for some kind of an analog form of representation, although the only thing that actually follows from the data is the plausibility that all magnitudes may be represented in some common manner (Gallistel, 1990).

There are many other phenomena involving the inspection of visual mental images that appear to parallel those that are found when real scenes are inspected, including the time it takes to judge the similarity of such imagined properties as color (Paivio and te Linde, 1980) or shape (Shepard and Chipman, 1970). Others are discussed in the remainder of this chapter. The parallel between imagery and vision has led a number of people (e.g., Finke, 1980; Shepard, 1978b) to propose that in mental imagery, visual information in memory is fed into the visual system in place of information coming from the eyes. But it should be noted that even if the visual system were involved in mental imagery in this way, it would not support the pictorial nature of mental images. As I noted in chapter 1, the idea that vision involves the construction of an extended image of a scene has been thoroughly discredited and that there is every reason to believe that vision generates symbolic representations. So mental imagery may involve the same kinds representations as does vision, and yet in neither case need these representations be pictorial, notwithstanding our intuitive impression that there are pictures in our heads. Clearly the picture-theorists wish to make a stronger point than that vision and mental imagery share some mechanisms. They wish to infer from the involvement of the visual system that images are something that can be "seen," which, in turn, would mean that they must be pictorial in nature. The claim that images function in this way is discussed in chapter 7, in connection with the use of neuroscience evidence in pursuit of the picture theory. In what follows I will describe some of the behavioral evidence for the involvement of vision in mental imagery, without specifically raising the question of whether the evidence addresses the pictorial nature of images.

6.5.1   Interference between imaging and visual perception

One of the earliest sources of experimental evidence that persuaded people that imagery involves the visual system is that the task of examining images can be disrupted by a subsidiary visual (or at least spatial) task. Brooks (1968) showed that reporting spatial properties from images is susceptible to interference when the response must be given by a spatial method (i.e., pointing) than a by verbal one. For example, if subjects are asked to describe the shape of the letter "F" by providing a list of right and left turns one would have to take in traveling around its periphery, their performance is worse if the response is to point to the left or right (or to the symbols L and R arranged in a table) than if it is to say the words "left" and "right." Segal and Fusella (1969, 1970) subsequently confirmed the greater interference between perception and imagery in various same-modality tasks and also showed that both sensitivity and response bias (i.e., both measures d' and β, derived from *Signal Detection Theory*) were affected. Segal and Fusella concluded that "imagery functions as an internal signal which is confused with the external signal" (p 458). This conclusion may be the correct one to draw. What it may imply, however, is that interference occurs between two tasks when the same type of representational contents are involved, or the same concepts are deployed. What do representations of visual patterns have in common with representations underlying mental images? One obvious answer is that they are both about visual patterns. Like sentences about visual patterns, they all involve concepts such as "bright," "red," "right angle," "parallel to," and so on. It is not surprising that two responses requiring the same conceptual vocabulary would interfere with each other. (That the linguistic output in the Brooks study is not as disruptive as pointing may simply show that spatial concepts are not relevant to *articulating* the words "left" or "right" once they have been selected for uttering, whereas these concepts *are* relevant to issuing the motor commands to move left or right.)

6.5.2 Visual illusions induced by superimposing mental images

Other studies suggesting that the visual system may be involved in mental imagery include ones showing that projecting images of certain patterns onto displays creates some of the well-known illusions, such as the Müller-Lyer illusion, the Pogendorff illusion, or the Herring illusion, or even the remarkable long-lasting orientation-contingent color aftereffect, called the McCollough effect.[10] As I have already suggested, studies that involve projecting images onto visual displays are special in that they provide an opportunity for the visual system to operate on the visual part of the input. In many cases the imagery-induced illusions can be explained simply by noting that in both vision and projected imagery the illusory effect is arguably related to an attention-directing process induced by part of the display. If that is so, then imagining that part as projected onto a display may reproduce the same attention manipulation, resulting in the same illusion. Take the following example of the Müller-Lyer effect. When viewed visually, a line appears longer if it has inward pointing arrowheads at each end (as shown on the right in figure 2.3). It has been argued that merely imagining the arrowheads produces the same effect. For example, Bernbaum and Chung (1981) showed subjects displays such as those illustrated in the top part of figure 6.9.

10. Many of these studies have serious methodological problems that I will not discuss here in detail. For example, a number of investigators have raised questions about possible experimenter-demand effects in many of these illusions (Predebon and Wenderoth, 1985; Reisberg and Morris, 1985). Few potential subjects have never seen illusions such as the Müller-Lyer (it is shown in virtually every introductory text in psychology, not to mention children's books), so even if they do not acknowledge familiarity with the illusion, chances are good that they have some foreknowledge of it. Also, the usual precautions against experimenter influence on this highly subjective measure were not taken (e.g., the experiments were not done using a double-blind procedure). The most remarkable of the illusions, the orientation-contingent color aftereffect, known as the McCollough effect, is perhaps less likely to lead to an experimenter-demand effect since not many people know of the phenomenon. Yet Finke and Schmidt (1977) reported that this effect is obtained when part of the input (a grid of lines) is merely imagined over the top of a visible colored background. But the Finke finding has been subject to a variety of interpretations as well as to criticisms on methodological grounds (Broerse and Crassini, 1981, 1984; Harris, 1982; Kunen and May, 1980, 1981; Zhou and May, 1993), so it will not be reviewed here. Finke himself (1989) appears to accept that the basis of the effect may be classical conditioning rather than a specifically visual mechanism.

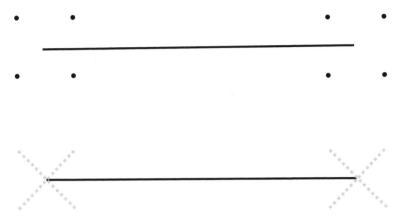

Figure 6.9
Example of figures used to induce the Müller-Lyer illusion from images. Imagine that the end points are connected to the inner or the outer pairs of dots in the top figure (as in the experiment by Bernbaum and Chung, 1981), or selectively attend to the inward or outward arrows in the bottom figure (as in the experiment by Ohkuma, 1986, and by Goryo, Robinson, and Wilson, 1984).

Subjects were asked to imagine the endpoints of the lines connected to either the outside or the inside pairs of dots in this display (when the endpoints are connected to the inside pair of dots they produce outward-pointing arrows, and when they are connected to the outside pair of dots they produce inward pointing arrows, as in the original Müller-Lyer illusion). Bernbaum and Chung found that adding imagined arrowheads also produced the illusion, with the inward-pointing arrows leading to the perception of a shorter line than the outward pointing arrows. Also Ohkuma (1986) found that merely instructing subjects to attend selectively to the inward- or outward-pointing arrows (as in the bottom of figure 6.9) produces the same result. I might note that such an effect is not only weak, but it is an ideal candidate for being a classical experimenter-demand effect of the sort discussed by Predebon and Wenderoth (1985). But for the sake of argument let us take these results as valid.

Consider first what may be involved in such illusions when the critical parts are actually viewed (as opposed to imagined), using the original Müller-Lyer illusion as our example. Explanations for this and similar illusions tend to fall into one of two categories. They either appeal to the detailed shapes of contours involved and to the assumption that these shapes lead to erroneous interpretations of the pattern in terms of 3D shapes, or they appeal to some general characteristics of the 2D envelope created by the display and the consequent distribution of attention or direction of gaze. Among the popular explanations that fall into the first category is one due to Richard Gregory (1968), known as the "inappropriate constancy scaling" theory. This theory claims that "Y" type (or inward-pointing) vertices, being generally associated with more distant concave corners of 3D rectilinear structures, are perceived as being further away, and therefore actually larger than they appear. This theory has been subject to a great deal of criticism and is unable to explain a number of findings, including why the illusion is obtained when the inducing elements at the ends of the lines are not rectilinear vertices but various sorts of forklike curves that do not lend themselves to a 3D interpretation (see the review in Nijhawan, 1991). Theories in the second category include ones that attribute the illusion to attention and to mechanisms involved in preparing eye-movement. For example, one theory (Virsu, 1971) claims that the illusion depends on the distance between the vertex and the center of gravity of the arrowhead and appeals to the tendency to move one's eyes to the center of gravity of a figure. The involvement of eye movements in the Müller-Lyer illusion has also been confirmed by Bolles (1969); Coren (1986); Festinger, White, and Allyn (1968); Hoenig (1972); and Virsu (1971). Another example of the envelope type of theory is the framing theory (Brigell, Uhlarik, and Goldhorn, 1977; Davies and Spencer, 1977), which uses the ratio of overall figure length to shaft length as predictor. Such envelope-based theories have generally fared better than shape-based theories not only on the Müller-Lyer illusion, but in most cases in which there are context effects on judgments of linear extent. What is important about this from our perspective is that these explanations do not actually appeal to pattern-perception mechanisms and therefore are compatible with attention-based explanations of the illusions. The "envelopes" of the figures in many of these cases can be altered by assigning attention (or visual indexes) to objects or places or regions in the display.

Further evidence that attention can play a central role in these illusions comes from studies that actually manipulate attention focus. For example, Goryo and colleagues (1984) have shown that if both sets of inducing elements (the outward and inward arrowheads) are present, observers selectively attend to one or the other and obtain the illusion appropriate to the one to which they attended. This is very similar to the effect demonstrated by Bernbaum and Chung (1981) but without requiring that any image be superimposed on the line. Coren and Porac (1983) also confirmed that attention alone could create, eliminate, or even reverse the Müller-Lyer illusion. In addition, the relevance of imagery-induction of the Müller-Lyer illusion to the claim that imagery involves the visual system is further cast into doubt when one recognizes that this illusion, like many other imagery-based phenomena, also appears in congenitally blind people (Patterson and Deffenbacher, 1972).

There have been a number of other claims of visual illusions caused (or modified) by mental imagery (e.g., Wallace, 1984a, 1984b). When such image-induced effects on illusions are not due to experimental-demand effects, as they may well be in some cases where results cannot be replicated under controlled conditions (Predebon and Wenderoth, 1985; Reisberg and Morris, 1985), they are all subject to the interpretation that the effect is mediated by the allocation of focal attention. Indeed, the attention-mediation of such effects was shown explicitly in the case of ambiguous motion-illusion by Watanabe and Shimojo (1998).

6.5.3 Imagined versus perceived motion

Another way to examine the possible involvement of the visual system in imagery is to select some phenomenon known to occur in the early stages of vision and ask whether it occurs in mental imagery. A good candidate is one that involves adaptation to motion, which is known to have a locus in early vision (in fact, in the visual cortex). When a region of the visual field receives extensive motion stimulation, an object presented in that region is seen to move in a direction opposite that of the inducing movement (the "waterfall illusion") and a moving object is seen as moving more slowly (presumably because the motion detection cells in visual cortex have become fatigued). This phenomenon is of special interest to us, since the adaptation is known to be retinotopic and therefore occurs in a retinotopically mapped part of the visual system. Convinced that the visual system is involved in mental imagery, Gilden, Blake, and Hurst (1995) set out to show that the motion of an imagined object is similarly affected by the aftereffect of a moving field. They had subjects gaze for 150 seconds at a square window on a screen containing a uniformly moving random texture. Then they showed subjects a point moving toward that window and disappearing behind what appeared to be an opaque surface, and they asked subjects to imagine the point continuing to move across the previously stimulated region and to report when the point would emerge at the other side of the surface. Gilden et al. did find an effect of motion adaptation on imagined motion, but it was not exactly the effect they had expected. They found that when the point was imagined as moving in the same direction as that of the inducing motion field (i.e., against the motion aftereffect) it appeared to slow down (it took longer to reach the other side of the region). However, when the point was imagined as moving in the direction opposite that of the inducing motion field (i.e., in the same direction as the motion aftereffect), the point appeared to speed up (it reached the other side in a shorter time). The latter effect is *not* what happens with real moving points. In visual motion adaptation, motion appears to slow down no matter which direction the inducing motion field moves, presumably because all motion-sensitive receptors had been habituated or fatigued. But, as Gilden et al. recognized, the effect they observed is exactly what one would expect if, rather than the imagined point moving uniformly across the screen, subjects imagined the point as being located at a series of static locations along the imagined path. This suggests a quite different mechanism underlying imagined motion. We know that people are very good at computing what is known as the time to contact (or "time to collision") of a uniformly moving object at a specified location. This is why we are so good at estimating when a baseball will arrive at various critical places (e.g., over the batter's box, at a particular place in the field). What may be going on in imagined motion is that people may simply be using the visual-indexing mechanism discussed earlier to pick out one or more marked places (e.g., elements of texture) along the path, and then computing the time to contact for each of these places.

Jonathan Cohen and I explicitly tested this idea (Pylyshyn and Cohen, 1999) by asking subjects to mentally extrapolate the motion of a small square that disappeared behind an apparently opaque surface (shown in figure 6.10). They were asked to imagine the smooth motion of the square in a dark room. At some unpredictable time in the course of this motion the square would actually appear, as though coming out through

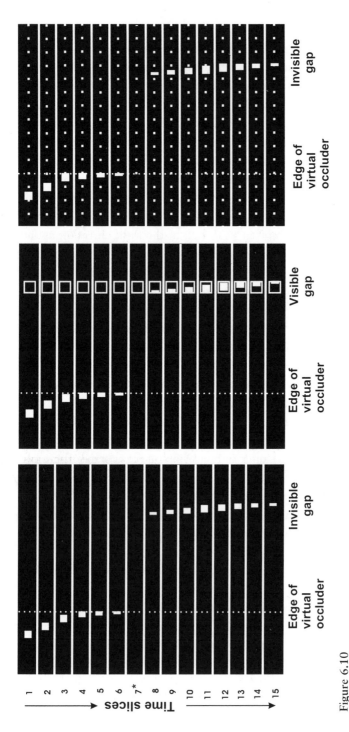

Figure 6.10
Illustration of displays used by Pylyshyn and Cohen (1999) to study how well people can imagine the continuing smooth motion of objects that go behind an occluding surface. Results showed that people were poor when no landmarks were visible (panel on left), but better when the gap where objects would reappear was visible (middle panel), or when landmarks were visible along the imagined path (third panel). These results suggest that in imagining smooth motion observers carry out a series of time-to-contact computations based on visible locations. (The time slice designated as 7* is not drawn to scale since it would take the object ad-ditional time to get to where it will reappear.)

a crack in the opaque surface, and then recede back through another crack, and subjects had to indicate whether it had appeared earlier or later than when their imagined square reached that crack. This task was carried out in several different conditions. In one condition, the location of the "cracks" where the square would appear and disappear was unknown (i.e., the cracks were invisible). In another condition, the location at which the square was to appear was known in advance: it was indicated by a small rectangular figure that served as a "window" through which, at the appropriate time, subjects would briefly view the square that was moving behind the surface (the way the squares appeared and disappeared in the window condition was identical to that in the no-window condition except that the outline of the window was not visible in the latter case). And finally, in one set of conditions, the imagined square moved through total darkness, whereas in the other set of conditions, the path was marked by a sparse set of dots that could be used as reference points to compute time to contact. As expected, the ability to estimate where the imagined square was at various times (measured in terms of decision time) was significantly improved when the location was specified in advance and also when there were visible markers along the path of imagined motion. Both of these findings confirm the suggestion that what subjects are doing when they report "imagining the smooth motion of a square" is selecting places at which to compute time to contact (a task at which people are very good; DeLucia and Liddell, 1998) and merely thinking that the imaginary moving square is at those places at the estimated times. According to this view, subjects are thinking the thought "now it is *here*" repeatedly for different visible objects (picked out by the visual indexing mechanism mentioned earlier), and synchronized to the independently computed arrival times.[11] This way of describing what is happening does not require the assumption that the visual system is involved; nor does it require the assumption that an

---

11. Note that this conclusion applies only to the voluntary movement of a locus of attention over a display, not to apparent motion, which has its locus in early vision. Shioiri et al., (2000) found that observers are good at estimating the location of a moving object along the path of apparent motion. This sort of motion, however, is different in many ways from the motion of an imagined focus of attention, as in mental scanning experiments (e.g., it is not cognitively penetrable—observers cannot change its speed or trajectory at will).

imagined square is actually moving through some mental space and occupying each successive position along a real spatial path. Indeed, there is no need to posit any sort of space except the visible one that serves as input to the time-to-contact computation.

6.5.4   Extracting novel information from images: Visual (re)perception or inference?

It is widely held that one of the purposes of mental images is to allow us to discover new visual properties or see new visual interpretations or reconstruals in imaginally presented information. It would therefore seem important to ask whether there is any evidence for such visual reconstruals. This empirical question turns out to be more difficult to answer univocally than one might have expected, for it is clear that one can draw *some* conclusions by examining images, even when those were not explicit in, say, the verbal description that led to your image. So, for example, if I ask you to imagine a square and then to imagine drawing in both diagonals, it does not seem surprising that you can tell that the diagonals cross or that they form an "X" shape. This does not seem clearly to qualify as an example showing that images are interpreted *visually*, since such an obvious conclusion could surely be derived from a description of a rectangle and of diagonals, and also it is a pattern that you have likely seen before. On the other hand, try the following example without looking ahead for the answer. Imagine two parallelograms, one directly above the other. Connect each vertex of the top figure to the corresponding vertex of the bottom one. What do you see? As you keep watching, what happens in your image? When presented visually, this figure consistently leads to certain phenomena that do not appear in mental imagery. The signature properties of spontaneous perception of certain line drawings as depicting three-dimensional objects and spontaneous reversals of ambiguous figures do not appear in this mental image.[12] (Now try drawing the figure and looking at it).

But what counts, in general, as a visual interpretation as opposed to an inference? I doubt that this question can be answered without a sharper sense of what is meant by the term "visual," a problem to which

---

12. This description accurately, if somewhat unconventionally, describes a Necker cube (see figure 1.7 for a visible counterpart).

I have already alluded. Since the everyday (pretheoretical) sense of "vision" clearly involves most of cognition, neither the question of the involvement of vision in imagery nor the question about visual reconstruals can be pursued nontrivially in terms of this broad notion of vision. At the very least we need a restricted sense of what is to count as vision or as a visual interpretation. I have argued, in chapters 2 and 3 (as well as in Pylyshyn, 1999) that there is good evidence for an independent visual module, which I referred to as "early vision." Because early vision is the part of the visual system that is unique to vision and does not involve other more general cognitive processes (such as accessing long-term memory and inference), it would be appropriate to frame experimental questions about the possible reinterpretation of images by examining phenomena that are characteristic of this system. Clearly, deciding whether two intersecting lines form an "X" is not one of these phenomena, nor is judging that when a "D" is placed on top of a "J" the result looks like an umbrella: you don't need to use the early-vision system in deciding that. All you need is an elementary inference based on the meaning of such phrases as "looks like an umbrella" (e.g., has a upwardly convex curved top attached below to a central vertical stroke— with or without a curved handle at the bottom). Thus, examples such as these simple figures (which were used in Finke, Pinker, and Farah, 1989) cannot decide the question of whether images are depictive or pictorial or, more important for present purposes, whether they are *visually* (re)interpreted.

Presenting information verbally and asking people to imagine the pattern being described is one way to get at the question of whether the interpretation can be classed as visual (as in the Necker cube example I cited above). Another way is to present a normally ambiguous pattern and then take it away and ask whether other new visual interpretations occur when the display is no longer there. This case, however, presents some special methodological problems. Not all ambiguities contained in pictures are visual ambiguities, and similarly, not all reinterpretations are visual reconstruals. For example, the sorts of visual puns embodied in some cartoons (most characteristically in so-called droodles, illustrated in figure 1.21 and available at http://www.droodles.com) do rely on ambiguities, but clearly not on ones that concern different visual organizations analyzed by the early-vision system. By contrast, the reversal of figures such as the classical Necker cube is at least in part the result of a reorganization that takes place in early vision. Do such reorganizations occur with visual images? To answer that question we would have to control for certain alternative explanations of apparently visual reinterpretations. For example, if a mental image appears to reverse, it might be because the observer knows of the two possible interpretations and simply replaces one of its interpretations with the other. This is the alternative view that many writers have preferred (Casey, 1976; Fodor, 1981). Another possibility, which applies when the image content is initially presented visually, might be that the observer actually computes two alternatives, but reports only one. This sort of simultaneous computing of two readings, which last for only a brief time, has been frequently reported in the case of sentence ambiguities. With lexically ambiguous sentences, it was shown that both interpretations are briefly available even though the person is aware of (and able to recall) only one of the senses. For example, Swinney (1979) showed that *both* senses of an ambiguous word such as "bug" (as in "There were many flies spiders and other *bugs* in the room" as opposed to "There were microphones, tape recorders, and other *bugs* in the room") primed associated words for a short time after they were heard in these two contextually disambiguated sentences (i.e., both "insect" and "spy" were read more quickly within a second or so of hearing "bug"). Similarly, in chapter 2 (as well as in Pylyshyn, 1999), I argued that notwithstanding the encapsulated nature of early vision, one of the ways that the cognitive system might still be able to affect the visual interpretation of ambiguous figures is if both possible interpretations are initially available so that the cognitive system can select among them based on their plausibility. Despite the methodological difficulties in obtaining a clear answer to the question of whether mental images allow visual reconstruals, a number of studies have provided converging evidence to suggest that no visual reconstruals occur from mental images.

Chambers and Reisberg (1985) were the first to put the question of the possibility of ambiguous mental images to an empirical test. They reported that no reversals or reinterpretations of any kind took place with mental images. Since that study was reported there has been a series of studies and arguments concerning whether images could be visually (re)interpreted. Reisberg and Chambers (1991) and Reisberg and Morris

(1985) used a variety of standard reversal figures and confirmed the Chambers and Reisberg finding that mental images of these figures did not reverse. Finke et al. (1989) have taken issue with these findings, citing their own experiments involving operations over images (e.g., the D–J umbrella examples that were mentioned briefly in section 6.1), but as I suggested above it is dubious that the reinterpretation of the superposition of such simple familiar figures should be counted as a *visual* reinterpretation. Moreover, even if the interpretations studied by Finke et al. were considered visual interpretations, there remains the serious problem of explaining why clear cases of visual interpretations, such as those studied by Chambers and Reisberg, do not occur with images.

Mary Peterson undertook a series of detailed explorations of the question of whether mental images can be ambiguous. Peterson and her colleagues (Peterson, 1993; Peterson et al., 1992) argued that certain kinds of reconstruals of mental images do take place. They first distinguished different types of image reinterpretations. In particular they distinguished what they called *reference-frame realignments* (in which one or more global directions are reassigned in the image, as in the Necker cube or rabbit-duck ambiguous figures) from what they called *reconstruals* (in which reinterpreting the figure involves assigning new meaning to its parts, as in the wife–mother-in-law or snail-elephant reversing figures). (Examples of two of Peterson's figures are shown in figure 6.11) I will refer to the latter as *part-based reconstruals* to differentiate them from other kinds of reconstruals (since their defining characteristic is that their parts take on a different meaning). A third type, figure-ground reversal (as in the Rubin vases), was acknowledged to occur rarely if ever with mental images (a finding that was also systematically confirmed by Slezak, 1995, using quite different displays). Peterson and her colleagues showed that reference-frame realignments do not occur in mental images unless they are cued by either explicit hints or implicit demonstration figures, whereas some part-based reconstruals occurred with 30 percent to 65 percent of the subjects.

Recall that our primary concern is not with whether any reinterpretations occur with mental images. The possibility of some reinterpretation depends on what information or content-cues are contained in the image, which is independent of the question of which mechanisms are used in processing it. What I am concerned with is whether the format

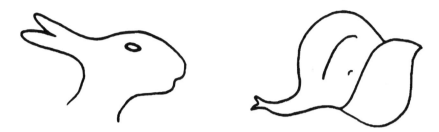

Figure 6.11
Ambiguous figures used by Peterson (1993) to study reconstruals from mental images. When these figures are perceived visually, the percepts tend to be bistable and change categories in a relatively sharp manner (e.g., duck-rabbit on the left and elephant-snail on the right). When these same figures are memorized and reconstrued from a mental image they tend to be reinterpreted in a wide variety of other ways, suggesting that local cues are being used to provide plausible reinterpretations, rather than reperceptions. (These figures are stylized versions of well-known illusions introduced by Jastrow, 1900, and by Fisher, 1976, respectively.)

of images is such that their interpretation and/or reinterpretation involves the specifically visual (i.e., the early-vision) system as opposed to the general inference system. The crucial question, therefore, is how Peterson's findings on reinterpreting mental images compare with the reinterpretations observed with ambiguous visual stimuli. The answer appears to be that even when reinterpretations occur with mental images, they are qualitatively different from those that occur with visual stimuli. For example, Peterson (1993) showed that although reference-frame reversals are dominant in vision they are rare in mental imagery, whereas the converse is true for part-based reconstruals. Also, the particular reconstruals observed with images tend to be different from those observed with the corresponding visual stimuli. Visual reconstruals tend to fall into major binary categories—in the case of the figures used by Peterson et al. these are the duck-rabbit, or the snail-elephant categories (see figure 6.11), whereas in the imagery case subjects provide a large number of other interpretations (which, at least to this observer, do not seem to be clear cases of distinctly different appearances—certainly not as clear as the cases of the Necker cube reversal or even the reconstruals discussed in the next paragraph). The number of subjects showing part-based reconstruals with mental images drops by half when only the particular interpretations observed in the visual case are counted. Rein-terpretation of mental images is also highly sensitive to hints and strate-gies, whereas there is reason to doubt that early vision is sensitive to such cognitive influences—as we saw on pages 76–82—although later stages clearly are.

The reason for these differences between imagery and vision is not clear, but they add credence to the suggestion that what is going on in the mental image reconstruals is not a perceptual (re)interpretation of an internally generated picture, but something else, perhaps the sort of infer-ence and shape-based memory-lookup that goes on in the decision stage of vision, after early vision has generated shape-descriptions. This is the stage at which beliefs about the perceived world are established, so we expect what happens at this stage to depend on inferences from prior knowledge and expectations, like all other cases of belief-fixation. It seems quite likely that parts of the highly ambiguous (though not clearly bistable) figures used by Peterson et al. might serve as cues for inferring or guessing at the identity of the whole figure (for illustrations of the other figures used, see Peterson, 1993). Alternatively, as suggested earlier, several possible forms might be computed by early vision (while the figures were viewed) and stored, and then during the image-recall phase a selection might be made from among them based on a search for a meaningful familiar shapes in long-term memory. While in some sense all of these are reinterpretations of the mental images, they do not all qualify as the sort of visual "reconstruals" of images that show that mental images are pictorial entities whose distinct perceptual organiza-tion (and reorganization) is determined by the early-vision system. Indeed, they seem more like the kind of free-association interpretations one gets from Rorschach inkblots.

The clearest source of evidence I am aware of that bears on the ques-tion of whether mental images can be reconstrued is provided by Peter Slezak (1991, 1992, 1995). Slezak asked subjects to memorize pictures such as those shown in figure 6.12. He then asked them to rotate the images clockwise by 90 degrees and to report what they looked like. None of his subjects was able to report the new imagined appearance, though they could easily report it by rotating the actual pictures. The problem was not with their recall or even their ability to rotate the simple images; it was with their ability to recognize the rotated image in their

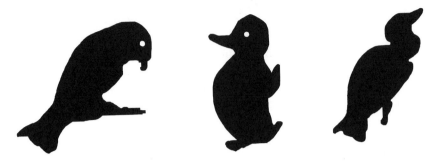

Figure 6.12
Memorize the shape of one or more of the figures, then close your eyes and imagine it rotated clockwise by 90 degrees (or even do it while viewing the figures). What do you see? Now try it by actually rotating the page. Peter Slezak reported that none of his subjects could see the second visual interpretations in these three examples, although they could easily see it if they drew the figure from memory and rotated the drawing. (From Slezak, 1991, 1995.)

mind's eye. Subjects had all the relevant information since they could draw the rotated figures from memory, and when they did, they usually recognized the rotated shape from their drawing! What is special about these examples is that the resulting appearance is so obvious—it comes as an "aha!" experience when carried out by real vision. Unlike the figures used by Finke et al. (1989), these shapes are not familiar, nor do they contain unique "landmark" features (which can be used to recognize the rotated pattern; see Hochberg and Gellman, 1977), and their appearance after the rotation could not easily be inferred from their description.

6.5.5 What about the experience of visualizing?

It may well be that the most persuasive reason for believing that mental imagery involves inner perception is the subjective one: Mental imagery is accompanied by an experience very similar to that of seeing. As I remarked at the beginning of this chapter, this sort of phenomenal experience is difficult to ignore. Yet studies of visual perception demonstrate that introspection is a highly suspect source of evidence about the nature of the underlying representation, because it trades on the failure to distinguish between the content of our experience (what we are imagining) and the causal entities in our mind–brain that are responsible for the way things appear in our imagination. There is a very strong temptation to reify the image content—to make what philosophers call the "intentional fallacy" (and what Titchener called the "stimulus error") of attributing to a mental state the properties of the world that it represents.

But the experience of imaging is not an experience that reveals the form of the image; rather, it reveals the content of the image. The experience of the image tells us what it is an image *of*. Because of this it is plausible that both vision and imagery lead to the same kind of experience because both are mediated by similar internal states. In fact, a common view, made explicit by Roger Shepard (1978b), is that imagining *X* is nothing but the activation of mental states normally associated with the visual perception of *X*, though without *X* being present. Shepard notes that because the image is not external, the experimenter cannot discover its shape or other visual properties. But if we *could* externalize it, by mapping from a brain state back to a stimulus, which could have been its distal cause, it would look like the scene illustrated by Shepard in figure 6.13 and figure 6.14.

Shepard recognized that even if the experience of mental imagery arises from the same brain states as occur in visual perception, this would not entail that the internal state is underwritten by pictorial, as opposed to symbolic, structures in the brain. However, the interpretation that Shepard presents in the above two figures does assume that a vision state and an imagery state carry sufficiently similar information that one

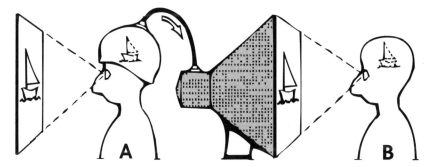

Figure 6.13
Illustration of a hypothetical mechanism (in a "thought experiment") that externalizes the brain states involved in visual perception by one person (A) so that another person (B) might have the same visual experience without the presence of the original visual stimulus. (From Shepard, 1978b.)

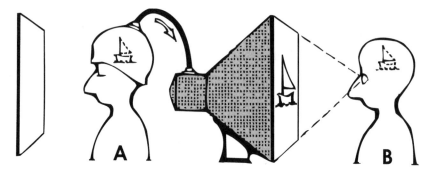

Figure 6.14
Illustration of how the apparatus introduced in the "thought experiment" of figure 6.13 could also be used to externalize a mental image as a visual display. (From Shepard, 1978b.) The point was to explore what it means for a mental image to be experienced as a percept or as a picture.

could, at least in principle, put another person's brain into the same state as that of a person having a mental image by providing the second person with appropriate *visual* stimulation. The proposal of a possible (though fanciful) way to externalize the visual experience of a person imagining some situation, assumes that a mental image and an actual display can be *informationally equivalent*. This turns out to be a very strong assumption, and one that is very unlikely to be true in general (as Shepard himself recognized; see note 13).

The situation shown in the above figures is clearly not possible in principle. In particular, B's brain could not, even in principle, be put into a state corresponding to A's having a mental image by providing inputs *through B's eyes*, using a display. Consider, for example, that in figure 6.13, A is able to examine the figure freely with eye movements as well as with covert movements of attention while B need not be scanning his display in synchrony or even scanning it at all. There is good reason to believe that without making the same voluntary eye movements and attentional scans, A and B would not have the same experience (see, e.g., O'Regan and Noë, 2002). B is in a position to examine the display freely, to scan it with eye movements and to selectively attend to parts of it. This assumes that the visual information about the scene in A's brain (which by assumption has been faithfully mapped onto the display that B sees) contains *all* the panoramic information needed to allow B to examine, scan, and interpret it—an assumption that we already found to be untenable since the information about a scene that is actually encoded by A is only a small part of the information that could be encoded given sufficient time. But B would have to be shown *all* the potential information to be able to scan the scene and thus to have the same experience as A (see section 1.4, as well as section 6.5.4, above).

The problem is that the experience of "seeing" is not informationally equivalent to *any* display because it must include potential as well as actual inputs. Part of the reason for this is that A is able to use visual indexes or some similar deictic mechanism to keep in contact with the display in order to access additional information as needed, thus ensuring that more of A's display is potentially available than is encoded or noticed at any point in time, whereas this potential does not apply to the display shown to B since that includes only the current state information. As I suggested in chapter 5, it is this capability to return to the display at will that confers the apparent panoramic and detailed pictorial feel on our perception of a scene.

Even more important is the fact that what A experiences is an *interpretation* of the stimulus; it is, for example, one view of an ambiguous display. Since what is presented on B's display is pictorial, and therefore uninterpreted, B is free to construe it differently from the way A construed it, even if it somehow accurately maps the contents of A's visual cortex. For example, suppose that in figure 6.13 A is looking at an ambiguous Necker cube (e.g., one of the Necker cubes shown in figure 1.7). A will see it in one of its two construals, so this will be the content of his phenomenological experience and, by assumption, of the state of his brain. But what will appear on B's display in that case? One cannot construct a pictorial image of the cube that already has one of its construals preselected (even if one were allowed to labels its parts). So then B is free to see a different construal of the Necker cube than A does, contradicting the assumption that the display has the possibility of conveying the phenomenological experience from A's brain to B's display. The situation in figure 6.14 has the same problem: When A imagines a Necker cube he imagines it with one or the other construal (recall that Peterson found no cases in which people could see reversals of the Necker cube in their image). Thus, again, B is in a position to have a different perceptual experience when the visual information is projected from A's brain to B's screen.

The problem arises because Shepard was attempting to "externalize" the contents of the experience of "seeing" (either seeing a visual scene or a seeing mental image), but the experience corresponds to having in mind an interpretation, not of having a raw unanalyzed array of light- and dark-colored regions.[13] As J. J. Gibson and many others before him have stressed, we do not experience patches of light and color; rather, we experience seeing people and tables and chairs—the ordinary familiar things that populate one's world, the recognition of which requires that we consult our long-term memory. That may be why the experiences of seeing and of having a mental image very likely correspond to activity at a high level of the visual process, after the stimulus is recognized and interpreted as something familiar (a number of authors, including Crick and Koch, 1995 and Stoerig, 1996, have suggested that the locus of our awareness occurs higher than primary visual cortex). So if the experience of seeing or of imagining is to be transmitted from A to B, then at the very least, it requires that the state of a much larger part of A's brain than his visual cortex be mapped onto B's brain. It would have to include parts where memory inference, and interpretation occur, and that part (even if it could be localized) could not be mapped to a picture.

In addition to these problems about conscious contents, it is also unlikely that the distinction between information-processing episodes of

13. Roger Shepard recognizes the inadequacy of the "externalization" view entailed by his figures 6.13 and 6.14, but he then goes on to say that this "deep structure" aspect of the percept is overplayed because most figures are not ambiguous and most people see the same things when presented with the same displays. But this concession misses the point since even if most people saw the same thing, it does not entail that the experience of having a mental image can be rendered on a display. It is in the nature of real displays that they are uninterpreted and therefore boundlessly ambiguous (as we saw earlier). Even if you could somehow create images that were unambiguous for most people most of the time, they would still need to be interpreted and the interpretation would not be equivalent to a display. This can be seen clearly in the case of experienced mental images because mental images are conceptual: one has a mental image under one's intended interpretation. One does not need to provide an interpretation of one's own image, and indeed one generally can't provide a new *visual* interpretation of one's mental image. This and related points will be discussed in chapter 7.

which we are conscious and those of which we have no awareness marks a scientific natural kind, the kind of demarcation that can help to focus our attention on the relevant causal variables. It could turn out that imagery is, after all, a special form of information processing that uses a special modular system, but that it overlaps only partially with episodes of which we are consciously aware as a kind of seeing. It *could* turn out that the correct analysis of the type of information processing involved in mental imagery does not distinguish between episodes of which we have a sensorylike awareness and those of which we do not. In other words, it could turn out that there is a theoretically interesting and distinct form of information processing that is sometimes accompanied by the phenomenology we associate with imagery and sometimes not. Already there has been talk of "unconscious imagery" and there is evidence that most experimental results obtained in studying imagery (such as the mental scanning results, the image size results, the mental rotation results, and others discussed earlier in this chapter) can be obtained with congenitally blind subjects (see, e.g., Barolo, Masini, and Antonietti, 1990; Cornoldi et al., 1993; Cornoldi, Calore, and Pra-Baldi, 1979; Craig, 1973; Dauterman, 1973; Dodds, 1983; Easton and Bentzen, 1987; Hampson and Duffy, 1984; Hans, 1974; Heller and Kennedy, 1990; Johnson, 1980; Jonides, Kahn, and Rozin, 1975; Kerr, 1983; Marmor and Zaback, 1976; Zimler and Keenan, 1983) as well as with subjects who profess little or no experience of mental imagery (see chapter 7 for more on the dissociation between imagery and vision). It is also significant that the status of reports of vividness of images is problematic. That is, subjective vividness does not appear to correlate with performance in a great many imagery tasks. For example, it has been reported that the ability to recall visual experiences is either uncorrelated (Berger and Gaunitz, 1977) or even negatively correlated with vividness of the experience (Chara and Hamm, 1989), although the confidence level of the reports is correlated with vividness (McKelvie, 1994) as is performance on tasks such as inducing visual illusions by superimposing imagined patterns over perceived ones (see pp. 337–340). Other tasks show differences between vivid and nonvivid imagers that are hard to interpret in terms of their use of mental images (see, e.g., Wallace, 1991).

In assessing the evidence from phenomenology one needs to seek objective corroborating evidence for informational differences between mental episodes accompanied by the experience of seeing and mental episodes that are accompanied by some other experience (or no conscious experience at all). A great many studies suggest that unconscious states play the same role in cognition, as do conscious states (e.g., stimuli of which we have no conscious awareness appear to influence perception and attention the same way as stimuli of which we are aware; see Merikle, Smilek, and Eastwood, 2001). But there are also some different information-processing and neurophysiological correlates of episodes accompanied by awareness (Dehaene and Naccache, 2001; Driver and Vuilleumier, 2001; Kanwisher, 2001). What I have argued, here and elsewhere, is just that we are not entitled to take the content of our experience as reflecting, in any direct way, the nature of the information-processing activity (what Pessoa, Thompson, and Noë, 1998 call the "analytical isomorphism" assumption). In particular, the evidence does not entitle us to conclude that episodes that we experience as *seeing in one's mind's eye* involve examining uninterpreted, spatially displayed depictive representations (i.e., pictures) using the early-vision system.

Finally, cognitive science has nothing illuminating to say about the subjective impression that we are experiencing a "seeing" or a "hearing" episode, since this is tied up with the deeply mysterious questions of consciousness. It is always very tempting to view our experience *as such* as playing a causal role—as having causal powers. We say that we scan our image or zoom in to see a small detail in it or that we remember a certain emotional crisis by thinking of it in a certain way (e.g., as having a spiral shape). I am sure that there is a sense in which all these are true reports. But this way of putting it suggests that how a cognitive episode is experienced *causes* a certain observable consequence, rather than the cause being some underlying physical state. Taken literally, such claims entail a dualist (or at least an interactionist) metaphysics. They claim that there can be causes that are not physical (i.e., that do not follow natural physical law). Although that is a coherent position one could take, it is not one that most writers on mental imagery would want to defend. What we would prefer to defend is the notion that underlying a certain type of experience are certain physical and biological properties and that these properties are the causes of the behavior. A particular experience, say, the experience of "seeing in the mind's eye," is not a possible natural property, so the statements that contain references to such experiences as causes are not literally what their authors want to claim. But if it's not literally the case that I behave in certain ways because of how I experience some mental episode, then I need a different way to talk about the causal sequence, a way that will not attribute causal properties to experiences the way that everyday discourse sometimes does; a way that does not mention that I do something or think something because it feels like I am seeing a picture in my mind's eye.

7

Seeing with the Mind's Eye: Part 2, The Search for a Spatial Display in the Brain

One of the most widely accepted claims about mental images is that they are "spatial," and among the most frequently cited demonstrations of this claim are the mental scanning experiments, which I discussed on pages 303–310. There I argued that it is unwarranted to conclude that, because it takes longer to scan across greater imagined distances, images must "preserve" metric spatial information (Kosslyn et al., 1978)—if by "preserving" distances one means that images *have* spatial properties such as size and distance, rather than simply that they encode such properties. Yet the alleged spatiality of mental images is central to the claim that images are *depictive* and thus unlike a language of thought.

The claim that images have spatial properties comports with one's intuitions about mental images, but it raises some interesting and subtle questions about what it means to *have* spatial properties, and whether there could be any sense to this notion apart from the literal claim that images are written on some physical surface, presumably on some surface in the brain. In what follows I will examine the claim that images are spatial and then examine the recent evidence that has been presented and interpreted as bearing on this question.

7.1 Real and "Functional" Space

One of the more seductive claims about images made by Kosslyn (e.g., in the quotation cited in section 6.4) and echoed by many other writers (e.g., Denis and Kosslyn, 1999; Prinz, 2002; Tye, 1991) is that images are laid out spatially in a *functional* rather than a physical space, where the notion of a functional space is introduced by example, as something like a matrix or array data structure in a computer. This is a seductive idea because it appears to allow us to claim that images are spatial without also committing us to claiming that they are laid out in real space in the brain or in some other physical medium. It also appears to give some meaning to the claim that images somehow incorporate (or "preserve") distance as well as size. Because the idea that images are somehow spatial has been so influential in theorizing about mental imagery, I will devote this chapter to a discussion of this claim and to some of the recent evidence cited in support of it. Before going into the evidence, however, I consider what it might mean to claim that images are spatial. Then I will argue that the appeal to a functional space is empty and merely restates the phenomena we are trying to explain.

The problem with the functional space proposal is that functional spaces do not have any particular properties intrinsically. Being functional, they are not subject to any natural laws and therefore can be assumed to have whatever properties are needed to account for the experimental data. Because a functional space has no intrinsic properties, any properties it has are stipulated or extrinsically assumed, and so it can accommodate any findings whatever. Or, to put it more positively, if the extrinsic assumptions provide any explanatory advantage at all, they can be equally well adjoined to a theory that assumes *any* form of representation, not just a pictorial one. They can, for example, be added to a theory that claims that the form of information underlying images is that of a language of thought. Despite this blatant inadequacy of the functional space proposal, the idea remains widely accepted in psychology and even in some quarters of philosophy. The reason for this seductive quality of the proposal is itself quite revealing, and so I will devote part of this chapter to discussing how the functional space idea connects with the literal space (the "display-in-the-head") hypothesis and how it maintains a strong pull on contemporary research on mental imagery, which itself has led to certain lines of investigation of mental imagery, particularly in neuroscience.

In the computational model of mental imagery described in Kosslyn et al., 1979, the inner "screen" on which images are "displayed" is a matrix of elements—a computer data structure that corresponds to a two-dimensional matrix. It functions like a two-dimensional display in several respects. Graphical elements, such as points, lines, contours, regions, and other components of figures are written on the matrix by filling designated cells that correspond to places on the image, defined in terms of quantized Cartesian coordinates (pairs of matrix indexes). The principles for generating figures are explicitly stated, as are principles for reading off figural properties (at least in principle, if not in an actual working system). For example, to examine a certain part of a figure after examining another part, the system has to move a locus of processing (corresponding to its focal attention) through intermediate points along the path from one cell of the matrix to the other. This is done by successively incrementing the (x and/or y) indexes. The matrix itself appears *intrinsically* to contain unfilled places that serve as potential locations of figural elements, so that empty places appear to be explicitly represented. As Kosslyn claims in the earlier quotation, in this kind of representation, "each part of an object is represented by a pattern of points, and the spatial relation among these patterns in the functional space correspond to the spatial relations among the parts themselves. . . . Not only is the shape of the represented parts immediately available to appropriate processes, but so is the shape of the empty space." In other words, empty places are explicitly displayed, along with filled places, so that regions between contours are formed and displayed as a natural consequence of displaying contours. This form of representation appears to embody the criteria for being a depictive representation as described in the quotation. In this way the model appears (at least in principle) to account in a natural way for much of the relevant data, as well as the qualitative aspects of our experience of imagining. What else could one ask for?

As we saw when we discussed the mental scanning results in section 6.3, to provide an explanation it is not enough that a model exhibit certain patterns of behaviors. We still need to say *why* these behaviors arise. As with all the examples I discussed earlier (including the mystery code-box example), it makes a great deal of difference whether a particular generalization holds because (a) the system uses its representations of the world, along with its reasoning capacity, to simulate some behavior it believes would occur in the imagined situation, or because (b) the principle that determines the behavior of the system is inherent in the mechanism or architecture of the system that displays and examines images. So we need to ask which of these is being claimed in the case of the matrix model (or any other functional space model) of the image. The answer is crucial to whether the model provides an explanation of the experimental findings or merely summarizes them, the way a table or other sorts of descriptive data summary might.

Here the image theorist is caught on the horns of a dilemma. On the one hand, the system (say, the one that uses a matrix data structure) might be viewed as a model of the architecture (or, equivalently, of the format or the medium) involved in mental imagery. If that is the case, its properties ought to remain fixed and they ought to explain the principles by which the imagery system works (and perhaps even provide some suggestions for how it might be implemented in the brain). This proposal (which we might call a "model of the architecture of mental imagery") can be subjected to empirical scrutiny, using, among other techniques, the criterion of cognitive penetrability. This architectural version of the functional space proposal entails that the observed properties will not change with changes in the person's beliefs about the task. On the other hand, the matrix model might be thought of as simply summarizing the pattern of people's behavior in particular circumstances (e.g., the increase in time to shift attention to more distant places in the image, or the increase in time to report details from a "smaller" image), with no commitment as to *why* this pattern of behavior arises. This purely descriptive view of the imagery model is compatible with the pattern being a result of what subjects understood the experimental task to be (e.g., that the task is to simulate as closely as possible what would happen in a situation in which they were looking at a real display) and their tacit knowledge of what would happen if they were to see certain things occur. Summarizing such a pattern of behavior is a perfectly legitimate goal for a theory, although it only meets the criterion that Chomsky calls "descriptive adequacy" as opposed to "explanatory adequacy." If that is how one views the matrix, however, one is then not entitled to draw conclusions about the nature and more specifically the format of mental images. It is clear from the writings of picture theorists that this is *not* what they have in mind; rather, they take their CRT model (or what I called their "picture theory") to be what we have called a *model of the architecture* of mental imagery (certainly this is explicitly claimed in Kosslyn, 1981).

Consider first the matrix model (Kosslyn, 1994) viewed as an architectural model. For now I will examine why such a model appears intuitively attractive and what in fact it assumes about the mental architecture underlying the use of mental imagery. Later I will consider whether the empirical facts are consistent with such a model. The conclusion I reach is that a matrix is attractive precisely because it *can* be (and typically is) viewed as a computer simulation of a real 2D surface, which is precisely the *literal* display-in-the-head assumption one was trying to avoid by talking of "functional space." Consider some reasons why a matrix appears to be spatial. It appears to have two dimensions, to explicitly have distances (if we identify distance with the number of cells lying between any two particular cells) as opposed to merely representing them (say, in some numerical code), and to explicitly have empty spaces. It also seems that a matrix can be "scanned": there is a natural sense in which it exemplifies topological properties, like that of "being adjacent," so that searching for an object by passing through intervening empty places makes sense. The trouble is that all these spatial notions—adjacency, distance, unfilled places, and scanning—are properties of a way of thinking about a matrix; they are not properties of the matrix as a data structure. Looked at as a data structure, cells (25, 43) and (25, 44) have nothing "adjacent" between them—except when we view them as points in a real space, as opposed to two discrete registers in the computer, which is what they are. What we think of quite naturally as two *locations* in space are nothing but two discrete symbols or register names (which, in the case of a computer, we refer to as "addresses," or even "locations" in memory, thus inviting a spatial metaphor). What makes them appear to be locations is not inherent in their being indexes of cells in a matrix data structure; it is a property that is tacitly introduced by our way of thinking about the data structure. For example, according to Kosslyn, "It is only by virtue of how this information is 'read' and processed that it comes to function as if it were arranged into an array (with some points being close, some far, some falling along a diagonal, and so on)" (1994, p. 5). But that isn't the way a matrix has to be used, *unless it is being used to simulate a real spatial surface or display*—and then it is not the matrix but the thing being simulated that has the spatial properties. In a matrix, one does not get to a particular cell by "moving" there from an "adjacent" cell—one simply retrieves the contents of the cell by its name (names happen to be pairs of numerals, but that is of no consequence—the pairs are converted to a single symbolic address anyway). Of course, when it is used as a model of space, accessing registers is constrained in the way it is constrained in physical space, that is, one gets to a cell by accessing a sequence of cells defined as whatever is between the currently accessed cell and the desired cell. But in that case it is this extrinsically stipulated constraint that is responsible for this way of accessing information, not the fact that it is a matrix; and of course the reason the extrinsic constraint is stipulated is because the theorist implicitly believes that the mental image is actually written on a physical surface, not a "functional" surface. This is the only possible motivation for what would otherwise be a totally arbitrary constraint.

Viewed in this way, the notion of a functional space has no explanatory role; it just has whatever properties we require it to have. If we wish the functional space to have the properties of real space, then we arrange for the relevant properties to be manifested. But then we cannot appeal to something we call a functional space to explain why it has those properties: it has those properties because we stipulated them. The spatial character of a matrix (or any other implementation of "functional space") is something that is stipulated or assumed *in addition* to the computational properties of the data structure. The critical fact here is that such an extrinsic postulate could be applied to *any* theory of mental images, including one that assumes that images are sentencelike symbolic structures. Indeed, there is nothing to prevent us from modeling an image as a set of sentences in some logical calculus and then, in addition, stipulating that to go from one place to another (however places are referenced, including the use of numerals as names) requires that we pass through "adjacent" places, where adjacency is defined in terms of the ordinal properties (or even metrical properties, if the evidence merits that assumption) of place names. If this sounds ad hoc, that's because *it is*. But the assumptions are no more ad hoc than they are when applied to a matrix formalism. For example, in a matrix data structure it is equally natural to go from one "place" to *any* other place (think of places as having names; you can go from a place named Q1 to a place named Q2 just by issuing those two names to the function that accesses cells in a matrix). If you want to restrict the movement, you have to do it by assuming a constraint that is extrinsic to the form of the matrix. Only if you view the matrix as a representation of a real (physical) two-dimensional display do you get a notion of "adjacent cell," and only if you confine operations on names to ones that move to adjacent cells defined in this manner do you get a notion of scanning. The same is true of the claim that matrices represent empty places. An empty place is just a variable name with no value: any form of computational model can make the assumption that there are names for unoccupied places (in fact, you don't even have to assume that these places exist prior to your making an inquiry about their contents—they don't, in some computer implementations of sparse matrices).

The point here is not that a matrix representation is wrong. It's just that it is neutral with respect to the question of whether it models intrinsic (i.e., architectural) properties of mental images—for example, the property that is responsible for many experimental results such as scanning—or merely summarizes the data that arise from people's knowledge of how things happen in the world (e.g., that when using mental images, people usually act as though they are observing things in the world). When appeal to the matrix appears to provide a natural and principled account of the spatial imagery phenomena (such as mental scanning and the effect of image size) it is invariably because the theorist is tacitly viewing it as a representation of a two-dimensional physical surface. In other words, the theory is principled if and only if it assumes that mental images are written on a physical surface. A real surface *has* the relevant properties because physical laws apply to it. For example, on a real physical surface, it takes time $t = d \div v$ to traverse a distance d at velocity v. This is guaranteed by a law of nature. In a functional space, the relation between d, v, and t is indeterminate: it has to be stipulated in terms of extrinsic constraints. On a real physical surface, the relative 2D distances between points remain fixed over certain kinds of transformations (e.g., rotation, translation, change of size) and the Euclidean axioms always hold of distances between those points. In particular, distances obey metrical axioms; for example, the triangle inequality must hold of the distances d between three elements x, y, and z so that $d(x, y) + d(y, z) \geq d(x, z)$. In a functional space none of these constraints is required to hold by virtue of the format or intrinsic nature of the representation (unless, once again, functional space is just a gloss for real space).

Of course, in principle it is possible to implement a model of space in another (analog) medium by mapping sets of properties of space onto sets of properties of the model medium (that's what an analog computer typically does). For example, one might use the relationship between voltage, resistance, and current flow (specified by Ohm's Law) to model the relationship between distance, speed, and time, respectively. Although in this case the properties of the model are different from the properties being modeled, they are nonetheless intrinsic properties— certain properties and relations in the model hold because of the physics of the analog medium. A system that follows Ohm's Law constitutes an analog model of a system consisting of the three properties involved in mental scanning (distance, speed, and time). That part is easy because it involves the relationship between only three variables. But it would be surprising if *all* properties of space could be modeled by something other than space itself. Notice that the above analog model of distance, speed, and time would fail to model lots of other aspects of space and motion, such as the principles that hold for distances and relative directions, or distances and areas. This is because Ohm's Law provides no natural quantity corresponding to, say, direction or area. One could, of course, define such quantities as area or trajectory in terms of some functions over time, distance, and current flow, but these would have to be calculated, as opposed to being measured directly in the model. It would also fail to model such interesting relationships as those embodied in the Pythagorean Theorem, the invariance of some properties or relations (such as area, relative distances, and relative angles) over certain transformations (such as rotation). It would clearly not be able to model such assumed image properties as the visibility of an object's features as a function of the size of the object. There are an unlimited number of such properties and relationships, which is why it's hard to think of any system of variables other than those intrinsic to space and time that could model them all. The problem of finding a non-Cartesian model of Euclidean space more appropriate as a psychological model is precisely what concerned the French philosopher Jean Nicod. His brilliant and ambitious early work on this problem (Nicod, 1970), discussed briefly on pages 372–373, did not go very far toward providing possible models of space that could be of use in understanding mental imagery.

But even though such considerations are relevant to the attempt to make sense of the intuitive picture theories of mental images, this entire discussion of analog representation is beside the point when it comes to explaining most mental imagery phenomena. The real question is not how to implement any particular model of space, but whether one should explain the apparent spatial character of images in terms of the architecture of mental imagery. My purpose in belaboring the issue of which constraints are imposed by format and which are imposed by extrinsic stipulations is simply to clarify the role that some functional space like a matrix *could* play, and thereby set the stage for the real issue, which is an empirical one; whether imagery findings arise from architectural properties at all. I have already described some of the empirical findings concerning mental scanning, (such as studies of mental scanning when the task is understood as imagining lights that go off in one place and simultaneously go on at another place, or in which the task is focused on aspects of retrieving information from an image that play down the question of how one gets from one place to another). Such findings show that no architectural model could explain the results, since the results depend on observers' beliefs. The same goes for the finding that it takes longer to answer questions about small visual details when the image is experienced as "small" than when it is experienced as "large." The way the data turn out in these cases shows that the imagery architecture of the mind does not impose constraints like those you would expect of a real spatial display, at least not in the case of these particular phenomena.

But what about other properties of spatial representations? Are the properties of represented space cognitively penetrable? Can we imagine space not having the properties it has? Kosslyn has claimed that the spatial property of the image display constrains what we can imagine. He says, "We predict that this component will not allow cognitive penetration: that a person's knowledge, beliefs, intentions, and so on, will not alter the spatial structure that we believe the display has. Thus we predict that a person cannot at will make his surface display four-dimensional or non-Euclidean" (Kosslyn et al., 1979, p. 549). But as I remarked at the beginning of chapter 6, the more likely reason why people cannot image a four-dimensional or non-Euclidean world is that they do not know what such a world would *look like*, and knowing what it would look like is essential to being able to carry out the task we call "imaging." According to this view, not knowing where the edges and shadows will fall is sufficient reason for failing to image it; there is no need to invoke properties of a "surface display."

It appears that we are not *required* to scan through adjacent places in getting from one place to another in an image: we can get there as quickly or as slowly as we wish, with or without visiting intermediate (empty or filled) places. In fact, as we saw earlier (pp. 340–344), recent work provides reason to doubt that we *can* smoothly scan a mental image (or even a real stationary scene) or visit more than a few places along the way, even if we want to. Rather, it looks as though the best we can do visually is estimate how long it would take an object traveling at a given speed to move between a few places we can literally see, and the best we can do in our mental image is to imagine *that an object is moving*; we can't imagine the object as being at a succession of imagined intermediate places along the way (at least not for more than a few such places). Since the spatial nature of mental images is such a well-entrenched belief, I will devote the next section to a discussion of what it would mean for images to be spatial, and also to a brief discussion of two potential reasons why in certain situations images may exhibit some nontrivial spatial properties without themselves being laid out on a spatial surface.

7.2   Why Do We Think That Images Are Spatial?

7.2.1   Physical properties of mental states: Crossing levels of explanation

In chapter 1, I mentioned the strong temptation to reify experiential properties like color, shape, or duration by attributing these properties to mental representations. This tempting mistake is to slip from saying that you have an image of a scene and that the scene has property *P* to the conclusion that the mental event or the formal object in your head itself has property *P*. The temptation is to equivocate between the two ambiguous senses of the phrase "an image of *X* with property *P*", namely, "an image of (*X* that has property *P*)" and "(an image of *X*) that has property *P*." In the first case *X*, a thing in the world, has the property, whereas in the second case the image of *X*, a thing in the head, is claimed to have the property. In referring to one's representational states (e.g., one's thoughts or images), the relevant properties are always properties of the thing one is imagining, not of the object that stands in for it—the representation itself. The degree of the temptation to reify properties varies with the particular property. It is fairly easy to see that an image of a cat does not have to be furry, an image of an orange need not be colored orange, or that an image of one object on top of another need not be made up of two parts, one of which is on top of the other. Nonetheless, it is a bit harder to accept that an image of a big thing need not be large (or larger than an image of a small thing), and harder still to appreciate that imagining a long-lasting event need not last long.

I once wrote a brief commentary (Pylyshyn, 1979a) in which I reflected on how freely we speak of the beginning, end, and duration of mental events—of the representations produced by perception or by imagination, for example. I wondered why we were not disposed to speak of other physical properties of mental events, such as their temperature, mass, or color. After all, these are all legitimate physical properties: if the result of perception is a physical state or event, which few people would deny, then why do we find it odd to ask what color or weight or temperature a percept is, somewhat less odd to ask how big it is or where it is, and completely natural to ask how long it took? The commentary did not elicit any response; people found it puzzling that I should even raise such a question when it is obvious that mental events have durations but not temperatures. But this should have been a puzzle. The reason we do not speak of the physical properties of mental events is not because we are closet dualists who believe that mental things are in a different realm than physical things, but because mental event *types* need not correspond to physical event *types*. To speak of an event type is to refer to an entire class of events among which we make no distinction for certain purposes. All the instances of the letter "a" on this page are considered equivalent for the purposes of reading, even though they may differ in size, font, and in other ways of interest to a typesetter—and they certainly differ in their location. Thus we speak of the letter *type* "a" of which there are many letter *tokens*, or instances of "a" on the page that are distinguishable in many ways. There is no answer to the question, What size is the letter "a" as such? It can be any size and still be the letter "a." But a mental event type has many event tokens each of which could have arbitrarily different physical properties—at least, they are not required to have any fixed property merely by virtue of being a member of a particular event type. When we ask whether a mental event (such as imagining a particular melody being played) has a particular duration, we are asking about the event-type, not the event-token.

There need be no answer to the question, What is the temperature of an imagined singing of "Happy Birthday"? though there is an answer to the question, How many words are there in an imagined singing of "Happy Birthday"? (at least according to the usual interpretation of what it means to "imagine X," namely, that to imagine X one must imagine, as best one can, each part of X in the right sequence and with roughly the right relative duration).

To make the idea of an event-type more concrete, consider the parallel case in computing. The event of computing a certain function (say, a square root function) is realized physically in a computer; therefore, it is a physical event. No doubt about that. Yet *where* it is carried out it is not relevant to its being that particular function, in part because it may occur anywhere in the machine and in fact will occur over widely dispersed locations from occasion to occasion. There is no physical location corresponding to the function *as such*, even though each token occurrence of such a function does take place somewhere or other. This is what we mean by an event type: it is what all occasions of the event (e.g., executing a square root function) have in common. Clearly all events of executing the square root have certain functional properties in common (namely, they all map 4 into 2, 9 into 3, 16 into 4, and so on). But does the square root function have a temperature? Perhaps. Nothing in principle prohibits all possible instances of executing a square root from being realized in some physical form that always has a certain temperature, though that would certainly be surprising inasmuch as it is not necessary that the instances share some common physical property—and it is not hard to provide a counterexample to any claim about the temperature of a particular function (e.g., by putting the computer in a freezer!). And even if there were such a property, it would very likely be an adventitious correlation that is highly unlikely to be of computational significance. The point is that the function is defined and has its significance in the arena of mathematical operations, not in the arena of physical processes, and the two are not type-equivalent. Now what about time: does the square root function have duration? The same answer applies. It does if every token occasion on which it occurs takes approximately the same amount of time (within some limits). It could also be that parts of the function (e.g., the basic arithmetic operations involved) have an actual duration that does not vary from token to token. But if the duration varies from occasion to occasion, then only token computations of that function have some particular duration. This is what I claimed in my commentary about the duration of mental events. The typical response my commentary evoked ("most people think that mental events have durations but Pylyshyn does not") shows how deeply the reification of time goes. The interesting thing about this reaction is not that people think it makes sense to speak of the duration of a mental event (it does, for tokens of the event), but that the intentional error is so deep that people do not notice that any assumption is being made.

If there is a temptation to reify time in the representation of temporally extended events, the temptation to reify space is at least as strong and has immediate implications for one's theory of mental imagery. The temptation to assume an inner display is linked to the fact that images are experienced as distributed in space (just as they are experienced as distributed in time). Because they are experienced as distributed in space, we find it natural to believe that there are "places" on the image—indeed it seems nearly inconceivable that an image should fail to have distinct places on it. This leads naturally to the belief that there must be a medium where "places" have a real existence. We feel there must be a form of representation underlying an image such that it makes sense to ask of some object X in the image: Where (in the image) is X? Or, How big is (the image of) X? Or, Where (in the image) are X's parts located relative to one another? If the space in question were not real, then in what sense could we ask where a particular feature is located in relation to other features? Moreover, we have seen that a feature's being at a particular place in relation to other features in a scene *does* have an effect on how the scene is perceived. We saw this in the examples given in chapter 1. It is the fact that the illusory line is seen to be (or is represented as being) in a certain place that creates the Pogendorff illusion, illustrated in figure 1.5.

Dan Dennett (1991) has written on the temptation to reify mental space and time and has pointed out, correctly in my view, that representing a certain spatial pattern does not require that one represent all its parts as distinct individual elements situated somewhere in space. For example, in representing a checkerboard one need not represent each of its squares at each possible location on the board (as assumed when one speaks of the image of the checkerboard being laid out in functional space). Dennett suggests that rather than explicitly representing each part of the imagined scene and each feature of the scene at once, the visual system may be just assigning coarse labels to regions ("more of the same here"). But this leaves a puzzle: Where is "here" and where is the coarse label placed, if not on the dubious inner display? Certainly "here" does not refer to a place on the retina or on the objects in the world (unless we are going around putting real labels on things!). The idea of labeling parts of a scene is ubiquitous and plays an important role in computational theories of vision, as we saw in chapter 3 (especially on pp. 99–106). But what is it that is being labeled? Can we label part of a representation or part of an experience? Many psychological theories of pattern detection (Ullman, 1984) and of visual attention (Watson and Humphreys, 1997; Yantis and Jones, 1991) speak of placing "tags" on certain stimulus objects (e.g., to tell us that the item has already been processed, as in counting). If the tags must be located at a precise location in the representation, then such theories must tacitly assume an inner display of some sort—or at least a representation in which it makes sense to refer to distinct *locations*. Is there any sense that can be made of talk of labeling or of tagging places in a scene that does not assume an inner image that reifies space?

Space has been subject to a great deal of analysis that began long before the debate over the nature of mental images surfaced in cognitive science. For a long time space was viewed as a sort of receptacle that contains matter without itself partaking in the laws of nature—a view that had to be abandoned with the acceptance of general relativity and the notion of non-Euclidean or curved space that is affected by gravity. Even with this change in status, space (along with time) retained its special place among physical properties. Immanuel Kant claimed that our intuitions of space and time were prior to our concepts of properties—that they were a priori categories of mind, presumably preconceptual and innate. The French mathematician, Henri Poincaré (1963), taking a more empirical stance, asked (and provided a partial answer to) the question of how we could ever learn that space has three dimensions, given our multidimensional and multimodal experience of it. And more recently, a brilliant young French doctoral candidate named Jean Nicod wrote a dissertation speculating on how we could construct a three-dimensional world from the sensory experiences available to us (1970). He put the problem differently. He took space itself to be a set of formal properties defined by the axioms of Euclidean geometry, and asked how the mind could develop a model of these axioms based on sensory experiences together with a small number of basic perceptual categories (primarily the notion of volumetric containment). Nicod's starting point is one we must take seriously. To say that something is spatial is to claim that it instantiates (or is a model of) the Euclidean axioms of plane geometry, at least in some approximate way (perhaps the model might be what is sometimes referred to as "locally Euclidean"). In addition, in speaking of something being spatial one usually implies that it is also metrical (or quantitative), which means that certain of its properties also fall under the metric axioms (see, e.g., Luce et al., 1995; Palmer, 1978).[1] Thus a rigorous way to think of the claim that images are spatial is as the claim that certain properties of images (not of *what* they represent, but of their inherent *form* or their material instantiation) fall under, or can be mapped onto, certain formal mathematical axioms.

But the claim that mental images have spatial properties in this formal sense is much stronger than the empirical facts warrant. Indeed, even visual space fails to meet many Euclidean requirements (Attneave, 1954; Luce et al., 1995; Suppes, 1995; Todd, Tittle, and Norman, 1995). What exactly one means by images having spatial properties is thus not very clear. Nonetheless there are some properties of imagery that most writers have in mind when they claim that images are spatial. Before I examine the possibility that images may be displayed on a real physical surface in the brain, I should stop to ask what reasons there are (other than the pervasive temptation to reify mental qualities discussed earlier) for thinking that some form (physical or otherwise) of space may be involved in representing spatial properties in mental imagery. There are obviously many reasons for thinking that mental images at least *encode* metrical spatial properties in some way. For example, distances on an image appear to map onto distance in the represented world in a systematic (and monotonic) way: people are able to make judgments of relative

---

1. In most formulations there are four metric axioms: If d is a metric (or distance) measure, then (1) $d(x, y) \geq 0$; (2) if $d(x, y) = 0$, then $x \equiv y$; (3) $d(x, y) = d(y, x)$; and (4) $d(x, z) \leq d(x, y) + d(y, z)$.

size and even some (limited) absolute judgments of size from their experienced images (Miller, 1956; Shiffrin and Nosofsky, 1994). Even if one agrees with the analysis I provided in chapter 6, that the scanning effect is attributable to a mental simulation of what would happen in the real visual situation, this still requires that relative distances be encoded and used in the simulation. The ability to represent relative spatial magnitudes is surely a necessary part of our ability to recall and reason about geometrical shapes, since shape is defined in terms of relative spatial dimensions. Consequently, it is reasonable to think that we require some encoding of spatial magnitudes when we think using mental images.

Spatial intuitions are very powerful and appear, at least prima facie, to be operative when we reason about space while relying on our mental images, just as they are when we reason with the aid of a diagram (a topic I pursue in section 8.3). If we are to shun the intuitively satisfying notion that we do this by drawing an inner picture in our mind, we will need some account of how we solve such problems at all. Nobody is yet in a position to provide a detailed account of this sort. On the other hand, neither are the proponents of the picture theory: even if there were real 2D diagrams in the head we would have no idea how they could be used. What we do know is that sooner or later the pictorial information has to be interpreted and transformed into a form that can enter into inferences, that is, a form that meets the requirements of compositionality and productivity discussed in chapter 8, section 8.2 (and taken up in detail in Fodor, 1975; Fodor and Pylyshyn, 1988).

The spatiality of images arises not only from the fact that we can retain distances and shapes in memory (often in visual memory). There are other properties of images that give them their apparent spatiality. Among these are the experiments discussed earlier (e.g., mental scanning), the more robust of which are those in which people "project" their image onto the world they are perceiving. These are discussed in the next section, where I suggest that although some spatial properties inferred from imagery experiments are real, they do not arise from the spatial nature of the images themselves. These spatial properties, I argue, can be attributed to the real spatial nature of the sensory world onto which they are "projected." Such properties inherited from perceived space, can also explain the way that images connect with the visual-motor system.

This derivative origin of image spatiality is discussed in the following sections.

7.3   Inheritance of Spatial Properties of Images from Perceived Space

In many imagery studies subjects are asked to imagine something while looking at a scene, thus at least phenomenologically superimposing or projecting an image onto the perceived world. Although it has been amply demonstrated (see the review in O'Regan and Lévy-Schoen, 1983) that true superposition of visual percepts does not occur when brief visual displays are presented in sequence, or across saccades, the impression that superposition occurs in cases of imagery remains strong. What happens, then, when a mental image (whether constructed or derived from memory) is superimposed on a scene? In many of these cases (e.g., Farah, 1989; Hayes, 1973; Podgorny and Shepard, 1978) a plausible answer is that one allocates attention to the scene according to a pattern guided by what is experienced as the projected image. A simpler way of putting this is that one simply *thinks* of imagined objects as being located in the same places as certain perceived ones. For example, in their 1978 study, Podgorny and Shepard asked subjects to imagine a letterlike figure projected onto a grid (such as shown in figure 7.1) and to indicate as quickly as possible whether a spot that was then displayed on the grid was located on or beside the imagined figure. In the visual version of the task when both the letter and the spot were displayed, subjects were faster when the spot was on the figure than when it was immediately beside it, faster when it was at certain stroke intersections (such as in the corners or the "T" junction) than when it was in the middle of a row or column, and so on. When subjects were asked to imagine the figure projected onto the empty grid, the pattern of reaction times obtained was very similar to the one obtained from the corresponding real display. This result was taken as showing that the visual system is involved in both the visual and the imaginal cases. But a more parsimonious account is that in "imagining" the figure in this task, observers merely attended to the rows and columns in which the imagined figure would have appeared. We know that people can indeed direct their attention, or assign a visual index, to each of several objects in a display or conform their attention to a particular shape. As I argued in chapter 5, either

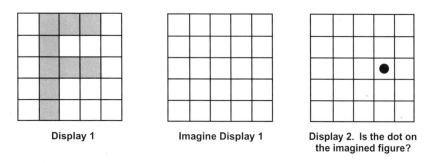

Display 1   Imagine Display 1   Display 2. Is the dot on
                                                   the imagined figure?

Figure 7.1
Observers were shown a simple figure (display 1), which they had to retain as a memory image superimposed on a grid after the pattern was extinguished. A second pattern (the dot in display 2) was then projected onto the same grid and observers had to indicate whether the dot was positioned on or off the imagined figure. The pattern of reaction times was found to be similar to that observed when the figure was actually present. What does this show about the form of the memory image? (Adapted from Podgorny and Shepard, 1978.)

focusing attention in this way or assigning several indexes to certain objects is all that is needed to generate the observed pattern of reaction times. In fact, using displays similar to those used in the Podgorny and Shepard (1978) study but examining the threshold for detecting spots of light, Farah (1989) showed that the instruction to simply *attend* to certain regions was more effective in enhancing detection in those regions than the instruction to superimpose an image over the region.

A similar analysis applies in the case of other tasks that involve responding to image properties when images are superimposed over a perceived scene. If, for example, you imagine the map used to study mental scanning (discussed in chapter 6) superimposed over one of the walls in the room you are in, you can use the visual features of the wall to anchor various objects in the imagined map. In this case, the increase in time it takes to access information from loci that are further apart is easily explained since the "images," or, more neutrally, "thoughts" of these objects *are actually* located further apart. What is special about such superposition cases is this: the world being viewed contains rigid 2D surfaces that embody the properties expressed by spatial axioms— Euclidean and other mathematical properties of metrical space literally apply to it—so the combined image/perception inherits these properties.

How does this happen? How does cognition obtain access to these spatial properties and apply them to the superimposed image?

What makes it possible for certain spatial properties to be inherited from a real scene is the visual indexing mechanism discussed in chapter 5. Using this mechanism, a person can pick out a small number of objects in a scene and associate mental contents (or thoughts) with them. So, for example, the person could think that particular token objects in a scene correspond to certain imagined objects in memory. As we saw in chapter 5, we can have thoughts such as "assume that this *<object-token-1>* is the beach, and that *<object-token-2>* is the lighthouse," where the italicized terms are pointers to visual objects that are picked out and referenced using visual indexes. We have already seen that such visual indexes allow thoughts about certain token properties to be connected to particular objects in a scene, the way that demonstrative terms like "this" or "that" do in natural language. Thus we can literally think, "*this* is the beach," "*this* is the lighthouse," and so on. Given this capability, something interesting happens. Because the scene obeys physical laws and geometrical axioms, the indexed objects systematically maintain their spatial relations, providing only that visual indexes remain bound to their scene objects. For example, if you indexed three points that just happened to be collinear, then regardless of what you had encoded about their relationship, they would always have an ordinal position along the line; the second point would bear the relation "between" to the other two, and so on. So if you subsequently *noticed* that they were collinear or that the "between" relation held among the three points, you would be guaranteed that it was consistent with the axioms of geometry and with their being on a rigid surface, whether or not you remembered or noticed that the points you had picked out had other properties and whether or not you knew that they maintained their fixed locations while you examined other properties of the scene. Such a guarantee would be underwritten, not by *your knowledge* of geometry (and, in particular, not by your knowledge of the formal properties of the relation "between"), but by the physical facts about the world you are looking at and the fact that your visual system is able to detect certain relations that hold among objects in that world. In other words, by picking out (i.e., indexing) certain objects in the world, and by binding certain thoughts to these objects, you are able to draw conclusions about their configuration by *visually* noticing these properties. Without such a display you would have to draw inferences based on the postulates of geometry.

This point connects directly with several of the phenomena that have been cited in support of the claim that mental images are spatial. For example, if you could individuate and refer to several objects in a visual scene, you could then associate certain objects or properties in memory with each of these perceived objects. Then you could literally move your attention (or even your gaze) from one to another of these places. Many other imagery phenomena might also be attributable to real vision operating over a display. For example, with real vision taking part in the imaging process one could deploy attention in a way that could produce certain visual illusions (as suggested on pp. 337–339). Such attentional phenomena are different from a real superimposition of an image over the scene. For example, in the scanning case all you need to be able to do is recall (from *some* representation of the scene) where point B was in relation to point A. The effect does not depend on a detailed picture being projected, only on attention and visual indexes being allocated in certain ways. By anchoring a small number of imagined objects to real objects in the world, the imaginal world inherits much of the geometry of the real world.

7.3.1 Scanning when no surface is visible

What if the scanning experiment were to be carried out in the dark or that there were no visible objects to correspond with the objects in your memory? One prediction is that you would have trouble with this task, since it is known that after a few minutes of looking at a featureless display (called a ganzfeld), vision becomes unstable and it even becomes difficult to keep track of where you are looking in relation to where you were looking earlier (Avant, 1965). Such featureless displays are rare—almost any surface has texture features, as can easily be seen, for example, in displays of first and second derivatives of image luminance that invariably show many clear discontinuities (e.g., in Marr, 1982). But what if you generate a new image of something without at the same time viewing a real scene? What if you imagine a scene with your eyes closed? The first thing that can be said is that the results in such cases are much less robust and more easily influenced by task strategies and beliefs. It is not even clear that mental scanning experiments can be carried out in total darkness since even viewing a single light in total darkness leads to illusory motion called the autokinetic effect (in which a stationary light appears to move around autonomously). As argued earlier (on pp. 341–343) there is also reason to believe that smooth imaginal scanning, in which the focus of the scan passes through intermediate points, is not possible under these conditions. Notwithstanding these problems, it may still be possible to generate the relevant time-distance relationships without having a spatially laid out scene either in the visible world or in your head. All you need is a way to represent magnitudes such as distance, speed, and time[2] and to use these to compute time-to-contact (as discussed on p. 343). There is no general theory of how such magnitudes are encoded, but we do know that they must be encoded with considerable precision, not only in humans but also in animals (Gallistel, 1990). But it may also be possible to simulate the relevant scanning times without carrying out time-to-contact computations using representing magnitudes—by doing something similar to what I suggested we do when we use real visible surfaces to provide the spatial distances over which we scan attention. We may do this by exploiting a more general "spatial sense' that involves modalities other than vision, for example, a proprioceptively sensed space or the space of potential motor movements. I explore this possibility in the next section.

7.3.2   The exploitation of proprioceptive or motor space
Where does the strong impression of the spatial nature of our images come from? What, other than the subjective experience of seeing our mental image laid out in space, prompts us to think that images are in

---

2. I have no quarrel with those who propose analog representations of magnitudes. This is a very different matter from the assumption that there is an analog representation of an entire system of magnitudes corresponding to space. The trouble is that unlike the hydraulic analog model of electric flow, an analog model of space-time would have to map many properties (including at least three dimensions orthoganal spatial plus time) and meet a large number of constraints, such as those embodied in Euclidean axioms. It would have to exhibit such general properties as the Pythagorean Theorem, the single point-of-view requirement discussed in Pinker and Finke (1980) and countless other properties of projective geometry (including the metrical axioms; see note 1). It is no wonder that nobody has proposed an analog model of space-time other than space-time itself.

some important sense spatial? One simple answer is that when we imagine a spatially distributed layout of objects and shapes, then something is indeed spatial, namely, the layouts and shapes that we are imagining. It is the things that we think *about*, not the patterns in our brain that we think *with*, that are spatial. This simple answer should carry more persuasive force than it typically does: just as when we imagine a round thing, or a green thing, or a furry thing, it is the thing we are imagining that has those properties, not our image. But there is one difference in the case of spatial properties of mental images: If you close your eyes and imagine a familiar spatial layout (say, a map of your city), you feel the image is "out there in front of you" in the sense that you can actually point to parts of it. But what are you actually pointing at when you do this? I have already suggested that when you do this while looking at a scene ("projecting" your image onto the visible world) you may be binding objects in your image to objects in the scene, thus providing the imagined objects with an actual location in the world so that they inherit the spatial properties of the real external space. Might it be that when you do this with eyes shut (or in the dark) you bind objects in your image to places in a *proprioceptively sensed* space? If that were so, there would once again be a real space over which scanning could occur, but as in the case of projecting images onto a perceived scene, the space would not be in the head; it would be real space in the world or in the body, sensed through proprioceptive, haptic, kinesthetic, auditory, or any other perceptual modality that was operating when your eyes were closed.

Our sense of space is extremely precise and fluent. It is used not only for dealing with concrete spatial patterns, but also for individuating and thinking of abstract ideas. In fact, sign languages (like American Sign Language) make use of locations in perceived space to individuate ideas and refer back to them. An entire topic can be located at a place in allocentric space, and then when the speaker wishes to refer to that topic he or she simply points to the empty space where the topic had been "deposited." You can easily demonstrate for yourself how good we are at localizing things in the space around us. Close your eyes and point to things in the room around you; you may find that you can point accurately and without hesitation—even to things behind you. Given this skill it seems plausible that we can utilize it for binding objects in our image to places in our immediate proprioceptive space, even in the absence of vision. What this would give you is the sensed spatial quality of images without requiring that images *have* space themselves. The difference between appealing to pictorial images and appealing to what I have been calling a *spatial sense* is that the latter does not assume any particular form of representation, only the skill to pick out locations that are currently being sensed, through whatever ambient inputs are available to calibrate locations.

Studies of the recall of locations have demonstrated a surprisingly facile skill that allows us to sense and recall where things are around us. Attneave and Farrar (1977) and Attneave and Pierce (1978) show that the ability to recall locations is extremely good and the accuracy is about the same whether the locations are in front of or behind the observer. When observers looked at a row of seven objects located in front of them and were later seated with their backs to where the objects had been, they could recall their relative locations almost as well as they could if they were asked to imagine them as being in front of them. It thus appears that observers could easily take one or another of two perspectives 180 degrees apart in recalling the locations of objects in a room. They could do this even without generating a detailed visual image of the objects. Attneave and Farrar (1977) report that when subjects were asked about the relative location of two objects, "the second object was located in space (subjects typically said) and the question was answered accordingly, before the object was clearly pictured. This is logically consistent with the report that images were evoked or constructed, rather than continuously present: one must decide *where* to draw the picture before drawing it." It seems that deciding where the item is occurs primitively, quickly, and accurately. Attneave and Farrar also report that when an image of the scene behind the subject's head did occur it was not accompanied by a sense of turning and looking. They remark, "This contradicts the view that a visual image must correspond to some possible visual input. . . . We are being told, in effect, that the *mind's eye* has a cycloramic, 360 degree field." This suggests that the representation of location in space is rather different, both phenomenologically and behaviorally, from visual images. The latter are usually assumed to have sensory and pictorial properties and to have a "visual angle" about the size of foveal vision (Kosslyn, 1978).

The study of the "sense of space" (a term chosen so as not to prejudge the question of whether the space is visual, proprioceptive, motoric, or completely amodal) has only recently been conducted under controlled conditions and has led to some unexpected findings. For example, it has been shown that although people have a robust sense of the space around them, this space tends to be calibrated primarily with respect to where the person is located at any moment. The reference point, where people perceive themselves as being, also depends on their motor activity; as they move about they automatically recalibrate their proprioceptive sense of space, even if they move about without benefit of vision. Rieser, Guth, and Hill (1986) had subjects view a set of target objects (which also served as alternative viewing points) and then had them either walk blindfolded to specified points or merely imagine walking to these points, and then to indicate (by pointing) the direction of other targets. They found that people were faster and more accurate when they had moved on their own volition to the designated locations, even though they did not have the benefit of visual information in doing so. This was also true for pure rotation. People who had rotated their body appeared to instantaneously recalibrate their orientation so they could point to the location of various targets, whereas when they merely imagined themselves to rotate, their localization of targets was slow and deliberate (Farrell and Robertson, 1998; Rieser, 1989).[3]

3. It is possible to make too much of the involvement of motor activity in mental imagery. I have suggested that we use our proprioceptive/motor space in deriving the spatial character of mental images. But others have suggested that the motor system is involved in transforming mental images as well. The role that motor mechanisms play in the transformation of visual images is far from clear, notwithstanding evidence of correlations between visual image transformations and activity in parts of the motor cortex (Cohen et al., 1996; Richter et al., 2000), or the influence of real motor actions on visual transformations (Wexler, Kosslyn, and Berthoz, 1998). Some of the cortical activity observed during both motor performance and the mental transformation of visual images may reflect the fact that these areas (e.g., posterior parietal cortex) compute some of the higher-level functions required for extrapolating trajectories, for tracking, for planning, and for visual-motor coordination (Anderson, et al., 1997). Since many of these functions also have to be computed in the course of anticipating movements visually, it is reasonable that the same areas might be active in both cases. Studying the interaction of imagery and the motor system is clearly important, but at present we are far from justified in concluding that dynamic visual imagery is carried out *by means of* the motor system (or that visual operations *exploit* motor

In his commentary on my paper on mental imagery, David Ingle (2002) describes his own case of long-term visual persistence (which he views as an extreme type of mental image). He observed that the location of his image remains fixed in allocentric space as he moves or turns around. But if he observes an object held in his hand, and closes his eyes, his image of the object moves when he moves his hand. This sort of anchoring of perceived location of an image to proprioceptively perceived locations is consistent with the notion that proprioceptive cues are used to locate images in real space. We will see another example of this principle in the next section when I discuss the finding that a visually guided motor skill (smooth pursuit), which responds only to perceived motion and not imagined motion, also responds to proprioceptively perceived motion.

The idea that the spatial quality of a mental image derives from its connection with proprioceptive and motor systems is further supported by the work of Ronald Finke (1979) on the interaction of mental images and visual-motor control (see below for details), and by findings regarding the role of motor activity in relation to locations of objects in mental images. The work was carried out to support a version of the picture theory of mental imagery, but as we will see, it does not require the involvement of anything pictorial; only the position of imagined objects in relation to the environment is relevant.

Consider the stimulus-response compatibility findings of Tlauka and McKenna (1998), which showed that when you respond using crossed and uncrossed hands, it takes longer to respond to features on the opposite side of your mental image. From this Tlauka and McKenna (1998) concluded that stimulus-response compatibility factors affect reactions to locations in images just as they do in real displays. But what the result actually shows is that observers orient to objects imagined to be in certain locations in (real) space just the way they would have if the objects actually were at those locations. Thus it is not surprising that the same phenomena are observed when observers react to objects in real

---

control mechanisms). This way of speaking suggests that our motor system can grasp and manipulate our images, a view that unfortunately reinforces the general tendency to reify the world that pervades much mental imagery theorizing.

displays as they do to objects merely imagined to be located "out there" in these same locations. We will have a closer look at this phenomenon again later.

The Finke (1979) studies are striking because they involve a detailed analysis of the interaction of imagery, visual-motor coordination, and "felt location" of objects. In a series of ingenious experiments, Finke showed that the well-known adaptation to displacing prisms could be obtained using imagery alone. In the original visual adaptation studies (see, for example, Howard, 1982), observers wore prism goggles that displaced the apparent location of everything in view by some fixed angle (e.g., 23 degrees). After wearing the goggles for some period of time, observers became adept at reaching for things (and also walking around). When the goggles were later removed, observers had the opposite experience—objects looked to be mislocated in the opposite direction to the way the prisms had shifted them in the adaptation phase. Finke's studies are of special interest to the present discussion because they illustrate the way in which projected images can work like real percepts in certain ways—in particular in respect to perceptual-motor coordination. They also illustrate the important role played by visual indexes in accounting for certain results in studies on mental imagery.

In one study, Finke (1979) asked subjects to imagine seeing their (hidden) hand as being in certain specified locations. The locations where he asked them to imagine their hand to be corresponded to the errors of displacement actually made by another subject who had worn displacing prisms. He found both the pattern of adaptation and the pattern of aftereffects exhibited by observers who only had imagined feedback to be similar to that exhibited by observers who actually wore displacing prisms. Now it is known that adaptation can occur as a result of solely verbally presented error information (Kelso et al., 1975; Uhlarik, 1973), though in that case (and in contrast with the case where the hand is continually viewed), the adaptation occurs more slowly and transfers completely to the nonadapted hand. Yet Finke found that in the case of imagined hand position, the adaptation, though significantly lower in magnitude, followed the pattern observed with the usual visual feedback of hand position. Moreover, when subjects were told that their hand was not where they imagined it to be, the adaptation effect was nonetheless governed by the imagined location, rather than by where they were told their hand was, and it followed the same pattern as that observed with visually presented error information about their erroneous hand position. When subjects did not move their arm, or if they just imagined moving their arm, the results were like those obtained when they were given only verbal feedback: slow adaptation effects that transfer to the nonadapted hand. From these results, Finke concluded that adaptation to imagined hand location taps into the visual system at the same "level" as that of visually presented information. But do these results really require that we appeal to the visual system, as understood in chapter 2, or can they be explained in terms of the orienting of attention to *real* places in a visual display?

The generally accepted view of what goes on in prism adaptation experiments is that there is a recalibration between where subjects are looking or visually attending and either where they feel their arm is located or the motor commands they must issue in order to move their arm correctly (the so-called reafferent signal). The exact way this happens has been the subject of some debate (Howard, 1982), but it is generally accepted that important factors include the discrepancy between the seen position and the felt position of the hand (or the discordance between visual and kinesthetic/proprioceptive location information). Significantly, such discordance does not require that the visual system recover any visual property of the hand other than its location. Indeed, in some studies of adaptation, subjects viewed a point source of light attached to their hand rather than the hand itself (Mather and Lackner, 1977) with little difference in the ensuing adaptation. But it also appears that where the subject attends is equally important (Canon, 1970, 1971). In some cases even an immobile hand can elicit adaptation, providing the subject visually attends to it (Mather and Lackner, 1981). Thus the imagery condition in Finke's study provides all that is needed for adaptation without making any assumptions about the nature of imagery. In particular, subjects direct their gaze toward a particular (erroneous) location where they are in effect told to pretend their hand is located, thus focusing attention on the discordance between this viewed location and their kinesthetic and proprioceptive sense of the position of their arm.

Ian Howard (1982) has provided a thorough discussion of the conditions under which more or less adaptation occurs. The most important requirement for adaptation is that the discordant information be salient for the subject, that it be attended, and that it be interpreted as a discordance between two measures of the position of the same limb. Thus anything that focuses more attention on the discordance and produces greater conviction that something is awry helps strengthen the adaptation effect. It makes sense, therefore, that merely telling subjects where their hand is would not produce the same degree of adaptation as asking them to *pretend that it actually is* at a particular location, which is what imagery instructions do.

It seems that there are a number of imagery-motor phenomena that depend only on orienting one's gaze or one's focal attention to certain perceived locations. The Finke study of adaptation of reaching is a plausible example of this sort of phenomenon, as is the Tlauka and Mckenna study of stimulus-response compatibility. None of these results requires that imagery feed into the visual-motor system. Indeed, these two cases involve *actual* visual perception of location (i.e., there really are some visible features located in the relevant locations). The only information that needs to be provided by the mental image for adaptation (as well as the stimulus-response compatibility effects) to occur is information about the location of some indexable visible features in the scene, where the hand can be imagined to be located (by binding the idea of the hand to a visible feature through the index). It does not require that the image provide shape, size, orientation, color, *or any other visual information*, other than the locations where things are imagined to be.

Rather than support the notion that imagery feeds into the visual-motor system at the same level as vision, the evidence we have considered provides support for the notion that vision and motor control are closely connected precisely because the spatiality of images derives directly from the spatiality of the real world that arises from the perceptual space provided by proprioceptive, kinesthetic, auditory, and other sense modalities. This connection of image locations with both proprioceptively sensed space and with potential actions of the motor system is much more important than has generally been recognized. It extends the earlier argument about imaginal space being inherited from vision to the proposal that imaginal space can be inherited from a wider range of space-sensing modalities. Just as we can direct our eyes or our attention to the visually perceived space when we examine images that are projected onto a visual scene, so we can move our hand from one imagined place to another, and when we do so we demonstrate the spatiality of images.[4]

7.4   The Search for a Real Spatial Display

There are many reasons for resisting the conclusion that images themselves are spatial. I have presented a number of arguments suggesting that many of the experimental findings that have led people to claim that images are spatial (or at least that they have "metrical" properties) can be explained more parsimoniously in terms of the use of tacit knowledge to simulate what would happen if observers actually saw the appropriate event actually taking place (e.g., if they were to examine a real map). I have also presented some arguments suggesting that the spatial character of images may derive from the way that imagined objects are attached (using FINST indexes) to perceived features in the world. When a visual surface is not available, sensed locations in proprioceptive or auditory space might be used instead. What will not do, as an explanation, is to appeal to a functional space, since the only way such an appeal can be explanatory is if the functional space is taken as a simulation of real space.

The only other alternative that still appears to be viable is the view that images appear spatial because they are actually realized in the brain on real 2D spatial displays. If we are convinced that images are different from other forms of thought and if we think that part of their difference is that they are laid out in space (or that they are "depictive"), then a reasonable strategy might be to take the bull by the horns and try to find a literal spatial medium in the brain. This approach at least has the virtue of making an explicit testable claim, which, despite its initial implausibility, would provide some explanatory advantage over an

4. In chapter 5, I discussed a theoretical mechanism for binding objects of thought to perceived objects in a scene. This mechanism is the FINST visual index. In the original paper that introduced this mechanism, I proposed a parallel mechanism that binds objects of thought (or of visual perception) to proprioceptively sensed objects or locations. These indexes are called *Anchors*, and they play an important role in perceptual-motor coordination along with FINST indexes.

elusive metaphor or an appeal to the misleading notion of a functional space. Despite the advantage of this approach, surprisingly few picture theorists have been willing to endorse the assumption that there is a literal spatial display in the brain. In recent years, however, much of the work directed at supporting the picture theory of mental imagery has been carried out within neuroscience, and much of it has involved the search for a spatial display (using new techniques such as neural imaging). The hope has been to find a 2D display along the lines of the CRT metaphor introduced several decades ago (Kosslyn et al., 1979). In what follows I will examine the recent neuroscience work from several perspectives, beginning with a general methodological discussion of the status of neuroscience evidence in the imagery debate.

7.4.1   Aside: Does biological evidence have a privileged status in this argument?

A number of writers seem to believe that neuroscientific evidence renders all previous behavioral evidence obsolete. Stephen Kosslyn himself laments the indecisive nature of mental imagery research of the previous twenty-five years and speaks of the new neuroscience-based research as finally being able to provide a clear and decisive answer to the nature of mental imagery (Kosslyn, 1994). Nothing could be further from the truth. It was behavioral and phenomenological considerations that raised the puzzle about mental imagery in the first place and that suggested the picture theory. And it is a careful consideration of that evidence and its alternative interpretations that has cast doubt on the picture theory. Even if we found real colored stereo pictures displayed on the visual cortex, the problems raised thus far in this and the previous chapter would remain and would continue to stand as evidence that these cortical pictures were not serving the function attributed to them. For example, the fact that phenomena such as mental scanning are cognitively penetrable is strong evidence that *whatever* might be displayed on the cortex it could not be what is responsible for the patterns of reaction times observed in the scanning studies, because, as I argued in section 6.3, those patterns reflect not properties of mental architecture but properties of what subjects know. Similarly, the question of what is responsible for the facilitation of recall and problem solving that accompanies the phenomenology of mental imagery requires a psychological process theory to link any proposals about the nature of mental images with actual perform-ance data. It is important to understand that the mere fact that the data are biological does not privilege those data in deciding the truth of a psy-chological process theory, especially one whose conceptual foundations are already shaky.

In examining the behavioral evidence so far, I have distinguished two types of claims about the representations underlying mental images. The first concerns the nature or the format of mental images and the second concerns the nature of the mechanism used in processing them. We saw that although these may be related questions, they are also largely inde-pendent, since it is logically possible for the visual system to be involved in both vision and mental imagery and yet in neither case use picture-like representations. Similarly, it is possible for representations to be topographically organized and yet have nothing to do with visual per-ception, nor with any depictive character of the representation. In a certain sense the physical instantiation of any cognitive representation *must* be topographically organized. Fodor and I (Fodor and Pylyshyn, 1988) have argued that any form of representation that is adequate as a basis for cognition must be compositional, in the sense that the content of a complex representation must derive from the content of its con-stituents and the rules by which the complex is put together (the way the meaning of a sentence is compositional and depends on the meaning of its constituents together with the way they are syntactically put together). But the physical instantiation of any representation that meets the requirement of compositionality will itself be compositional (Pylyshyn, 1984a, pp. 54–69; 1991b). In the case of symbolic representations, parts of expressions are mapped recursively onto parts of physical states and syntactic relations are mapped onto physical relations. As a result, there is a real sense in which the criteria in the Kosslyn quotation on page 328 are met by any compositional physical symbol system, not just a depictive one. Note that in a digital computer, representations are both compositional and topographically distributed and yet are generally not thought to be depictive, whereas when they are supposed to be depic-tive, as when they encode images (especially when they use bitmapped codes, such as GIF, JPEG, or BMP), their topographical distribution does not mirror the physical layout of the picture. Thus the question of the spatial distribution of images, the question of whether they are depictive, and the question of whether they are connected with vision are logically independent. In the present state of neuroscience, it remains highly unclear how information-processing mechanisms, representations, and other theoretical entities map onto brain structures, and consequently it is unclear how such evidence can address the question of the format of thought, including the format of mental images. In what follows I will look at some of the evidence as it applies to the study of mental imagery. In the course of this review it will become clear that what neuroscience research is being directed toward is what it is best at: locating patterns of activity in the brain. As a result, the technique appears to be well suited for testing the literal picture-in-the-head theory of mental imagery.

As we saw earlier, the question of whether mental imagery uses the visual system is intimately tied to the question of what constitutes the uniquely visual system. If the question is merely whether some mechanisms used in vision are also used in visual imagery, then the answer is clearly *yes*, for the uninteresting reason that they both involve accessing memory and making inferences. The involvement of visual mechanisms in mental imagery is of interest to picture theorists primarily because of the possibility that the role played by the early-vision system in processing mental images will vindicate a version of the picture theory by showing that imagery does indeed make use of a special sort of spatial display (this is explicitly the claim in Kosslyn, 1994). The question that naturally arises is whether we can make a case for this view by examining the neuroscientific evidence concerning which areas of the brain are involved in mental imagery and in visual perception. It is to this question that I now turn, beginning with an examination of the evidence of neural activity cited in support of the claim that mental images are realized in a topographic or spatial display in the brain, and then considering some of the clinical evidence from brain damage.

7.4.2   The argument from differential activity in the brain

An argument along the following lines has been made in the recent neuroscience literature (Kosslyn, Pascual-Leone, et al., 1999; Kosslyn, et al., 1995). Primary visual cortex (area 17) is known to be organized retinotopically (at least in monkey brain). So if the retinotopic visual area were active when subjects generate mental images,[5] it would suggest that (1) the early-vision system is involved in some aspect of processing visual

5. At present, one of the primary sources of evidence from experimental neuroscience of brain activity during mental imagery comes from neural imaging (particularly PET, but more recently fMRI). This fairly recent technique, which is extremely important in clinical neurology, relies on assumptions about the relation between blood flow and metabolism, and between metabolism and cognitive processing in the brain. Yet it is far from clear what kind of neural activity is indicated by increased blood flow; whether, for example, it indicates activation or inhibition (e.g., the active attempt to suppress otherwise disrupting visual activity); whether it is associated with the same activity that is responsible for the sorts of behavioral measures discussed earlier (e.g., reaction time functions), whether it is related to the experience of "seeing," or something entirely different. It is even problematic whether increased cerebral flood flow indicates increased information-processing activity (Fidelman, 1994; Haier et al., 1988). There is also concern that the widely used subtractive technique (in which the activity map associated with a control condition is subtracted from the activity map associated with an experimental condition) has problems of its own (Sergent, 1994), as well as being predicated on the assumption that the function under study is a modular one that involves activity in the same particular brain region each time it occurs (Sarter, Berntson, and Cacioppo, 1996). Even processes known to be functionally modular, such as the syntactic aspect of language processing, often give inconsistent neural imaging results (Démonet, Wise, and Frackowiak, 1993), so we ought to be wary when drawing conclusions about functions like mental imagery, which the empirical data give us every reason to believe is nonmodular. Problems such as these may eventually be resolved by better technologies for more precise localization and measurement of brain activity in time and space. But the value of neuroscience data will increase even more when we develop a better understanding of the questions that we need to address. For the time being we should treat neural imaging evidence the way we treat all other essentially correlational evidence, such as reaction time, error rate, or ERP—as indirect indexes whose validity needs to be independently established, rather than as direct measures of the variables of primary interest. Even the use of the intrusive method of transcranial magnetic stimulation (rTMS), which gets around the problem of purely correlational evidence by effectively disabling an area of the cortex, has its own problems and cannot be assumed to provide direct evidence of causal mechanisms. For example, in a recent paper (Kosslyn, Pascual-Leone, et al., 1999) showed that if area 17 is temporarily impaired using rTMS, performance on an imagery task is adversely affected (relative to the condition when they do not receive rTMS), which Kosslyn et al. interpreted as showing that the activation of area 17 plays a causal role in imagery. However, this result must be treated as highly provisional since the nature and scope of the disruption produced by the rTMS is not well established and the study in question lacks the appropriate controls for this critical question; in particular, there is no control condition measuring the decrement in performance for similar tasks *not* involving imagery.

mental images, and (2) during episodes of mental imagery the visual system receives inputs in the form of a retinotopic display. In other words, in mental imagery the cognitive system generates a display that is laid out in a spatial or "depictive" form (i.e., like a two-dimensional picture) in primary visual cortex, and this display is then interpreted by the early-vision system.

Writers espousing the picture theory routinely cite evidence showing that the early-vision area of the brain is organized retinotopically. For example, one of the most widely cited papers is a study by Tootell et al. (1982), which shows that there is a pattern of activation in monkey visual cortex that closely resembles a pattern of lights that the monkey viewed. Tootell et al. trained macaques to stare at the center of a pattern of flashing lights while the monkeys were injected with radioactively tagged 2-deoxydextroglucose (2-DG), whose absorption is related to metabolic activity. Then the animal was sacrificed and a record of 2-DG absorption in its cortex was developed. This record showed a retinotopic pattern in V1 that corresponded closely to the pattern of lights (except for a cortical magnification distortion). In other words, it showed a *picture* in visual cortex of the pattern that the monkey had received on its retina, written in the ink of metabolic activity, as shown in figure 7.2. This led many people to conclude that a picture, corresponding to what we see, appears in primary visual cortex during visual perception. Although no such maps have been found during mental imagery, there can be no doubt that this is what the picture theorists believe is there and is responsible for both the imagery experience and the empirical findings reported when mental images are being used.

The idea that, in mental imagery, cognition provides input into the early-vision system that is then "perceived" and given a (possibly new) interpretation is very much in keeping with the views developed earlier from behavioral evidence. It is also in keeping with the subjectively satisfying picture theory of mental imagery. Given this background, it is no surprise that those who hold the picture theory would receive any evidence of the involvement of early vision in mental imagery with a great deal of enthusiasm. Evidence such as that of Tootell et al. has been hailed as the critical evidence that shows how vision and imagery are related: they both involve generating an image in primary visual cortex, which is processed by the visual system. We have already seen some reasons to

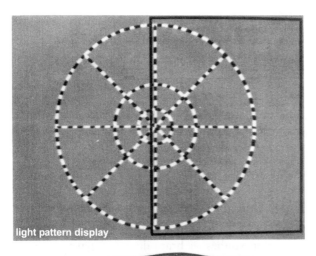

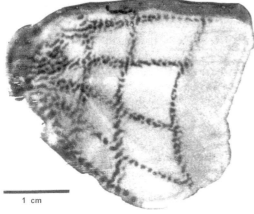

Figure 7.2
The top photograph (A) shows the stimulus used by Tootell et al. (1982) to demonstrate the retinotopic organization of the visual cortex in the macaque. The monkey stared at the top pattern, formed by flashing lights, while it was injected with a radioactively tagged tracer. Figure B shows the pattern of radioactivity recorded on the macaque's primary visual cortex. (Reprinted with permission from Tootell, et al., 1982. Copyright 1982, American Association for the Advancement of Science.)

doubt the picture theory, so one might perhaps wonder what the neuro-scientific results tell us about either vision or imagery. The relevance of the Tootell et al. results to the picture theory of mental imagery will be discussed in section 7.5 (especially pp. 407–409).

With this sketch as background, we can now ask whether there is indeed evidence for the critical involvement of early vision in mental imagery and, if so, what that would tell us. There appears to be some evidence that mental imagery involves activity in areas of striate cortex associated with vision, though the question of whether it is necessary or sufficient for mental imagery is far from being univocally answered. Most of this evidence has come from studies using neural imaging (e.g., Positron Emission Tomography or PET brain scans) to monitor regional cerebral blood flow, or from studies of brain-damaged patients. Some neural imaging studies report activity in topographically organized cortical areas (Kosslyn, Pascual-Leone et al., 1999; Kosslyn et al., 1995), but most have reported that only later visual areas, the so-called visual association areas, are active in mental imagery (Charlot et al., 1992; Cocude, Mellet, and Denis, 1999; D'Esposito et al., 1997; Fletcher, et al., 1996; Goldenberg, Mullbacher, and Nowak, 1995; Howard et al., 1998; Mellet et al., 1998; Mellet et al., 1996; Roland and Gulyas, 1994b; Roland and Gulyas, 1995; Silbersweig and Stern, 1998); but see the review in Farah, 1995, and some of the published debate on this topic (Farah, 1994; Roland and Gulyas, 1994a, 1994b). There is some reason to think that the activity associated with mental imagery occurs at many loci, including higher levels of the visual stream (Mellet et al., 1998).

To support the "cortical display" version of the picture theory it is important not only to show that some part of the visual system is involved in imagery, but also that the areas involved are the topographically mapped areas of cortex and that their involvement is of the right kind. In particular, it is important that the topographic organization reflect the spatial properties of the phenomenal image. Few neuroscience studies meet this criterion, even when they show that the visual areas are activated during mental imagery. One of the few examples of a finding that has been assumed to meet this criterion was reported in Kosslyn et al., 1995. This paper describes findings that relate a specifically spatial property of mental images (their size) to a pattern of neural activity. It showed that "smaller" mental images (mental images that the observer subjectively experiences as occupying a smaller portion of the available "mental display") are associated with more activity in the posterior part of the medial occipital region, while "larger" images are associated with more activity in the anterior parts of the region. Since this pattern is similar to the pattern of activation produced by small and large retinal images, respectively, it has been taken to support the claim that the activation of visual cortical areas during mental imagery corresponds to the activation of a cortical display that maps represented space onto cortical space. For this reason Kosslyn et al. (1995, p. 496) feel entitled to conclude that the findings "indicate that visual mental imagery involves 'depictive' representations, not solely languagelike descriptions."

But this conclusion is premature, for the spatial distribution of brain activity is not the kind that would explain the phenomenological and behavioral findings concerning image size and image distances. Even if the cortical activity that shows up in the PET brain scans corresponds to a mental image, the evidence shows only that a mental image experienced as being larger involves activity that is located in areas where larger retinal images would be projected. But in the case of vision, the reason that larger retinal images activate the regions they do is related to the way that the visual fibers project from the periphery of the retina to the occipital cortex. Thus the PET result is not the same as finding that a pattern of activation maps the size of a mental image onto a metrical spatial property of its cortical representation (Fox et al., 1986). In particular, the PET data do not show that image size is mapped onto some function of the size of the active cortical region. On reflection it might not be surprising that properties such as mental image size do not map monotonically onto the size of the activated region, yet this is exactly what would have to happen if the activity pattern is to serve as the basis for explaining such phenomena as mental scanning. A literal metrical mapping is required if the cortical display is to explain image scanning and image size effects. The mapping does not have to be linear, but it does have to be a continuous mapping (up to the grain of neuronal cells) that preserves local topology—such as a mapping known as a homeomorphism or a locally affine transformation. This is what it means to claim (as Kosslyn does in Kosslyn et al., 1978) that images "preserve metrical information."

A cortical display that preserves at least a monotonic function of magnitudes is required if the display is to account for the imagery data reviewed earlier. For example, the explanation for why it takes less time to notice features in a large image than in a small one is that it is easier for the mind's eye to "see" a feature in large cortical display. One could not attribute that result to the fact that some of the mental image is located in the more anterior part of the medial occipital cortex. The property of being located in one part of the visual cortex rather than another simply does not bear on any of the findings regarding the spatial nature of mental images discussed earlier (e.g., the mental scanning result). Consequently, the PET data cannot be interpreted as supporting the picture theory of mental imagery, nor do they in any way help to make the case for a cortical display theory of mental image representation. Those of us who eschew dualism are perfectly prepared to accept that *something* different happens in the brain when a different phenomenal experience occurs; consequently, we take it for granted that something different must occur in the brain when a larger image is experienced. The point has never been to dispute the view that psychological properties are supervenient on physical properties, but only to question the claim that the content of an image maps onto the brain in a way that helps explain the imagery results (e.g., mental scanning times, image-size effects on information access, and other metrical effects) and perhaps even the subjective content of mental images. If it had turned out that greater phenomenal distances were mapped monotonically onto greater cortical distance it might have left room for a possible cortical display account of some of the classical imagery findings (though it would still have left many questions unanswered); but a merely different locus of brain activity is no help in explaining metrical effects.

7.4.3   The argument from clinical cases of brain damage

Another source of evidence that has drawn the interest of picture theorists is found in studies on brain-damaged patients.[6] If the specifically

---

6. Problems comparable to those faced by neural imaging studies (see note 5) also arise with the use of data from clinical populations (Trojano and Grossi, 1994). It is hard enough to find "pure" cases in which the lesions are highly localized and their locations accurately known, but when such patients are found, the evidence is even less clear in supporting the involvement of the earliest (topographically organized) areas of visual cortex (Roland and Gulyas, 1994b).

visual areas of the brain are responsible for mental imagery, then it follows that damage to those areas should impair both vision and imagery functions in similar ways. In particular, if the damage is to a cortical display one should find similar patterns of deficits in both vision and imagery. A number of cases of parallel deficits in imagery and vision have indeed been reported. For example, Farah, Soso, and Dasheiff (1992) report that a patient who developed tunnel vision after unilateral occipital lobectomy also developed a reduction in the maximum size of her images (as determined by asking how close an image of a familiar object, such as a chair or an automobile, could be before it overflowed the edge of her image). If the cortical display were involved in both vision and imagery, and if the peripheral parts of the display were damaged, then it might explain the parallel deficits. Although it is certainly possible that tunnel vision and tunnel imagery could have a common underlying neural basis, the Farah et al. finding does not show that this basis has anything to do with a topographical mapping of the mental image onto spatial properties of a neural display. In fact, in this case there is a possible explanation for the reported finding that need not even involve the visual system, let alone a cortical screen. If one accepts the proposal that many imagery phenomena, such as those associated with different sizes of mental images, generally arise from the implicit task requirement of simulating aspects of what things would look like, then it is possible that the patient was merely reporting how a visual scenes looked to her after her surgery. In this study the patient had nearly a year of post-surgery recovery time before the imagery testing took place. During this time she would have become familiar with how things looked to her now, and was therefore in a position to simulate her visual experience by producing the relevant phenomena when asked to image certain things (e.g., to answer appropriately when asked at what distance some familiar object would overflow her vision). As I have often pointed out, this would not be a case of the patient being disingenuous or being influenced by the experimenter, which Farah et al. were also at pains to deny, but of the patient doing her best to carry out the required task, namely, to "imagine how it would look."

The clinical phenomenon of visual or hemispatial *neglect* has also often been cited in support of the cortical display theory. In a famous (1978) paper, Bisiach and Luzzatti reported two patients who had the classical syndrome of visual neglect, in which they tended not to report details on one side of a scene (in this case the left side). Bisiach and Luzzatti found that both patients also tended to omit reporting details from the left side of their mental images. More interestingly, this did not appear to be a problem of memory, since they could recall the details that appeared to be missing in the left side of their image if they were asked to imagine turning around and then to report their image of the scene viewed from the opposite perspective. This is indeed an interesting phenomenon and is frequently cited in favor of a cortical-screen view of mental imagery (after all, it's hard to think why a symbolic representation would favor one side of a scene over another). The explanation in terms of a cortical display appears to be straightforward: if one side of the display is damaged then one would expect both visual perception and visual imagery to be subject to neglect on the same side. However, it has since turned out that visual neglect and imaginal neglect are dissociable. There are patients who neglect one side of a visual scene but do not neglect one side of their image, patients who neglect one side of their image but do not neglect one side of a visual scene, and even patients who neglect one side of a visual scene and neglect the other side of their image (Beschin, Basso, and Sala, 2000).

Notwithstanding the problems of replicating the original finding with other patients, the idea that what is damaged in visual neglect is one side of a display seems too simplistic;[7] it does not account for the dissociation between visual and imaginal neglect (Beschin et al., 2000; Coslett, 1997), for the amodal nature of neglect (the deficit shows up in audition as well as vision; Marshall, 2001; Pavani, Ladavas, and Driver, 2002), for the fact that "neglected" stimuli typically provide some implicit information (Driver and Vuilleumier, 2001; McGlinchey-Berroth et al., 1996; Schweinberger and Stief, 2001), for the characteristic response-bias factors in neglect (Bisiach et al., 1998; Vuilleumier and Rafal, 1999) or for the fact that higher-level strategic factors appear to play a central role

7. Kosslyn (1994) does not explicitly claim that the "depictive display" is damaged in cases of neglect, preferring instead to speak of the parallels between the vision and imagery systems. But to be consistent he *should* claim that the display is damaged, since one of the reasons for assuming a display is that it allows one to explain spatial properties of imagery by appealing to spatial properties of the display. Simply saying that it shows that vision and imagery use the same mechanisms does not confer any advantage to the depictive theory, since that claim can be made with equal naturalness by *any* theory of imagery format.

in the neglect syndrome (Behrmann and Tipper, 1999; Bisiach et al., 1998; Landis, 2000; Rode, Rossetti, and Biosson, 2001). The "damaged display" view also does not account for the large number of cases of object-centered neglect (Behrmann and Tipper, 1999; Tipper and Behrmann, 1996), in which patients neglect one "side" of an object viewed from an object-centered frame of reference (so that, for example, the ending of words are neglected regardless of whether they are on the left or the right or up or down). Moreover, as Bartolomeo and Chokron (2002) have documented (and reiterate in their commentary on Pylyshyn, 2002), the primary deficit in neglect is best viewed as the failure of stimuli on the neglect side to attract attention.

Unlike the tunnel imagery case described above, most cases of imaginal neglect are unlikely to be due to tacit knowledge. Deficits such as neglect, whether in vision or in imagery, represent a failure to orient to one side or the other. But the critical question is "one side or the other of what?" As in the example of stimulus-response compatibility or imagery-induced perceptual motor adaptation (discussed on pp. 379–387), the direction of orientation may be better viewed as a direction in relation to objects in the world, rather than a direction in relation to objects in an image. Orienting is a world-directed response. When apparently attending to the left side of an image, patients may actually be orienting toward the left side of the perceived world (or perhaps of their body). Even with eyes closed we can perceive the spatial layout of objects before us through nonvisual modalities, and we also have accurate recall, at least for a short time, of the location of things in the visual world around us, and it may be that attention orients toward these world-locations. As I suggested earlier (section 7.3), it may be generally the case that the perception of physical space outside the head gives imagery its apparent spatial character and that it does so by virtue of how mental contents are associated with (or bound to) objects or locations in the perceived world. The ability to bind objects of thought to the location of perceived (or recalled) external objects might allow us to orient to the objects in our image (using the visual-index mechanism discussed in chapter 5, or the generalization of this mechanism I called *Anchors*; see note 4). If something like this were true, it would provide a natural account of such parallels between image space and visual space as arise in some of the neglect cases.

Despite studies such as those described, the preponderance of clinical findings concerning mental imagery and vision shows that the capacity for visual imagery and the capacity for vision are often dissociated in cases of brain damage (see the review in Bartolomeo, 2002). This has been shown by the presence of normal imagery in patients with such visual deficits as cortical blindness (Chatterjee and Southwood, 1995; Dalman, Verhagen, and Huygen, 1997; Goldenberg et al., 1995; Shuren et al., 1996), dyschromatopsia (Bartolomeo, Bachoud-levi, and Denes, 1997; De Vreese, 1991; Howard et al., 1998), visual agnosia (Behrmann, Moscovitch, and Winocur, 1994; Behrmann, Winocur, and Moscovitch, 1992; Jankowiak et al., 1992; Servos and Goodale, 1995) and visual neglect (Beschin et al., 1997, review the evidence for a double dissociation of neglect in vision and imagery). The case for independence of imagery and vision is made all the stronger by the extensive evidence that blind people show virtually all the psychophysical phenomena associated with experiments on mental imagery, and may even report rather similar experiences of "seeing" shapes and textures as do sighted people. There is even some evidence suggesting that what characterizes patients who show a deficit with certain kinds of imagery-generation tasks (e.g., imagining the color of an object) is that they lack the relevant knowledge of the appearance of objects (Goldenberg, 1992; Goldenberg and Artner, 1991). On the other hand, insofar as blind people know (in a factual way) what objects are like (including aspects that are essential to their "appearance," such as their shape, size, orientation, as well as other features that show up clearly in vision, such as smoothness), it is not surprising that they should exhibit some of the same psychophysical behaviors in relation to these properties. The pervasive evidence of the dissociation between imagery ability and visual ability is one of the sources of evidence most damaging to the view that having a mental image involves using the visual system to "see" some state of the brain.

7.5   What Would It Mean if All the Neurophysiological Claims Turned Out to Be True?

Despite their problems, results such as those of Kosslyn et al. and Farah et al. (discussed above) have been widely interpreted as showing that topographical picturelike displays are generated on the surface of the visual cortex during mental imagery and that it is *by means of this spatial display* that images are processed, patterns perceived, and the results of mental imagery experiments produced. In other words, these results have been taken to support the view that mental images are *literally two-dimensional displays* projected onto primary visual cortex. Since this idea comports with the experience we have that when we are imagining we are examining a display in out head, it has become the accepted view in cognitive science and even among philosophers who favor an empiricist view of mental states (e.g., Prinz, 2002). I have already suggested some reasons why neuroscience evidence does not warrant such a strong conclusion (and that a weaker conclusion about functional space is inadequate to support the claims of a special depictive form of representation for mental images).

If we are to take seriously the view of picture theorists who propose to take literally the cortical display interpretation of mental imagery, we need to understand the role that could possibly be played by such a literal picture on the surface of the visual cortex. Suppose that one day it is discovered that when people entertain a visual image there really is a picture displayed on the visual cortex and the picture has all the spatial and depictive properties claimed for it (such as in the Kosslyn passage, quoted on p. 328). What would be the implications of such a finding? Would the claim that such a cortical picture is causally responsible for the phenomenology and psychophysics of mental imagery be consistent with the large body of experimental evidence regarding the function of mental imagery (e.g., all the evidence collected in Kosslyn, 1980, 1983, 1994)? Equally important, what would we need to assume about the cognitive system (i.e., about the function carried out by the "mind's eye") for this sort of theory to work? What would the existence of a cortical display tell us about the nature and role of mental images in cognition? We have known at least since Kepler (see n. 1, p. 7) that there is a literal image on our retinas when we perceive, and early neuroanatomy suggested there is probably some transformed version of this very image on our visual cortex; yet knowing this did not make us any wiser about how vision works. Indeed, ruminating on the existence of such an image just raised problems such as why we do not see the world as upside down, given that the image on the retinas is upside down. It also led many psychologists to try to answer such questions as why we perceive objects to be roughly veridical in size despite differences in their retinal size, why we see a large colored panoramic view of the world when our eyes provide only a small peephole of high-resolution colored information, why the world appears to be stable despite the rapid movement of our retinal image, and so on. These and other similar puzzles arising from the discrepancy between properties of our retinal image and properties of our percept led many people to assume that these discrepancies could be overcome by presenting the mind with a corrected panoramic display, built up during visual perception. As we saw in chapter 1, there is now overwhelming evidence against that proposal. This proposed panoramic display was a blind alley into which we were led by a strong tendency to reify our subjective impressions. The temptation to concretize a literal image in both vision and imagery, as well as the concomitant assumption of an equally literal "mind's eye," may be very strong, but it leads us at every turn into blind alleys.

Even if it were shown that there is a picture displayed on the surface of the visual cortex during episodes of mental imagery, it would be hard to justify the leap from such a finding to a picture theory of mental imagery—one that explains the phenomenology and the psychophysics of mental imagery with the claim that people project a picture on their cortex and that they reason by visually examining this picture. I have already considered many reasons, both conceptual and empirical, to doubt the picture theory of mental imagery. In the rest of section 7.5 I summarize a few of the reasons why a cortical-display version of the picture theory is equally unsatisfactory.

7.5.1 The "mind's eye" must be very different from a real eye

Some of the psychophysical evidence that is cited in support of a picture theory of mental imagery suggests a similarity between the mind's eye and the real eye that is so remarkable that it ought to be an embarrassment to the picture theorists.[8] Such evidence not only suggests that the

---

8. To this point, Kosslyn, Thomson, and Ganis (2002) reply, "These characteristics have been empirically demonstrated—which hardly seems a reason for embarrassment. Like it or not, that's the way the studies came out. The depictive theories made such predictions, which were successful." Perhaps some people do not embarrass easily, but the fact that the data came out that way *ought* to be embarrassing to someone who believes that the data tell us about the format of images (or the architecture of the imagery system), since for these people it would entail that the "mind's eye" is a duplicate of our real eye. It also ought to be embarrassing because the tacit knowledge explanation, which avoids this extravagant conclusion, provides a better account.

visual system is involved in imagery and that it examines a pictorial display, but it appears to attribute to the "mind's eye" many of the properties of our real eyes. For example, it seems that the mind's eye has a visual angle like that of a real eye (Kosslyn, 1978) and that it has a field of resolution that is also similar to that of our eyes; it drops off with eccentricity and inscribes an elliptical acuity profile similar to that of our real eyes (Finke and Kosslyn, 1980; Finke and Kurtzman, 1981a). It even appears that the mind's eye exhibits the "oblique effect" in which the discriminability of closely spaced horizontal and vertical lines is superior to that of oblique lines (Kosslyn, Sukel, and Bly, 1999). Since in the case of the eye, such properties arise from the structure of our retinas and the way they map onto the cortex, it would appear to suggest that the mind's eye is similarly constructed. Does the mind's eye then have the same color profile as that of our eyes—and perhaps a blind spot as well? Does it exhibit afterimages? And would you be surprised if experiments showed that they did? Of course, the observed parallels could be just a coincidence, or it could be that the distribution of neurons and connections in the visual cortex has come to reflect the type of information it receives from the eye. But it is also possible that such phenomena reflect what people have implicitly come to *know* about how things appear to them, a knowledge that the experiments invite them to use in simulating what would happen in a visual situation that parallels the imagined one. Such a possibility is made all the more plausible in view of the fact that the instructions in these imagery experiments explicitly ask observers to "imagine" a certain visual situation—to place themselves in certain circumstances and to consider what it would look like to see things, say, located off to the side in their peripheral vision. (I have often wondered whether people who wear thick-framed glasses would have a smaller field of vision in their mind's eye.)

The picture we are being offered, of the mind's eye gazing on a display projected onto the visual cortex, is one that should arouse our suspicion. It comes uncomfortably close to the idea that properties of the external world, as well as many of the properties of the peripheral parts of the visual system, are internalized in the imagery system. But if such properties were built into the architecture, our mental imagery would not be as plastic and cognitively penetrable as it is. If the mind's eye really had to move around in its socket (if such a notion is even coherent) we would not be able to jump from place to place in extracting information from our mental image the way we can. And if images really were pictures on the cortex, the theory might well not have discharged the need for an intelligent agent to interpret them, notwithstanding claims that the system has been implemented on a computer (which is far from being the case, since a working model would require that all of vision be simulated). Even if there were a computer implementation of a high-performance system that behaved like a person examining a mental image, it would still not guarantee that what was claimed about the system, viewed as a model of the mind/brain, was true. As Slezak (1995) has pointed out, labels on boxes in a software flowchart (such as "visual buffer," "attention window," or "pattern recognition") constitute empirical claims that must be independently justified. They also constitute explanatory debts that have yet to be discharged, to use Dan Dennett's illuminating terminology (1978). Certain kinds of claims entail missing and unexplained intelligent processes, and the hyperrealistic mind's eye we are being invited to accept may well be such a claim.[9]

7.5.2   The capacity for imagery is independent of the capacity for vision

The notion that viewing a mental image is very like seeing a scene must contend with a great deal of evidence showing that the capacity for visual imagery is independent of the capacity for visual perception (as we saw on p. 400). Indeed, there is evidence for double-dissociations in the kind of damage observed in vision and in mental imagery (see the reviews in Bartolomeo and Chokron, 2002; Beschin et al., 1997). If the early-vision areas are the site of mental images and their topographical form

---

9. This example is reminiscent of a story I first heard from Hilary Putnam. It seems there was an inventor who bored his friends with unremitting stories about how he had invented a perpetual motion machine. When his friends stopped paying attention to him he insisted that he had actually constructed such a machine and would be happy to show it to them. So they followed him into his workshop where they were greeted by a wondrous array of mechanical devices, gears, levers, hydraulic pumps, and electrical bits and pieces. They stood looking at all this display in rapt amazement until one of them remarked to the inventor that, amazing though all this was, he noticed that nothing was actually moving. "Oh that," replied the unruffled inventor, "I am awaiting delivery of one back-ordered little piece that fits right here and goes back and forth forever."

is responsible for the mental imagery results discussed earlier, it is hard to see why congenitally blind people produce the same imagery results (such as scanning times) as sighted people (Carpenter and Eisenberg, 1978; Zimler and Keenan, 1983). Cortically blind patients can also report imagery, while some people who fail to report imagery have normal sight (Chatterjee and Southwood, 1995; Dalman et al., 1997; Goldenberg et al., 1995). Similarly, cerebral achromatopsia can be dissociated from the capacity to have colorful images (Bartolomeo et al., 1997; Shuren et al., 1996), hemispatial neglect can be manifested independently in vision and imagery (Beschin et al., 1997; Coslett, 1997; Guariglia et al., 1993), and visual agnosia can occur with intact mental imagery ability (Behrmann et al., 1994; Behrmann et al., 1992; Servos and Goodale, 1995). Although there have been attempts to explain these dissociations by attributing some of the lack of overlap to an "image-generation" phase that is presumably involved only in imagery (see the recent review in Behrmann, 2000), this image-generation proposal does not account for much of the evidence for the independence of imagery and vision. In particular, it cannot explain how one can have spared imagery in the presence of such visual impairments as total cortical blindness.

7.5.3   Images are not two-dimensional displays

The conclusion that many people have drawn from the neural imaging evidence cited earlier, as well as from the retinotopic nature of the areas that are activated, is that images are two-dimensional retinotopic displays (since the topographical mappings found in visual cortex are at best two-dimensional mappings of the retina). But even if a two-dimensional display were activated during episodes of imagining, it could not possibly correspond to what we mean by a mental image. The psychophysical evidence shows that mental images are, if anything, three-dimensional inasmuch as the phenomenology is that of seeing a three-dimensional scene. Moreover, similar mental scanning results are obtained in depth as in two dimensions (Pinker, 1980), and the phenomenon of "mental rotation"—one of the most popular demonstrations of visual imagery—is indifferent as to whether rotation occurs in the plane of the display or in depth (Shepard and Metzler, 1971). Neither can the retinotopic "display" in visual cortex be three-dimensional. The spatial properties of the perceived world are not reflected in a volumetric topographical organization in the brain: as we penetrate deeper into the columnar structure of the cortical surface, we do not find a representation of the third dimension of the scene, as we would have to if the cortical display were to explain image-scanning and image-rotation results.

Images also represent other properties besides spatial relations. For example, images must represent the motion of objects. People have assumed that once you have a way to "depict" relative locations you automatically have a way to depict motion. The naive assumption is that motion is depicted as changing location, so that the motion of objects is represented by images that are themselves moving on the cortical display (although it is not clear what to do about motion in depth). But there is evidence that motion is encoded as a property distinct from a sequence of changes in location. For example, people who are motion-blind or suffer from cerebral akinetopsia are still able to tell that objects are in different locations at different times and can even detect motion in tactile and auditory modalities (see, e.g., Heywood and Zihl, 1999).

Depicting translation and rotation requires depicting that the shape of rigid objects remains invariant. Consider the well-known example of mental rotation. What rotates in mental rotation? If the actual shape is to be depicted over a smooth succession of orientations, what ensures that the shape is retained—that the parts move in a way that ensures that their locations relative to other parts of the object remain fixed? In real rotation this is guaranteed by the object's rigidity. Since nothing rigid is rotating in mental rotation, what enforces this rigidity constraint? What is it about a cortical display or a spatial (or depictive) format that makes rotation seem like a natural transformation, while other transformations seem odd (e.g., the transformation of a 3D object into its 3D mirror image, or its enantiomorph)? These questions have a natural answer in the represented domain, that is, in the world of rigid objects. So perhaps what enforces the constraint is knowing that it holds in the world of rigid objects. What ought to be clear is that the maintenance of the shape of a figure as it rotates (as well as the figure's passage through intermediate locations) does not follow from the mere fact of its being represented on a 2D surface. Yet people continue to cite the spatial nature of image representations to explain mental rotation.[10]

Mental images represent not only spatial properties, but also the color, luminance, and shape of objects. Are these also to be found displayed literally on the surface of the visual cortex? If not, how do we reconcile the apparently direct spatial mapping of 2D spatial properties with a completely different form of mapping for depth and for other contents of images of which we are equally vividly aware?

7.5.4   Images are not retinotopic

The cortical display view of mental imagery assumes that mental images consist in the activation of a pattern that is the same as the pattern activated by the corresponding visual percept. It follows, then, that such a pattern corresponds to the retinotopic projection of a corresponding visual scene. This assumption is a direct consequence of viewing a mental image the same as a visual image that is believed to occur in visual perception, which is why the finding of Tootell et al. (1982) is always cited in discussions of the nature of mental images (see pp. 392–394). But such a retinotopic pattern does not correspond to a mental image as the latter is understood in the psychological literature, and it is not what we "see" in our "mind's eye." A mental image covers a much larger region than the fovea and may even cover the region behind the head (as Attneave

---

10. For example, in his critical discussion of the idea that representations underlying mental images may be "propositional," Prinz says, "If visual-image rotation uses a spatial medium of the kind that Kosslyn envisions, then images must traverse intermediate positions when they rotate from one position to another. The propositional system can be designed to represent intermediate positions during rotation, but that is not obligatory. If we assume that a spatial medium is used for imagery, we can predict the response latency for mental rotation tasks" (2002, p. 118). But Prinz does not tell us why it is obligatory in a "spatial medium" that "images must traverse intermediate positions" or what he thinks is passing through intermediate positions in the mental rotation task. Passing through intermediate positions is obligatory if an actual rigid object is moving or rotating. If a representation of an object or an experience (a phenomenal object) is rotating, the laws of physics do not apply, so nothing is obligatory except by stipulation. And stipulating that the mental image must pass through intermediate positions occurs only because its referent (a real rigid object) would have done so. It seems that even philosophers are caught up in the intentional fallacy.

suggests in the passage quoted on p. 328). David Ingle has also pointed out (Ingle, 2002) that since mental images (particularly memory images) typically remain fixed in allocentric coordinates, they must correspond to processes further along the visual pathway than areas 17 or 18. Cells whose receptive fields remain fixed in allocentric coordinates are found in inferotemporal cortex or in parietal cortex, but these areas are not mapped in terms of a 2D map the way cells are in visual cortex. Moreover, Ingle argues, since mental images contain recognized and localized objects, images must be located after the "two visual systems" converge, such as in prefrontal cortex, where there is no evidence for a topographical organization.

There is some inconsistency in how picture theorists describe the cortical display. On the one hand, the only evidence for a clearly topographical representational structure in cortex is the retinotopic structure in early vision. Information higher up in the visual stream tends not to be topographically organized (at least in a way that reflects visual space). Consequently, proponents of the cortical display view cite evidence such as presented by Tootell et al., as well as evidence of activity in the retinotopically mapped visual cortex during mental imagery. On the other hand, among the reasons put forward for the existence of a cortical display (Kosslyn, 1994, chap. 4) is that it is needed to explain the stability of our perception during eye movements and the invariance of recognition with movements of the retinal image (Kosslyn and Sussman, 1995, also assume that amodal completion and "filling in" occur in this cortical display). But for that to be the case, the image would have to be panoramic rather than retinotopic: it would have to display the larger stable view constructed from the sequence of saccades. Unfortunately, there is no evidence at all to support that kind of cortical display. Indeed, as we saw in section 1.4, there is every reason to believe that vision does not achieve stability and completeness by accumulating information in a spatially extended inner display. There is a great deal of evidence showing that visual stability and saccadic integration are not mediated by any kind of inner display (Blackmore et al., 1995; Irwin, 1991; McConkie and Currie, 1996; O'Regan, 1992). For example, information from successive fixations cannot be superimposed on a central image as required by this view.

Recent evidence also shows that there is no central repository where visual information is enriched and accumulated to form a detailed panoramic view of a scene, of the sort we typically experience. For example, work on change blindness shows that the visual system stores very little information about a scene between fixations, unless attention has been drawn to it (Rensink, 2000; Rensink et al., 1997; Simons, 1996). Thus it appears that there is no panoramic pictorial display. On the other hand, the proposal that mental images are displayed on a retinotopic display, although consistent with neuroanatomical data, is inconsistent with the findings of mental imagery experiments as well as with the phenomenology of mental imagery. Both these sources of data conflict with the assumption that only retinotopic (and particularly foveal) information is displayed. Thus there appears to be little support for either a retinotopic or a panoramic display as the basis for mental imagery.

7.5.5   Images do not provide inputs to the visuomotor system

I have suggested that mental images get their spatial character because the objects that one imagines are bound (by means of indexes) to perceived locations in real space, including information from proprioception and other perceptual modalities. As a result, imagined locations are tied to real space and hence provide the basis for a certain kind of spatiomotor coordination. According to the account I have been giving, the only thing that engages the motor system are the perceived locations to which imagined objects are bound (and that's what the location of objects in an image *means*). A more interesting question is whether anything more than location is involved when images interact with the motor system. For example, is there is any evidence to suggest that an image can engage the motor system in terms of more detailed properties of the image content, the way that real vision engages the motor system?

When we look in detail at cases that involve more than just the location of imagined objects, we find that images do not interact with the perceptual-motor system in a way that is characteristic of visual interaction with the perceptual motor system. To show this we need to examine certain signature properties of the visual control of movements, rather than cases where the control may actually be mediated by spatial attention or visual indexing of the sort introduced in chapter 5. One clear example of the strictly visual control of motor action is the type of eye movement called *smooth pursuit*. People can track the motion of slowly moving objects with a characteristic smooth movement of the eyes. There are also reports that under certain circumstances people can track the voluntary (and perhaps even involuntary) movement of their hand in the dark by smooth pursuit (Mather and Lackner, 1980). They can also track the motion of objects that are partially hidden from view (Steinbach, 1976) and even the induced (apparent) motion of a point produced by a moving surrounding frame (Wyatt and Pola, 1979). In other words, they can engage in the smooth pursuit of inputs generated by the early-vision system and perhaps the proprioceptive system as well. Yet what people cannot do is smoothly pursue the movement of imagined objects. In fact, it appears to be impossible even to voluntarily initiate smooth pursuit tracking without a moving stimulus (Kowler, 1990).

There are also significant differences between the way that other parts of the motor system interact with vision and the way they interact with mental images. Consider the visual control of reaching and grasping. Although we can reach out to grasp an imagined object, when we do so we are essentially reaching toward a location and mimicking a grasping gesture. The movement we execute resembles a *pantomiming* movement rather than a movement generated under visual control. The latter exhibits certain quite specific trajectory properties not shared by pantomimed reaching (Goodale et al., 1994). For example, the time and magnitude of peak velocity, the maximum height of the hand, and the maximum grip aperture are all significantly different when reaching for imagined than for perceived objects. Rather, reaching and grasping gestures toward imagined objects exhibit the pattern observed when subjects deliberately pantomime a reaching and grasping motion. Such differences provide strong reasons to doubt that imagery can serve as input into the dorsal stream of the early-vision system, where the visuomotor control process begins. What the evidence does support is the claim that the *locations* of imagined objects can have observable consequences on motor behavior. But these results are best accommodated by the independently motivated assumption that observers can associate (bind) imagined objects to real perceived objects or orientations using either visual indexes (FINSTs), when they can see the environment, or proprioceptive indexes (*Anchors*), when their eyes are closed.

There is considerable evidence that the visuomotor system is itself an encapsulated system (Milner and Goodale, 1995), which, like the early-vision system, is able to respond only to information arriving from the eyes, often including visual information that is not available to consciousness. As with the visual system, only certain limited kinds of modulations of its characteristic behavior can be imposed by cognition. When we examine signature properties of the encapsulated visuomotor system, we find that mental images do not engage this system the way that visual inputs do.

7.5.6   Examining a mental image is very different from visually perceiving a display

In accessing information from a real scene, we have the freedom to examine it in any order, and we may even access several aspects in parallel. But this is not true of accessing information from mental images. Take the following simple examples. Imagine a familiar printed word (e.g., your name) and try reading or spelling it backward from your image. Write down a 3 × 3 matrix of letters and read them in various orders. Now memorize the matrix and try doing the same from your image of the matrix. Unlike in vision, some orders (e.g., along the diagonals of the matrix) are extremely difficult to scan on the image. If one scans one's image the way it is alleged one does in the mental scanning experiments, there is no reason why one should not be able to scan the matrix freely. Of course, one can always account for these phenomena by positing various properties specific to a mental image generated from memory, such as assuming a limit on the number of elements that can be drawn, or assuming that elements decay. Such assumptions are completely ad hoc. For example, in many imagery studies visual information is not found to fade rapidly (Ishai and Sagi, 1995) nor does it appear to fade in the case of images used to investigate mental scanning phenomena (which, like the map used by Kosslyn et al., 1978, is more complex than a 3 × 3 matrix of letters). Moreover, the hypothesized fading rates of different parts of an image have to be tuned post hoc to account for the fact that it is the conceptual as opposed to the graphical structure of the image that determines how the image can be read and manipulated (i.e., to account for the fact that it is how one interprets the image, rather than its geometry, that determines its apparent fading). For example, it is how figures are conceptualized that determines the difficulty of an image-superposition task (illustrated in figure 1.24), or how quickly figures can be "mentally rotated" (illustrated in figure 6.8).

The fact that mental images represent the conceptual content of a scene (either recalled from memory or constructed during certain tasks) explains why images are distorted or transformed over time in characteristic ways (see the examples on pp. 28–36), why they can't be visually (re)interpreted, and why they can fail to be determinate in ways that no picture can fail to be determinate (Pylyshyn, 1973, 1978). For example, no picture can fail to have a size or shape or can fail to indicate which of two adjacent items is to the left and which to the right, or can fail to have exactly *n* objects (for some *n*), whereas mental images can be indeterminate in these and many other ways. Imagine throwing a ball in the air; then ask yourself about incidental perceptual properties of the event, such as the color or weight of the ball and whether it was spinning, the appearance of the background against which you saw the ball rise, how long it took the ball to reach the peak of its trajectory or to fall back to earth, and so on. As I argued in section 1.4, when recollected images are incorrect, they are invariably incorrect in conceptual ways (some discrete object is missing or mislocated or its properties are incorrectly conjoined); an incorrectly recalled image is not like a photograph that has an arbitrary piece torn off.

Not surprisingly, there are also many ways of patching up a picture theory to accommodate the fact that image contents are interpreted rather than strictly iconic. For example, one can allow images to be tagged as having certain properties (perhaps including the property of not being based on real perception), or one can assume that parts of images have to be refreshed from time to time from conceptual representations stored in memory, thus bringing in conceptual factors through an image-generation function. With each of these accommodations, however, the depictive format has less and less of an explanatory role to play, because the work is being done elsewhere. It becomes like an animated computer display whose behavior is determined by an extrinsic encoding of the principles that govern the animation, rather than by intrinsic properties of the display itself.

There are two basic problems with the assumption that the contents of a mental image are like the contents of a picture and therefore not conceptualized. The first problem is that both the contents of an image and the dynamic properties that an image has can be whatever you wish them to be, and the fact that you have a choice means that you must at some stage have had some conceptualized content in mind—you must have had an interpretation in mind. Thus, no matter what content you put into your image representation, you do so under a particular description or conceptualization or intended interpretation. For example, if you decide to imagine a rectangle as such, you know that whatever sort of representation you construct you do so with the knowledge that it is meant to be a "rectangle," so you couldn't mistake it for, say, a square or a parallelogram—as you might if it were a real uninterpreted figure. And you couldn't mistake your image of a wire cube for its perceptually reversed interpretation, or your image of two parallelograms above one another with corresponding vertices joined as a Necker cube (as in the example discussed on p. 344), even though in each case you might if you drew it.

There is, however, one caveat to the above claims about the content of images. The choice of image content is subject to the understanding that to "mentally image" something generally means to imagine that you are seeing it. Consequently, this means that certain aspects will tend to be assigned some value or other (as opposed to being left indefinite). For example, if asked to "imagine a printed word," it would be reasonable (though not obligatory) for you to imagine a sequence of letter-shapes, which in turn invites you to choose upper- or lowercase letters and maybe even a particular font. None of these choices is mandatory (and indefinitely many visual properties will not get assigned a value, e.g., the nature of the background on which the letters are imagined), yet failing to assign some properties of shape may tend to suggest that you are not following the instruction (including the self-instruction) to *imagine seeing* a printed word (after all, if you saw a printed word it would have letters with particular shapes).

The second and related problem is that no display is informationally equivalent to *a mental image*. This is a point I discussed in chapter 6 (on pp. 350–357) in connection with Shepard's conjecture that the mental state corresponding to having a mental image could in principle be externalized as a picture, in such a way that a person who saw the picture would be in a similar mental state as the person who had the mental image. The reason this would not work is that no visual stimulus carries information about the picture's interpretation. By contrast, mental images *are* the interpretation and are therefore conceptual. As Kosslyn put it, mental images contain "previously digested information" (1994, p. 329). What is even more significant is that there is no reason to believe that they contain anything else.

The above examples illustrate a general problem with the view that examining an image is just like seeing a display. A few other examples where this parallel fails are outlined below.

Images do not have the signature properties of early vision Because vision (at least early vision) is encapsulated, it works according to different principles from those of rational reasoning. It provides interpretations of visual patterns according to certain rules, such as those I listed on page 107. In particular, it has signature properties such as the properties discussed in Hochberg (1968): certain line drawings are automatically interpreted as three-dimensional constructions, certain patterns are ambiguous and result in involuntary reversals or changes in perspective, and certain sequences of images lead to the automatic perception of motion. If we create a mental image from a description (as in the example I presented on page 344 where I described a Necker cube, in terms of two identical joined parallelograms), we do not find such phenomena as spontaneous interpretation of these 2D shapes as 3D objects, spontaneous reversals of bistable figures, amodal completion or subjective contours (Slezak, 1995), visual illusions, or the incremental construction of visual interpretations and reinterpretations over time as different aspects are noticed. This is just what one would expect if the mental image is an interpretation of some possible scene, as opposed to an uninterpreted image of one.

Perceiving an actual retinotopic pattern is different from having a mental image An interesting test would be if one could compare the case where a pattern was projected onto the cortical display with the case where one merely imagined the same pattern. This is not an experiment that we are in a position to carry out at this time. But we can come close. Because of the retinotopic mapping from retina to primary visual cortex we can create a known pattern of activity on the cortex by projecting the pattern on the retina. We can do that, without running into problems with eye movement, by creating an afterimage on the retina. When we do we find an interesting difference between the visual appearance of a pattern projected onto the retinotopic cortical display and the appearance of the same pattern when it occurs in a mental image. Images on the retina, and presumably on the retinotopically mapped visual cortex, are subject to Emmert's law: retinotopic images superimposed onto a visual scene change their apparent size depending on the distance of the background against which they are viewed. The farther away the background is, the larger the afterimage appears. By contrast, mental images imagined over a perceived scene do not change their apparent size depending on the distance of the background, providing strong evidence that mental images are not identical to images projected onto the retinotopic layers of the cortex. (Compare the Emmert's Law prediction based on the assumption that images are displayed on the visual cortex with the claim I presented earlier, concerning what happens when we "project" a mental image onto a real scene. I claimed that we do not superimpose two images, but rather simply think of the objects in our image as being located at places in the world occupied by some visible feature or object that we pick out and index. If the indexing view is correct, then we would not expect the distance of the background to make any difference initially, since we are free to pick features whose locations correspond to where we want certain imagined elements to be. But once we have locked our imagined elements onto features in this way, if the background begins to recede then we might expect the apparent size of the image to shrink as the distance between indexed features diminishes. So I would not expect a mental image to obey Emmert's law as the background recedes. If anything, I might expect the opposite: Emmert's law says that a retinal/cortical image looks bigger on a more distant background whereas the indexing view says that the size of the image shrinks because the distance between indexed elements diminishes as the background recedes. Of course, I also maintain that your image has whatever properties you wish it to have, so perhaps your belief in the fixed size of the imagined scene overrides the shrinking distances between indexed elements. In either case I clearly do not expect Emmert's law to hold for mental images.)

It appears that if having a mental image consists in certain activity in the visual cortex, this activity does not function as a *display* of that image, in the sense in which a picture or a TV screen is such a display. In particular, a pattern of cortical activity is not something that must be visually interpreted, the way that the electronic activity on the TV screen must be visually interpreted. As to whether the activity is in some other way similar to the activity involved in visual perception, this remains an open question. The assumption that is being questioned in not whether entertaining mental images has *some* connection with visual perception, it is the assumption that entertaining a mental image consists in visually interpreting some special form of representation, in particular a form of representation that is picturelike or, as some people prefer to call it, "depictive." Although the term depictive is not well defined beyond its metaphorical connection to pictures, it is intended to suggest that the image is preperceptual or preconceptual, and therefore in need of interpretation by the usual early-vision processes. This is why people have been concerned to show that activity associated with mental imagery occurs in areas of the cortex known to be retinotopically mapped. But, as I argued earlier, just because there is activity in an area that is retinotopically mapped is not sufficient reason to conclude either that the mental images themselves are retinotopically mapped in a way that preserves spatial properties, or that if they are, they serve as input to a visual system that perceives them in a way determined by their retinotopic shape. These assumptions, rather than the mere involvement of parts of the visual system, have been the contentious assumptions in the mental imagery debate, at least since my first critique in Pylyshyn (1973).

7.5.7   What has neuroscientific evidence done for the "imagery debate"?

Where, then, does the "imagery debate" stand? That all depends on what you think the debate is about. If it is supposed to be about whether reasoning using mental imagery is somehow different from reasoning without it, who can doubt that it is? If it is about whether in some sense imagery involves the visual system, the answer there too must be *yes*, since imagery involves similar experiences to those produced by (and, as far as we know, only by) activity in some part of the visual system (though not in V1, according to many writers, including Crick and Koch,

1995). The big open question is, *In what way* is the visual system involved? Answering that is likely to require a better functional taxonomy of the visual system and better alternative proposals for how nondeductive (image-based) reasoning might proceed. It is much too early and much too simplistic to claim that the visual system is deployed in visual imagery by allowing us to *look at* a reconstructed retinotopic input of the sort that comes from the eye (or at least at some topographically faithful remapping of this input).

Is the debate about whether images are depictive as opposed to descriptive, as Kosslyn (1994) claims? That all depends on what you mean by "depictive." Is any accurate representation of geometrical, spatial, metrical, or visual properties depictive? If so, any precise linguistic description of how something looks is thereby depictive. Does being depictive require that the form of the representation be spatial? As I have suggested, that depends on what restrictions are placed on "being spatial." Does being spatial require that images "preserve metrical spatial information," as has been claimed (Kosslyn et al., 1978)? Again that depends on what it means to "preserve" metrical space. If it means that the image must faithfully *represent* metrical spatial information, then any form of representation will have to do that to the extent that it can be shown that people do encode and recall such information. But any system of numerals (especially an extensible one such as the variable precision floating point number system, or the Dewey Decimal system used in libraries), as well any analog medium, can represent magnitudes as precisely as needed. If the claim that images preserve metrical spatial information means that an image *uses spatial magnitudes to represent spatial magnitudes* (by mapping magnitudes in a monotonic manner), then this is a literal form of the picture theory that I have argued is incompatible with the available evidence.

The neuropsychological evidence I have briefly examined, although interesting in its own right, does not appear capable of resolving the issue about the nature of mental images, largely because the questions have not been formulated appropriately and the options are not well understood. One major problem is that we are not only attempting to account for certain behavioral and neurophysiological facts, but we are attempting to do so in a way that remains faithful to certain intuitions and subjective experiences. It is not obvious that all these constraints can be satisfied simultaneously. There is no a priori reason why an adequate theory of mental imagery will map onto conscious experience in any direct and satisfactory way. Indeed, if the history of other sciences and even of other parts of cognitive science (e.g., linguistics or computational vision) is any indication, the eventual theory is likely to be at odds with our subjective experience and we will simply have to live with that fact, the way physics has had to live with the fact that the mystery of action-at-a-distance does not have a reductive explanation.

The typical response I have received to arguments such as those raised in this chapter is that the critique takes the picture theory too literally and that nobody really believes that there are actual pictures in the brain. Almost every article I have seen by advocates of the picture theory is at pains to point out that images are not in every way like pictures. For example, Kosslyn states, "Images contain 'previously digested' information" (1994, p. 329), and Denis and Kosslyn state, "No claim was made that visual images themselves have spatial extent, or that they occupy metrically defined portions of the brain" (1999). But then how do they explain the increase in time to scan greater image distances or to report details in smaller images? The explanations of these phenomena *require a literal sense of "spatial extent."* Otherwise the depictive theory is indistinguishable from what I have called the null hypothesis (see the discussion of the "functional space" alternative in section 7.1). And how, if one forswears the literal view of a cortical display, is one supposed to interpret the concern about whether imagery activates topographical areas of the visual cortex, or the claim that such activation establishes that images, unlike other forms of representation, are "depictive"? The problem is that while the literal picture-theory or cortical display theory is what provides the explanatory force and the intuitive appeal, it is always the picture *metaphor* that people retreat to in the face of the implausibility of the literal version of the story. This is the strategy of claiming a decisive advantage for the depictive theory because it has the properties referred to in the quotation on page 328, that it is located in the topographically organized areas of visual cortex, "preserves metrical information" and so on, and then, in the face of the theory's implausibility, systematically retreating from the part of the claim that is doing the work—the literal spatial layout. As Bertrand Russell once said about the advantage of postulating what you would like to prove, such a strategy "has many advantages; they are the same as the advantages of theft over honest toil" (1918/1985, p. 71).

7.6   What, if Anything, Is Special about Mental Imagery?

Notwithstanding the skepticism displayed in this book concerning many contemporary views of vision and mental imagery, I believe that visual science has made considerable progress in the past few decades. The trap we have had trouble avoiding is that of taking our introspections at face value, as showing us what vision is like and what its products are. Whatever form the representations generated by vision may take, they are very likely to be similar to those generated when we are engaged in visual imagining. Moreover, those representations may well be different from those generated when we reason about more abstract ideas. What we still do not have is a good idea of how such perceptually based representations are different from ones that are not accompanied by sensory experiences (though we have had numerous inadequate ideas). It may be worth speculating on the ways in which these may be different, and I will do so in the next chapter. But first let me review and try to be as explicit as I can about what it is that I do (and do not) claim about mental images.

7.6.1   What I am not claiming: Some misconceptions about objections to the picture theory

There has been a great deal of misunderstanding of the position that I have taken in the past on the nature of thought and of mental imagery (e.g., in Pylyshyn, 1973, 1981b, 1984b). For example, here are a few of the questions on which critics of picture theories have been widely misunderstood.

Do mental images really exist or are they merely "epiphenomenal"? Prior to the development of an adequate theory of mental imagery, the term "mental image" is only the name for the experience of "seeing" without the presence of the object being seen. Nobody can deny the existence of such an experience. Moreover, the content of the experience is a source of evidence that we rely on, along with a great many other sources, in formulating a theory of the what goes on during certain kinds of episodes of information processing—episodes are typically, though not necessarily, accompanied by the experience of "seeing" in one's "mind's eye." The claim that mental images are epiphenomenal is at the very least ambiguous: it corresponds either to the claim that we are deluded about what we experience—that we do not experience an image as something that is "seen," which is absurd, or to the claim that a scientific theory of mental imagery will not incorporate things that are like what we experience when we have a mental image, which is almost certainly true. That's because our experience is not the experience of seeing a mental event, but rather the experience of seeing a possible perceptual world. The objects of our experience are things in the world (perhaps nonexistent things, but nonetheless things whose proper place is in a world outside the head). Consequently, no theory of information processing will mirror our phenomenal experience by hypothesizing the existence of objects inside the brain that are the same as the objects of our experience. Nor will a neurological theory do so. To claim that mental images are epiphenomenal is to confuse an explanatory theoretical construct with the experience of having a mental image (see Block, 1981).

Is the form of representation underlying mental images propositional? It is certainly possible (and even quite plausible) that the content of both images and visual percepts can be adequately encoded in a propositional (or more precisely, quasi-sentential or quasi-logical, or symbolic) form of some sort.[11] Indeed, such an encoding would help explain the conceptual properties exhibited not only by mental images, but also by perception itself (as I suggested, for example, in Pylyshyn, 1973, as well as in chapter 1). But until someone produces a detailed theory that accounts for some significant imagery phenomena using a propositional encoding, this proposal serves primarily to illustrate some of the constraints on an adequate form of representation. Thus an important use of the idea that images are encoded in propositional form is as a foil against which to

11. I am using the term "propositional" in its common though somewhat informal sense, to mean any languagelike symbolic encoding for which a formal syntax and rules of inference are available and which has a truth value (i.e., propositions are either true or false, or some other value if you have a multivalued or fuzzy logic). In other words, by "proposition" I really mean a statement in a logical calculus of some sort, such as the predicate calculus.

test various proposals for image representations. There is something special about propositional representations. Thanks to the work in formal logic and computation theory over the last half-century, we know some important things about what have been called formal languages that we don't know about other forms of representation. Such propositional symbolic representations have a well-defined combinatorial syntax, together with a semantic theory and a proof theory and, if not a theory of other types of inference (e.g., inductive, abductive, heuristic), at least some indication of how semantic properties might be preserved over certain syntactic transformations. In other words, we know some of the essential formal (semantic and syntactic) properties of logical calculi, as ways of encoding knowledge. Consequently, such a system of encoding constitutes an appropriate baseline against which to compare other theories of the encoding of mental images. When a theory of mental imagery is proposed we can ask, Can it explain anything that a quasi-linguistic theory would not be able to explain (and vice versa)? If not, nothing is gained by accepting the proposal and a great deal is lost, such as the entire apparatus of inference as developed in formal logic and continued in nonclassical logics such as the nonmonotonic logics studied in artificial intelligence.

Is there anything special about the representations underlying visual imagery, or are they the same as representations for verbal or other forms of reasoning?   Putting aside the difficulty of distinguishing "types of representation," there appears to be every reason to think that *something* is special about the sort of reasoning that is accompanied by the experience of mental imagery—something that distinguishes it from other forms of reasoning. The relevant question to ask about some particular proposal for what is special about mental images is not whether it comports with our intuitions, but whether it can be empirically sustained. And here I do claim that every concrete proposal I have seen of what constitutes this special ingredient that is present in the case of mental images and absent from other forms of thought is either demonstrably false or ambiguous or incoherent (or all three). The proposals have typically been along such lines as that images are picturelike or that they "preserve the metrical properties of the objects they depict." But "preserve" can be taken to mean either that the representations have metrical properties or that they somehow represent them. The difference between these two senses is fundamental: the first is a claim about the form or the physical property of the system of codes used to represent magnitudes such as distance, whereas the second is simply a claim concerning what properties of the world can be represented (i.e., it is a claim about the representational capacity of the system of codes). The second is obviously much weaker than the first since, for example, it is fulfilled universally by human languages (since all languages spoken in industrialized parts of the world have a productive system of names for magnitudes, such as the numerals). The first claim (that images have metrical properties) can be taken either as a formal mathematical claim (i.e., the system of codes has a formal property that supports the metrical axioms), which is often put in terms of the claim that images are encoded as analogs, or as a literal claim that images are laid out in physical space in the brain. Since an analog theory of imagery (or of space) has yet to be developed (see note 2) I have concentrated entirely on the picture theory in the last two chapters. Also, in view of the cognitive penetrability of most imagery phenomena, there is good reason to doubt that an all-analog representation of imagery will do (as we saw in section 7.1).

Is the visual system involved in manipulating and interpreting mental images? The claim that imagery and vision are closely linked and use the same mechanisms may or may not be true, or even meaningful, depending on how broadly one takes the notion of "visual system." If by "visual system" one means any process concerned with interpreting visual information, including the processes involved in allocating attention and recognizing visual objects, then the claim is almost certainly true. But it is true for the uninteresting reason that much of what happens in this extended sense of vision is a form of reasoning that will thus naturally also apply to reasoning using mental images. If, however, the claim is that what I have called "early vision"—the part of the visual system, discussed in chapters 2 and 3, that is unique to vision and is cognitively impenetrable—then there is good reason to doubt that these mechanisms are involved in the examination of mental images.

Is the imagery debate over?   To call the arguments about the nature of mental imagery a "debate" is to suggest that there is disagreement about a well-defined set of options. This is far from the case. The dispute, as I understand it, has not been about which "side" has a better theory, but about whether particular proposals that have been put forward are conceptually coherent or empirically valid. While arguments have ranged from the conceptual to the methodological (e.g., arguments concerning the interpretation of particular experimental findings), the basic problem remains that those who claim to have a theory of mental imagery are burdened by ill-defined constructs and shifting assumptions.

The focus of the discussion about mental imagery has changed in the past decade and there has been a great deal more evidence brought into the discussion, especially evidence from clinical neurology and from various forms of brain imaging (such as PET, MRI, fMRI) and recently also from an intrusive technique of disabling part of the brain using transcranial magnetic stimulation (rTMS). Yet this increase in the empirical base, welcome though it is, cannot offset the fact that the questions and options under discussion continue to be ill formed. No matter how much objective reliable evidence is introduced, the "debate" cannot be resolved until the nature of the claims is made clear. There is, at the present time, an enormous gap between the evidence and the models and claims being made about the real nature of mental images.

7.6.2 What constraints should be met by a theory of mental imagery?

In the absence of an adequate theory of mental imagery, it is useful to consider some plausible constraints on representations that might underlie images. The following speculative list includes some of the ideas I have discussed throughout this and the previous chapter:

Image representations contain information about the appearance of things, so they use the vocabulary of visual properties (e.g., color, brightness, shape, texture, and so on). This is a very different claim from the empiricist claim, going back to Hume, that the vocabulary *consists of sensations*—a claim recently revived and repackaged in modern dress by many writers (Barsalou, 1999; Prinz, 2002).

Image representations contain information about the relative location of things, so they use the vocabulary of geometrical relations (above, inside, beside, to the right of, and so on). Indeed, there is reason to think that representing spatial properties is a more fundamental characteristic of what we call images than is representing properties of appearance (Farah, et al., 1988), but that such representation can be done without invoking a spatial medium, by relying on the spatial properties of immediately perceived space.

Image representations typically refer to individual things; they represent *token* individuals (things or objects, or whatever early vision delivers). The content of an image may also ascribe properties to these tokens, but they generally do not contain quantified assertions. For example, they might assert $Q(x_1)$, $Q(x_2)$, . . . , $Q(x_n)$ for n distinct individual xs instead of the general assertion "There are n things that have property Q." Image representations can, however, represent abstract properties, such as that X *caused* Y, something that no picture could do in a direct manner (without some iconic convention that would, in effect, serve to label parts of the image). Since a mental image constitutes an interpretation it can represent abstract properties without such conventions simply because the person who has the image knows the intention or the conceptualization under which it was created. (This, however, means that part of what an image denotes is offstage in the intention and does not appear in the part of the representation experienced as a picture. This fact plays a role in the claim that I will discuss on pp. 432–436, that one cannot think in images alone.)

Image representations lack explicit quantifiers. Images are not able to express such assertions as that *all* things in an image are Xs, or that *some* of the things in the scene are Ys and so on, although they can represent some or all individuals in the image as being Xs. Representing a content that is quantified (e.g., there is an unspecified individual who has property P, or all individuals that have property P also have property Q) can be accomplished only by adding symbolic tags that may be interpreted to have the meaning of a quantifier—which is to say, an image *qua image* can represent quantified or generalized properties only by means that are essentially nonpictorial.

Image representations lack explicit disjunctions. Images are not able to express such assertions as that either individual X or individual Y has property P, or that individual Y has either property P or property Q. The closest one can come to this is to have two images, one with only X and one with only Y.

Image representations lack explicit negation. Images cannot directly represent the fact that there are no Xs or that none of the Xs have property *P*. Rather, negation is expressed indirectly by the absence of certain things in the image, together with the implicit assumption that all relevant things are included.

Image representations provide access paths that make getting from one item or property to another more direct for some items and properties than for others. Relations such as *adjacent to* may have a privileged position in terms of providing more direct access paths than, say, *same size as*, so that it is easier to get a locus of processing from one individual to an individual that is represented as adjacent to it, than to another individual that is the same size.

Image representations may lend themselves to certain kinds of transformations in preference to other kinds of transformations. Without assuming any particular format for images, it might be that carrying out certain transformations on them is more natural than other transformation. This may have to do with which properties are encoded (e.g., orientation may be encoded independently of shape), or it may have to do with computational complexity issues. It may also be simpler to carry out certain operations in a certain sequence. For example, to compare two shapes that differ in orientation, it might be computationally cheaper (or even necessary given limited resources) to go through the computation of the representation of the shape at intermediate orientations (see pp. 320–321 for a brief discussion of why this might be so).

The information about individuals in a mental image can be associated with individuals in a perceived scene. This is what allows images to inherit spatial properties of visually perceived scenes. As I suggested in section 7.3, we can think about particular imagined individuals and use indexes to bind them to objects in a scene we are viewing. Doing so keeps their relative locations fixed so long as the background scene is fixed and rigid, and it ensures that other implicit relations between bound objects hold (e.g., if three imagined objects are bound to three collinear scene objects, the location of the middle imagined object could be visually perceived to be "between" the other two imagined objects.) On pages 379–387, I proposed that something like this might even be possible when the scene is perceived not visually but in some other modality (e.g., acoustically, proprioceptively, or kinesthetically). This simple assumption allows us to explain the apparent ability to project an image onto a scene so that the combined image-and-scene behaves in certain ways like a superimposed image-percept scene.

With a little thought this list could be extended. These proposed characteristics of or constraints on mental images are quite different from those proposed by picture theorists. None of the current theoretical ideas about the nature of mental imagery takes these desiderata seriously. Mental pictures do have some of the properties on this list, but they also have serious drawbacks. The only theory I am aware of that deals with this aspect of reasoning from images and that appears, prima facie, to have some properties listed above is a system of formal representation proposed by Levesque (1986). Levesque describes an expressively weaker, but more efficient, form of logic that he refers to as "vivid representations." This proposal has the merit of recognizing that we can have forms of representation that are more limited in what they can express but that have the special feature that they allow certain conclusions to be drawn rapidly, essentially by a form of pattern-matching. Like images, they do not allow one to express negation directly (e.g., the only way that they can represent the proposition "there are no red squares in the scene" is by representing a scene that contains no red squares) or disjunction (e.g., they can represent the proposition "the squares are either red or large" only by allowing two possible representations, one with red squares and one with large squares, to both be treated as true), and they do not allow quantification (e.g., they can represent the proposition "all squares are red" only by explicitly representing each square, however many there are, and asserting of each one that it is red). Like images, they cannot express the fact that there are five objects in the scene, except by representing each of the objects, of which there would have to be five in all. I had also informally proposed a similar set of ideas in speculating about what might be special about representations underlying imagery, as opposed to representations underlying other kinds of thoughts (Pylyshyn, 1978). These are, admittedly, small steps toward a formalism for representing mental images. They do not suggest why such representations should be accompanied by the experience of seeing, although they do have the virtue of being limited in some of the same ways that images are.

8

Seeing with the Mind's Eye: Part 3, Visual Thinking

8.1 Different "Styles" of Thinking

One of the most widely accepted ideas about reasoning and problem solving is that there are different styles of thinking and that these styles are most clearly characterized in terms of whether people are "visual" or "verbal" thinkers (or sometimes "concrete" or "abstract" thinkers). There is little doubt that people differ in a number of ways with respect to their habitual or preferred style of thought and their approach to problem solving. There is surely also something to the observation that some people tend to think in a way that is in some sense more "visual" in that their thoughts more often concern the appearance of things and may be accompanied by visionlike experiences. The problem is in spelling out this difference in a way that takes it out of the realm of subjective experience and connects it with a scientific theory.

Describing some people's style of thinking as visual may imply any one of several things: it may suggest that they prefer to use visual aids (models, mockups, diagrams, etc.) when they solve problems, or that they prefer to solve problems that are related to how something looks, or that they use their visual skill in some internal way (presumably by working with mental images) even when they don't have something concrete to look at. It is perfectly reasonable to say that some people prefer to think about appearances, just as it is perfectly reasonable to say that some people prefer to talk about appearances. But that in itself tells you nothing about the format of their thoughts. Pictures presumably depict appearances. But sentences such as "he looks tired" or "she looks good in her new hairdo" or "the big red ball is behind the blue door" also refer to appearances. Terms like "red" refer to a visual property. But these are all properties of things being described, not of sentences or of thoughts or of mental images. It is the content that is visual, not the form itself.

If I am right that thought does not in any way consist in examining mental pictures, then neither does it consist in listening to mental sentences in an inner dialogue, as introspection suggests. Here we come, once again, to the conflicting demands of one's conscious experience and those of a scientific theory that has explanatory power. It is to this conflict that I now turn.

8.2   Form and Content of Thoughts: What We Think with and What We Think about

8.2.1   The illusion that we experience the *form* of our thoughts

Ever since the use of mentalistic terms (such as "know," "believe," "think," "want," and so on) became once again permissible in psychology and philosophy after a long dry period of behaviorism, people have found it completely natural to assume that we have conscious access not only to the content of our thoughts, but also to the form that they take. Thus we find it natural to suppose that our thoughts take the form of either inner dialogue (thinking in words) or of imagining a visual scene (seeing an image in our "mind's eye").[1]

This homily has been translated into what is known as the "dual code" theory of mental representations (which was developed most extensively in the work of Allan Paivio; see Paivio, 1986). The dual code idea infects our interpretation of self-reports of thought. Most people—including great thinkers like Einstein, Maxwell, Faraday, Helmholtz, Galton, Watt, Tesla, and others (see, e.g., the review in Shepard, 1978a)—maintain that their deepest thoughts are "devoid of words." For example, Shepard

---

1. Notice that when you experience something, you invariably experience it as something *sensory*. Try imagining an experience that is not an experience of perceiving something—of seeing, hearing, feeling, smelling, or tasting. Even inner feelings like pain or queasiness, or emotions such as anger, are experienced in terms of some perceptual sensation (in fact, the James-Lange theory of emotions equates emotions with perceived bodily states). Given this universal property of conscious experience (for which there is no explanation), it is no surprise that when we experience our thoughts we experience them as seeing or hearing or some other perceptual modality (touch, taste, proprioception): what else *could* we experience them as?

quotes Einstein's prologue to Planck's book (Planck, 1933) as saying, "There is no logical way to the discovery of these elemental laws. There is only the way of intuition, which is helped by a feeling for the order lying behind the appearance." Taken together with the tacit assumption that thoughts must be either in words or in pictures (and perhaps also the assumption that any "logical" thoughts must be in words), such reports lead to the conclusion that the thoughts these famous people had were expressed in mental pictures and that these sorts of pictorial thoughts are the real source of their creativity (I will take up the question of the relation between mental imagery and creativity on pp. 469–474).

Of course, one also allows for the possibility that a person might think in terms of auditory, tactile, or other kinds of sensations, even though these may be less central for most people. But what about the possibility that the form of thoughts is not only unconscious, but is something that never could be made conscious? Many people have assumed that such an idea is nearly incoherent (see, e.g., Searle, 1990). Notwithstanding the widespread influence of Freud's idea of the unconscious, it is still generally assumed that thoughts are the sorts of things that, although they might occasionally slip by unconsciously, nonetheless *could* in principle be made conscious, and moreover if they were conscious they would be experienced as something we hear or see or otherwise perceive. Indeed, Western philosophy has generally made the awareness of one's thoughts the basis on which one justifies the ascription of particular contents to them: you know what your thoughts are about because they are *your* thoughts and you have privileged access to them through your conscious awareness. If that were not the case, the argument goes, there would be no basis for ascribing one content as opposed to some other content to a thought (for a discussion of why we need to appeal to contents at all, and for a different view of how we might ascribe content, see Pylyshyn, 1984a).

I will not quarrel with the idea that we have privileged access to the content of our thoughts, nor will I try to define what it means for thoughts to be conscious. What I claim, however, is that there is every reason to believe that (a) the form of one's thoughts is something that has to be inferred indirectly, just as one infers the form of matter in physics and chemistry, without prejudging the scientific issue based on how we experience our own thoughts; and (b) what one is aware of—the form and content of one's conscious thoughts—cannot be what plays the causal role in reasoning. In other words, what we are aware of, such as the inner dialogue of one's thoughts or the pictures one sees in one's "mind's eye," cannot be what is responsible for people having the thoughts they have and making the inferences they make. The reason for taking this view is that the content of one's experience is demonstrably insufficient to encompass the content of our thoughts. The sorts of things of which one is aware, such as the words or sentences of an "inner dialogue" or the "mental pictures" one imagines, greatly underdetermine what one is thinking at the time one has those experiences. Consequently, something other than more words or more images must be going on— or so I will argue in the remainder of this section.

8.2.2   Do we think in words?

Consider an example where one appears to be thinking in words. As I type these sentences I think to myself, "I'd better hurry and finish this section or I will be late for my meeting." This is a pretty innocuous thought with little apparent hidden meaning. But look at it more closely. If I "said" that sentence to myself in my inner dialogue, I meant something far more than what appears in the sequence of words. I knew which particular text on my computer screen I meant when I thought "this section," I knew how much time would have to pass (roughly) for it to count as being "late" for a meeting, I knew which meeting I had in mind when I only thought "my meeting," and I knew what counts as "hurrying" when typing a section of text, as opposed to running a race. And for that matter I knew what "I" referred to, although the sentence I imagined thinking did not specify who that was ("I" refers to different people at different times).

In fact, sentences *never* say all that their speakers mean. The sentences of your inner dialogue follow such Gricean maxims (Grice, 1975) as "make your statement as informative as required but not more informative than required" (in other words, don't express what you think your hearer already knows). More generally, a statement in a discourse is assumed by all parties to be relevant and to be as informative as appropriate. And sentences follow such maxims just as dependably in inner dialogue as they do in external conversation. But if the sentences do not express all that I know or intend, then what I know or intend must take some other form—a form of which I have no conscious awareness. It is no help to say, as one might in discussing an actual overt conversation, that the hearer of the sentence infers the missing parts, because in inner dialogue the speaker and hearer are the same. And if the speaker knows something that remains unexpressed in the sentences of the inner dialogue, it just goes to show that the inner dialogue is not doing the work one assumed it was doing. The imagined inner dialogue leaves many unstated things to the imagination of the inner speaker and hearer, whereas, as Steven Pinker puts it, "The 'language of thought' in which knowledge is couched can leave nothing to the imagination, because it *is* the imagination" (1997, p. 70). If we think in language then there is nowhere else for the unexpressed parts of the thought to hide.

The problem of expressing the entire content of your thoughts in sentences is even deeper than might appear from this discussion. It was already known in the early history of logic that sentences are too ambiguous to serve as the vehicles of reasoning. For this reason, logicians had to devise more precise formalisms to express the distinct meanings that a sentence could have. So they invented mathematical systems of symbolic logic, such as the predicate calculus. For example, sentences like "Every man loves a woman" can express at least two distinct senses (one in which for each man there is some woman that he loves, and the other in which there is a woman such that every man loves her), thus making it necessary to introduce such syntactic mechanisms as quantifiers and brackets to express these distinct meanings.

But the problem with the idea that natural language serves as the vehicle of thought is deeper than the problem posed by the existence of syntactic ambiguities or by the importance of unspoken context in determining the meanings of sentences in inner a dialogue. Words and phrases appear to cut the world up more coarsely than does thought. There are many concepts for which there is no corresponding word (though presumably for many of them there *could* be an appropriate word). But, even more important, one can have thoughts when one is perceiving something whose contents *cannot* be expressed in words, not even for one's own private purposes. The outstanding examples of such thoughts are ones that we have already encountered in chapter 5: they are thoughts with a demonstrative (or indexical) component. I can, for example, think a thought such as "This pencil is yellow," where I am able to pick out an individual and claim of it that it is a pencil and that it is yellow. The object that my visual indexing system picks out is the very object about which I am having the thought and of which I am predicating certain properties. The resulting predication forms part of the content of my thought, yet it cannot be expressed, linguistically or otherwise since it concerns an object that I am directly picking out from the world that I perceive at this very moment and in this very context.

For that matter, most of the properties of the object I am seeing and which can enter into my thoughts cannot be expressed, linguistically or otherwise. For example, I can have the perfectly clear and well-formed thought *"This* is the *same* color as *that,"* where the content of my thoughts in some important sense includes the color, as well as the proposition that the two *things* I have mentally picked out are the *same* color. Yet I cannot express this thought in language—not because I don't know the correct words, but because I needn't even have a category or concept for an important part of what I am thinking, namely, what is being referred to by the demonstrative "that," as well as its particular color. Some thoughts, in other words, can contain *unconceptualized contents*. This, in turn, means that the grain of thoughts, or the possible distinctions between their contents, is even finer than that of one's *potential* linguistic vocabulary (assuming that one's vocabulary is necessarily confined to the things for which one has concepts).

The idea that natural language cannot be the medium of thought because of inherent ambiguity and instability, in relation to the specificity of the contents it expresses, has been noted by many writers. Block (2001) has recently argued that there is also an inherent difference in grain between thoughts and experiences: we can have visual experiences at a finer grain than the grain of our thoughts. Sperber and Wilson (1998) make a similar point. They argue that there must be many more concepts than there are words and that, unlike concepts, the meaning of a particular word token may depend on many pragmatic factors. Fodor (2001) makes the same point in arguing that language only approximates the compositionality and systematicity required of thought (see also the discussion of systematicity and compositionality on pp. 437–439).

8.2.3   Do we think in pictures?

Suppose we concede that sensory contents can be finer grained than verbal ones and thus that we can represent properties visually that we cannot describe verbally. This suggests that mental states must include sensory contents as well as verbal contents, which is the basic premise of the dual code view of mental representations, as well as the "perceptual symbol system" idea championed by Barsalou (1999). In the case of visual properties, we might postulate that these could take the form of visual mental images. But visual images are just as inadequate in their expressive power as are sentences. Just as the idea that we think in sentences is inadequate because the bulk of the information remains elsewhere, so too is the idea that we think in mental pictures: both face the same indeterminacy problem. Consider a simple example in which a visual image allows one to solve a certain problem.

People find it easy to solve what are called three-term series problems by imagining that the objects described in the problem are located in an array where the spatial relations between them represent their relative standing on some measure. A typical problem goes like this. "John is taller than Mary but shorter than Susan. Who is tallest (shortest)?" (Instead of "taller" one can substitute "smarter," "richer," and many other such relations.) To solve this problem, all you have to do is place a tag representing John at a fixed location in an image. Then when you hear that John is taller than Mary you locate a tag for Mary below the one for John in a vertical stack, and when you hear that John is shorter than Susan you locate a tag for Susan above the one for John, to yield an image such as figure 8.1. You solve the "who is shortest" problem by finding the lowest tag in the image (and similarly for answering "tallest" or "all who are taller than" questions).

De Soto, London, and Handel (1965) refer to this way of solving problems as using "spatial paralogic" (see also Huttenlocher, 1968). Despite the simplicity of this example, it has inspired a great deal of research. For example, the exact wording has been shown to have a strong effect, which suggests that linguistic processes—translating from sentences to some other form of representation—may account for why problems worded in one way are easier than ones worded in another (Clark, 1969). But even here one might ask whether other sorts of cognitive representations are involved, besides those in the image and/or the sentences experienced by the person solving this problem. A moment's thought will reveal that there is much more going on than just inspecting the image. Right at the start, in hearing the sentence "John is taller than Mary but shorter than Susan," the hearer must figure out what are the missing

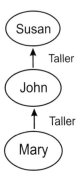

Figure 8.1
If elements in the three-term series problem are imagined as arranged in a vertical array, the answers to the problem may be obtained by merely examining the array.

parts of the sentence: the subject and verb of the second clause are missing and must be restored in the course of the grammatical analysis of the sentence. In fact, by some analyses even more words are missing in the surface structure ("John is taller that Mary but shorter than Susan" means "John is taller than Mary ⟨is tall⟩ but ⟨John⟩ ⟨is⟩ shorter than Susan <is short>"). This involves appealing to grammatical rules (in this case, deletion rules)—the processing of which is never conscious.

Following this grammatical analysis, there is still the question of how the problem statement is converted into instructions for "mental drawing." Notice that to know that a vertical array is an appropriate structure to use in this problem, the person must already have done some reasoning. Only relationships that have the formal property known as *transitivity* are candidates for such a structure. If the problem had been about the relation "likes," then the structure would have been inappropriate (since "Mary likes John" and "John likes Susan" does not entail that "Mary likes Susan"). How do subjects solve all these preliminary problems? Through what *conscious* imaginal or verbal steps do they go? Obviously they do not do it in language since the issue is how they understand the language, and they don't do it in pictures since the question is about deciding what pictures to construct and how to interpret them.

This characterization of the problem-solving process also assumes many properties of the imaged array. Where do these assumptions come from and how are they justified? For example, according to the account given, a symbol for Mary (call it *Mary*) is placed below *John* in a vertical stack. Next, *Susan* is placed above *John*. This appears also to locate *Susan* above *Mary* in the stack. Why? For that to be true, two further things must be true of the image. One is that it must be the case that some operations on the image do not change certain relations that are already there. In the case of an array written on a board, when you add an item above a stack of two items already there, the two items generally keep the same relations as they had before the addition. That is so at least partly because the board is rigid and some geometrical relations on a rigid board remain fixed when new objects and relations are added. But even this is not always the case. For example, a graphical representation of the two-placed relations "directly above" or "next to" do change when another object is inserted between them. Thus, if the instructions had led you to place *Mary* "directly below" *John* and the next instruction also led you to place *Susan* "directly below" *John*, the relation between *John* and *Mary* would be changed (or become indeterminate) as a result of the new addition (*Mary* may no longer be "directly below" *John*). (For more examples, see section 8.4.)

This might seem like a trivial matter that is easily corrected, but it turns out to be the tip of a large iceberg called the "frame problem" (see, e.g., Ford and Pylyshyn, 1996; Pylyshyn, 1987). When one carries out actions in one's mind, as opposed to executing those actions on the world, the problem of determining, given what one knows, what will change and what will remain fixed is in general intractable. That's because what can change is whatever may be relevant to the action, and the general problem of relevance is itself intractable; any belief can be relevant to any action so long as there is a possible chain of reasoning that could connect them. Such a chain always exists, since one can in principle have beliefs that conjoin any pair of other beliefs. One could have the belief "if P_j then P_k" for any possible pair of beliefs P_j and P_k, and so if P_a is relevant to action a, then there may a chain from any belief P_j to action a.

For example, suppose that you have the belief (P_1) that to leave the room (i.e., to be located outside the room) you should open the door, and the belief (P_2) that to open the door you must be near the door. If you also have the apparently unrelated belief (apparently unrelated because it does not involve any of the concepts of the first belief, such as *door, inside,* etc.) that there is a security system triggered by movements that locks all means of egress (P_3), then the link between P_1 and the goal of being outside the room is blocked. This information may be implicit in your knowledge, but inferring it could mean checking every belief in your entire database of beliefs—an intractable task, given the nearly unbounded size of your entire belief set (for more on the frame problem see the essays in Pylyshyn, 1987).

Even if you could correctly solve the problem of whether or not an already present relation in the image changes when an action (including checking the image for the presence of some property) is performed, there is then the problem of interpreting the resulting image. Consider figure 8.1 to be an exact rendering of the image from which you reason this problem through (notwithstanding the argument on pp. 350–357 that this can't be done in principle). Why do the size and shape of the ellipses and the size and font of the names not enter into the conclusion? What determines which relations are relevant and how to read them off the image? Also, in this example, the same meaningful relation ("taller than") occurs in different geometrical guises. Although the diagram shows John being taller than Mary, Susan being taller than John, and Susan being taller than Mary, it does not show each of these in terms of the same geometrical relationship (e.g., the symbols for Mary and Susan are further apart and there is an intervening item in the array). Reading off this relationship requires knowing that the presence of an intermediate item does not affect the relationship between the two items in question (unlike, e.g., the relationship "adjacent to"). This is a property that is not represented in the image or anywhere else in consciousness.

In each of these examples, reasoning is involved that is neither represented in the diagram, nor contained in an inner dialogue. The point of this mundane example is that the things of which we are aware—the words and mental images—are never sufficient for the function attributed to them. In every case, more is going on, as it were, "offstage." And what more is going on is, at least in certain cases, patently not expressible as a sentence or a picture. Yet, despite this important point, it is also true that pictures can enhance thinking in important ways (which I will take up in section 8.3), because vision, when directed to real diagrams, often provides operations that can be used to draw inferences more simply than by using rules of logic. This is especially true when reasoning about spatial properties, as in geometry.

8.2.4 What form must thoughts have?

Fodor (1975) presents a tightly argued case that thought must be encoded in what he calls a "language of thought" or LOT. Of course, LOT cannot be a natural language, such as English, for the reasons presented above. Also, a great many highly intelligent organisms, such as prelinguistic children and higher primates, do not have any language and yet they are clearly capable of thought. Any vehicle of thought must have certain properties. One of these properties is *productivity*. Since the number of thoughts we can have is in principle unbounded (except for practical considerations such as one's mortality and boredom), thoughts must be constructed from simple elements called concepts (as Humboldt put it, our representational capacity is capable of "infinite use of finite means".)[2]

Moreover, the meaning of a complex thought must be derived from the meaning of its constituent parts, which means that thoughts must be *compositional*. All the meaning of a complex thought must come from the meaning of its canonically distinguishable parts, together with the rules of composition (or syntax) of LOT; it cannot come from any other source. Even more important, thoughts must have the property that Fodor and Pylyshyn (1988) call *systematicity*. This means that if an organism is capable of thought at all it must be capable of having sets of related thoughts. If it can think, say, "Mary hit the ball" and it can think "John baked a cake," then it can also think "John hit the ball" and "Mary baked a cake" and even "John hit the cake" and "Mary baked the ball." Of course, it is unlikely to think the latter two because these would be bizarre events, but the point is that the system for encoding thoughts encodes complexes from simples. Once that system is in place and the constituent concepts are available, the capacity to form the complex thoughts is inherently there.

In Fodor and Pylyshyn (1988), we argued that inference also requires compositionality of the system of representation. Rules of inference are schemas; they tell you how to draw a conclusion from premises by recognizing the constituents of a structured representation and transforming them in ways that preserve truth (or some other semantic property,

---

2. This idea was made famous in the early 1960s by Noam Chomsky. For more on the Chomskian revolution in cognitive science see http://mitpress2.mit.edu/e-books/chomsky.

such as plausibility). For example, if you have a thought with the content "It is dark and cold and raining," you are entitled to conclude "It is raining" (or "It is cold" or "It is dark"). This follows from the rule of conjunction elimination: from "P & Q" infer "P" (or infer "Q"). In this rule the "P" and "Q" can be replaced by arbitrarily complex expressions. For example, in a particular case the position occupied by "Q" might instead be occupied by "R and (S or T)" in which case one would be entitled to infer from the expression "P and (R and (S or T))" that "P" or that "R and (S or T)." Take a thought such as the one given earlier ("It is dark and cold and raining"). Since any intelligent creature could infer from the thought "it is dark and cold and raining" that "it is raining" it must also be able to infer from "it is cold and raining" that "it is raining." In other words, there is systematicity in what you are able to infer from complex thoughts: if you can make one sort of inference, you are thereby also able to make other sorts of inferences (especially simpler ones as in the example here).

None of this analysis depends on exactly how the beliefs are encoded except that they must have recognizable parts that determine the meaning of the whole, and these parts, in turn, are what determine what can be inferred. These sorts of considerations are what lead one to the view that whatever form thoughts may take they must meet the condition of systematicity, from which it follows that they are bound to have constituents and to be compositional. This makes them rather more like a language than a picture or any other fused form of representation that does not recognize semantically interpreted parts, such as that proposed by the "connectionist" approach to modeling mind (for a more detailed exposition of this point, see Fodor and Pylyshyn, 1988).

Notwithstanding the argument presented above, the requirement of compositionality does not prevent there being analog components in representations. For example, there is no prohibition against individual terms in the vocabulary of LOT being drawn from an infinite set, as they might be if they constituted what Goodman (1968) calls a "dense symbol system." Although such arcane symbol systems are not prohibited, it is still an open question what would be gained from assuming them. We know, more or less, what can be done with discrete symbol systems (pretty much all of logic and computer science is concerned with such systems), but there are only hints as to what would be gained by admitting other sorts of symbols into LOT.

One can also augment LOT be adding nonlinguistic (or nonconceptual) elements in several ways. For example nonlinguistic entities can function in thought by providing external elements or models that can be used in reasoning. We are all familiar with the usefulness of diagrams, charts, graphs, and other visual aids in conveying ideas. Before considering the possibility that parts of thought may be carried by nonsymbolic means, we need to look at why real diagrams might be useful in reasoning and ask whether those functions can be obtained from imagined diagrams.

8.3   How Can Visual Displays Help Us to Reason?

8.3.1   Diagrams as logical systems that exploit visual operations

To accept the conditions on the format of reasoning is not to deny that thinking about some kinds of problems can be enhanced by the use of vision—real vision of real displays. Some kinds of problem solving—say, proving theorems in plane geometry—appear to proceed more efficiently when we are able to use displays or diagrams as a prosthetic to aid in thinking. Although the mathematician David Hilbert showed that Euclidean geometry using diagrams and based on Euclid's axioms (as put forward in his *Elements*) is not rigorous in that it makes hidden assumptions (particularly about the existence of points and lines that are drawn according to the compass-and-straightedge requirement), it is difficult to imagine proving a theorem in plane geometry without drawing a figure. But consider the assumptions that go into some of the simplest proofs from Euclid. To prove his First Proposition, Euclid used one diagram and accompanying text. The proposition says that an equilateral triangle can be constructed on a given line AB using only compass and straightedge. The construction is obvious from the diagram (figure 8.2): Draw a circle with one end of the line (A) as center and then another circle centered on the other end of the line (B). Then join the point where they intersect to each end of the line. It is an equilateral triangle by construction.

The trouble with this "proof," as many people have noted, is that it assumes without proof that the two circles *will* intersect—an assumption

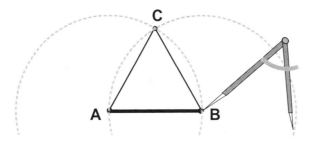

Figure 8.2
This figure illustrates Euclid's First Proposition: an equilateral triangle can be constructed on a given line using only compass and straightedge. You can see how to draw the circles and connect the resulting points from this illustration. Euclid's original proof was hardly more than this graphical presentation. Is this a rigorous proof?

that does not follow from any of Euclid's "elements" or axioms. Since Hilbert, the general consensus has been that diagrams can be dispensed with, or even must be dispensed with to provide rigorous proofs of Euclidean theorems. Hilbert provided an axiomatization of Euclidean geometry that was nonfigural and did not use geometrical constructions; using these axioms he was able to make Euclid's propositions rigorous and free from hidden assumptions.

The question of whether diagrams are merely heuristic or can provide a rigorous means of proving theorems has been controversial over the years. But the question has recently been revived. A number of writers (e.g., Allwein and Barwise, 1996) have argued that diagrammatic reasoning can be made rigorous while retaining its diagrammatic character. Miller (2001) developed an axiomatic system (EG) that treats elements of diagrams as syntactic objects and proves theorems about them that are nearly as simple and transparent as conventional Euclidean proofs. The system has even been implemented as a computer program (called CDEG, for computerized diagrammatic Euclidean geometry). Although this system reasons with syntactic objects that correspond to parts of diagrams, it does not conjecture possibilities based on appearances and thus lacks one of the important aspects of human diagrammatic reasoning. Miller was interested in providing a sound formal system, as simple as that based on Euclidean postulates, to support the use of diagrams to explore geometrical relationships, and in this he was eminently successful. Our goal in this section, however, is to examine how diagrams and the human visual system together could form a more powerful system for reasoning than unaided cognition (or perhaps than reasoning aided by a notepad for writing down formulas or for keeping track of cases).

The visual system is one of our most developed and exquisite cognitive faculties, and we make use of it in many more ways than recognizing familiar objects and guiding our movements. For example, we are able to convert many abstract problems into spatial form, as we do when we reason using Venn diagrams, graphs, and other modes of spatial representation (including the example illustrated in figure 8.1). Venn diagrams (which are one of the more successful of a wide range of logic-encoding diagrams discussed by Gardner, 1982) allow one not only to illustrate relations between sets or between propositions (the two are interdefinable) but also to aid reasoning. The Venn diagram representation of sets, an example of which is shown in figure 8.3, illustrates that certain properties of the visual system (e.g., the ease with which it detects whether one region overlaps another or whether some designated element is inside a particular region) can be exploited to facilitate reasoning. Such externalizations exploit the perceptual system (usually, though not necessarily, vision) to help us recognize patterns. In accepting that vision can play this role we need make no assumptions about the form of our thoughts, only about how we are able to map from perceived patterns to thoughts in the pursuit of problem-solving goals. Thinking while seeing allows our thoughts to exploit important properties of space without assuming that the form of our thought is itself spatial.

Venn diagrams and other graphical forms of inference are more than just mental crutches; they allow rigorous proofs to be formulated, as Allwein and Barwise (1996) and Jamnek (2001) have shown. But for this to occur, the graphical form, together with the appropriate operations and interpretations placed on them, must be isomorphic to normative rules of logic. The study of such graphical forms has been a serious pursuit since at least the time of Ramon Lull, an early thirteenth-century scholar. Lull invented an influential method, called *Ars Magna*, that consisted of a set of geometrical figures and mechanisms for guiding reasoning. Gardner (1982) provides a fascinating discussion of such devices, which include the diagrammatic inventions of Leonhard Euler, Sir William Hamilton, Allan Marquand, Johann Lambert, Charles Peirce, Lewis Carroll (Charles Dodgson), and Gerrit Marie Mes.

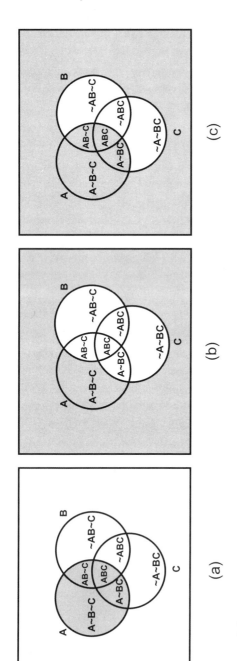

(a)   (b)   (c)

Figure 8.3
This figure illustrates the use of Venn diagrams to represent the sets A, B, C. Panel (a) shows the set of elements that are in A, by shading everything in the circle labeled A. Panel (b) shows the set of elements that are not in B and also not in C (i.e., everything in not-B, the complement set of B, denoted ~B, and also in not-C, or in the complement set of C, denoted ~C). We do this by shading everything (the universal set) *except* the elements that are in B or in C. Notice that being in not-B *and* being in not-C is equivalent to not being in either B or C—i.e., ~B~C = (~B *and* ~C) = ~(B *or* C), which illustrates how we can go from viewing the diagram in terms of set membership to viewing it in terms of the truth of propositions. Panel (c) shows the set of elements that are in not-B and in not-C (as in panel b), but it also includes those elements that are in A. Panel (c) is similar to panel (a) except that the elements it represents also include elements that are not in any of the named sets A, or B or C, as shown by shading the background. Relations among set memberships such as these can easily be seen by examining these figures, which help us to visualize sets and operations on them.

But diagrams and other sorts of figures can be useful even when they are not embodied in a rigorous system of valid reasoning. Indeed, the use of diagrams in proofs of plane geometry is of this nonrigorous sort. So the question remains, How and why can diagrams be useful as heuristics in such cases? Clearly, there is something about vision that provides functions that are not as readily available in other forms of reasoning. And if that is so, then perhaps mental imagery provides similar functions. It is worth considering, therefore, what vision might contribute to reasoning and perhaps also to creative reasoning.

8.3.2 Diagrams as guides for derivational milestones (lemmas)

Consider the following example, in which drawing the right diagram makes it easy and transparent to prove one of the most important theorems in plane geometry: the Pythagorean Theorem.

Figure 8.4 shows a right angle triangle (shaded) with sides a, b, and hypotenuse c. To prove that the square on c is the sum of squares on a and b, we begin by drawing a square on side c. Then we extend the sides a and b until they both equal $a + b$ and we draw a square on these sides (the area of this square is $a + b$ times $a + b$). Without going through the individual steps one can readily prove that the original triangle is reduplicated 4 times inside this large square (by checking the angles, verify that each of the triangles in the corners is similar to the original triangle; and because each has hypotenuse of length c, they are congruent to the original triangle). Thus we see that the large square, whose area is $(a + b)^2$, is made up of the square on c plus 4 triangles. Therefore, to get the area of the square on c, we subtract the 4 copies of the original triangle that fit between the square on c and the outer square on $a + b$. Since the area of each of those 4 triangles is $\frac{1}{2}ab$, we have the following equation: $c^2 = (a + b)^2 - (4 \times \frac{1}{2}ab) = a^2 + b^2 + 2ab - 2ab = a^2 + b^2$.

This proof, though easier to describe, is not as elegant as some of others that do not use algebra[3] (there are at least 367 published proofs, many of which require only folding and shearing and overlaying parts of the constructed figures; see the references in Dunham, 1994), but it does illustrate the importance of construction in geometrical proofs.

---

3. A selection of proofs of the Pythagorean Theorem, many of them animated and interactive, can be viewed at http://www.cut-the-knot.com/pythagoras/.

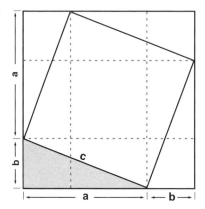

Figure 8.4
Illustration of how construction helps to prove a theorem in plane geometry, in this case the important theorem of Pythagoras. The construction is described in the text, but even without the details, one should be able to see the possibility of a proof since if we take the area of the square inscribed on the hypotenuse of the shaded triangle, and add to it four copies of the original triangle, which fit neatly in the corners, we get the area of the large square whose sides are known—so at least we have some visible relationship among the right parts of the puzzle. Writing this relationship down algebraically solves the problem easily. It is also possible to solve the problem in this graphical way without algebra, by using only draw, copy, rotate, and move operations.

Without drawing the square on c and on $a + b$ the proof would be extremely difficult and in fact would likely have been impossible in Euclid's time. So what purpose do the constructions serve? In Euclid's geometry the constraints on construction defined the rules of plane geometry: all problems could be paraphrased into the form, "using only a compass and straightedge, show that. . . ." The constraints placed on construction constituted one of Euclid's 5 "postulates." But beyond that, selecting which intermediate figures to construct is like deciding which lemmas to prove in the course of proving the main theorem. In addition, the visual detection of similarity and congruence (as we saw in figure 8.4) provides the important guidance in conjecturing lemmas and developing the proof.[4]

4. Barwise and Etchemendy (1996) use the same diagram but view its construction differently. They start off with the original triangle and construct a square on its hypotenuse. Then they explicitly replicate the triangle three times and move it into the positions shown in figure 8.4. The proof then proceeds by

The way in which diagrams and other visual aids help us to formulate and solve problems is far from understood. The following characteristics of vision are surely important to that pursuit:

(1) Vision provides primitive operations for a number of functions, such as shape recognition and the detection of relational properties like the "inclusion" of certain regions within other regions (in fact, recognizing this particular relation formed the basic operation out of which Jean Nicod hoped to build his "sensory geometry"; see Nicod, 1970). Primitive detection operations such as these are important, for example, in exploiting Venn diagrams. The usefulness of diagrams, graphs, charts, and other visual devices relies on the fact that people are good at visually detecting certain geometrical relations (as we saw in the discussion of "visual routines" in chapter 5).

(2) Another important property of vision, which has received considerable attention in recent years, is that it appears to keep track of where information is located in the world rather than encoding it all in memory, thus in effect providing what amounts to a very large memory. The idea that vision uses "the external world as memory" was argued forcefully by O'Regan (1992) and supported by findings of Ballard et al. (1997). Ballard and colleagues showed that in carrying out a simple task such as constructing a copy of a pattern of colored blocks, observers encoded very little in each glance (essentially only information about one block), preferring instead to return their gaze over and over to the model figure that they were copying.

In chapter 5 I argued for the general importance of keeping track of information in the world that had not yet been encoded (or conceptualized), and I proposed the mechanism of visual indexes (or FINSTs) to allow gaze or focal attention to return to certain parts of a figure whose properties had yet to be encoded. Thus, although there is now considerable evidence that surprisingly little of a scene is recalled from a single glance (Rensink, O'Regan, and Clark, 2000; Simons and Levin, 1997)—

---

showing that these triangles fit snugly in place by using the fact that three angles of a triangle sum to a straight line. Replicating and moving or rotating a triangle are operations that clearly would have little meaning without a diagram.

unless the observer happens to fixate or attend to a particular part of the scene (Henderson and Hollingworth, 1999; Rensink et al., 1997)—a great deal of information is potentially (as well as phenomenologically) available. (To anticipate the discussion in the next section I might note here that the mechanism of visual indexing can be exploited only when perceiving a real scene, not when accessing information from a mental image.)

(3) Vision routinely goes beyond the information given; a percept is invariably a generalization of the individual properties of a unique stimulus. In fact, any recognition of a pattern is just such a generalization: we do not see something as a chair except that we generalize the particular shape in front of us by putting it in the same category as an unlimited number of other shapes, namely, all the shapes we see *as* chairs. The naturalness of such visual generalization is an essential part of reasoning with diagrams and will be discussed in the next section.

8.3.3   Diagrams as a way of exploiting visual generalizations

When we draw diagrams and examine them to determine whether some general property holds, we do not just rely on whether we detect an instance of that property in the particular diagram; we often appear to "see" what properties will *necessarily* hold of any resulting construction. For example, if you want to know where the intersection of two lines will be if they are drawn inside a rectangle according to a certain specification, you have but to draw an *arbitrary* rectangle and then draw *arbitrary* lines in it meeting the specifications, and you can quite often see not only the location of the intersection of particular pair of lines that you drew, but also where the intersection must fall for *any* pairs of lines in *any* rectangle that meet the given specifications. For example, you can tell that if you draw a line from each of the two bottom vertices of any rectangle to any point on the opposite vertical side, then (a) these two lines will always intersect and (b) the intersection will always lie below the horizontal midline of the rectangle. You can see that by just looking at a particular instance, as in figure 8.5.

How you turn a particular instance of a figure into a universal generalization is far from obvious (although one can certainly come up with plausible hypotheses for particular cases). Going from a particular to a

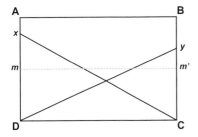

Figure 8.5
You can "see" from this figure that if lines (D-y, C-x) are drawn from the bottom vertices to any point on the opposite side, the lines will meet at or below the midline (m-m') of the rectangle, and that this will be true for any possible lines drawn to this specification and in any possible rectangle. What is it about the visual system that generalizes from particulars to universals?

universal is no doubt related to how one reasons abductively in general, but it appears in this case that the visual system is involved essentially. Its involvement, moreover, goes beyond merely recognizing that a certain pattern or property is present in a particular instance of the drawing. Visual perception appears to be the source of the generalization in the first instance.

How does vision make the jump from a particular instance to a generalization? One could visually encode general properties by such devices as annotations added to a diagram in various ways to show some general property. Sometimes these annotations are diagrammatic and so do not appear to be annotations. For example, we could represent graphically the infinite family of lines implied by the drawing in figure 8.5 (say, as a fan-shaped region, such as in figure 8.6). This would still be a particular token shape, except that we would know to interpret the shaded area as a set of possible lines, much as we would interpret a label. We would thus be relying on an interpretation (which might be quite natural, as in this case) to represent a quantified proposition such as "all lines lying in the region bounded by. . . ." In this case, the representation contains more information than the original drawing (it contains the limits of possible line locations) and would in part be "read" like a descriptive annotation.

The use of this sort of implicit annotation (where visual properties are used not to depict a visual or spatial property, but to bias the way spatial

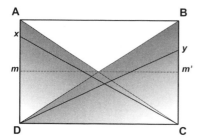

Figure 8.6
One way to think of the class of all lines from D to an arbitrary point on the opposite side is to imagine a fan-shaped area representing all such lines. Such an apparently pictorial way of representing a class is no different from providing an annotation that would be interpreted by the viewer, much the way a symbol would be. In this case, however, the annotation has to refer to sets of locations within the figure, so it is best if it is superimposed on the figure or, as in this case, is presented as a part of the figure. The diagrammatic form of the annotation is particularly useful because it provides a natural way to refer to particular visual objects and locations.

properties are interpreted by the viewer) is quite common in graphs and is often the only way that noncommittal or vague information can be depicted graphically (see chapter 1, especially note 7). It is also one of the techniques adopted in many practical schemes for graphing (or "visualizing") information. Such schemes emphasize selecting the most natural and perspicuous visual properties for conveying various types of secondary or annotation information, such as the use of certain visual dimensions for conveying magnitudes and relationships between magnitudes (this has been superbly exploited by Tufte, 1990, in his examples of visual communication). For example, practical schemes consider a variety of image properties, from physical size to brightness and color, as potential dimensions to convey both magnitudes and their location (e.g., on a map). Norman (1988, 1991) illustrates how things can go wrong if relative magnitudes are depicted on a map using a nonmetrical visual property, such as texture.

But it may be misleading to view the process by which diagrams depict general properties as equivalent to adding annotations. The process of going from a particular to a universal is inherent in how vision works—how it parses a complex figure into subparts and how it represents and recognizes patterns. For example, in section 3.1 we saw that perception of 3D objects makes essential use of the distinction between accidental and nonaccidental properties. Accidental properties are ones that depend on the precise viewpoint and disappear when the viewer makes the smallest movement. For example, two lines in an image could be aligned or could be coterminous (connected) entirely by accident. They could correspond to two randomly situated lines in 3D seen from a particular point of view that just happens to align them or cause their endpoints to be at the same place on the 2D image (as illustrated in figure 3.3). Yet the probability of this happening by accident (i.e., the probability of the 2D image containing two linearly aligned or coterminous line segments when the lines are actually not aligned or coterminous in the scene) is vanishingly small and could be easily detected by a slight change in viewpoint. Consequently, the visual system always interprets such occurrences as nonaccidental (the principles by which the visual system provides nonaccidental interpretations of image features are discussed in chapter 3, especially pp. 94–96). In making such an interpretation, the visual system appears to jump to a conclusion about a universal property from a single instance. Such apparent abductive leaps are characteristic of vision and may form the basis for how vision helps us to reason: it provides nondemonstrative inferences on matters pertaining to shape (especially 3D shape, which has been studied most).

Although it is not viewed in exactly these terms, the study of computational vision—and in particular, the study of object recognition and representation—centers precisely on the problem of how vision generalizes from particulars, or from token image shapes, to classes of image shapes. When we "recognize an object," we map some of the geometrical properties of the token proximal image onto properties that the object *class* possesses. That's because "recognizing an object" is, in part, to assign the image to a category, and in part it is to provide a representation of the shape that all members of the category possess. I say "in part" because this is only part of the story. In a sense, vision strips off the properties that are specific to the image token to focus on the properties of the general object class, but it generally does not throw this information away. It usually represents some of these particulars separately, for example as parameters. This is what various schemes for object representation do; they allow us to factor apart various aspects of the object shape.

For example, a scheme may factor out the object's size and orientation (using some natural axis) and then represent these as separate aspects of the object's shape. It may also encode the way in which the shape deviates from a simple core pattern. Several object-perception methods use what are called "deformable models" to represent a general shape. One common method is based on wrapping a mathematically simple skin over the shape, using a formalism called a "superquadric" (Pentland, 1986). Many such schemes for representing object shapes have been used in robot vision. One of the most widely adopted is the generalized cylinder (or generalized cone) representation, initially proposed by Binford (1971) and developed further by Marr (1982). This representation characterizes 3D objects in terms of structures of cylinders whose primary axes can be curved and whose radii can vary across the length of the cylinder. In other words, every shape is described as some set of interconnected and deformed cylinders. This form of representation has been adopted as part of a theory of object-recognition known as recognition-by-parts, developed by Irving Biederman (1987, 1995).

Another interesting example of a core-plus-deformation scheme for object representation was proposed by Michael Leyton (1992). In Leyton's theory, an object's core representation is a highly symmetric shape (for example, a sphere), and the transformations represent various ways that this simple core shape might have been transformed to yield the observed shape. The transformations in Leyton's theory are not just a mathematically compact way of representing shapes, but are chosen to reflect various salient ways in which *physical* processes might operate to transform the core shape. Hence the representation can been viewed as providing a reconstruction of the object's causal history of physical deformations. The shape transformations include those produced by physical forces such as stretching, squeezing, twisting, skewing, and so on, as well as other factors, such as biological processes like growth. They also reflect optical processes such as those involved in the projection of light from object to image, which result in perspective transformations.

There are many ways of representing shapes in terms of some canonical shape plus some parameters, or shape plus transformations. For our purposes I wish simply to note that choosing a form of representation, such as the one based on the generalized cylinder, establishes a pattern of generalization. For example, in the recognition-by-parts technique (which is based on deformed cylinders), a shape generalizes more readily to objects that have the same relational structure of cylindrical axes than to those that do not, more readily to objects with the same profile of axis diameters than those that do not, and so on. Biederman's recognition-by-parts system inherently generalizes shapes in just this way, as he showed experimentally by examining patterns of confusion in the recall of shapes (O'Kane et al., 1997). In particular, the system is relatively insensitive to size (Biederman and Cooper, 1992), viewpoint (Biederman and Bar, 1999), and rotation in depth (Biederman and Gerhardstein, 1993). To the extent that the theory is a valid description of what early vision computes, it embodies a scheme of visual generalization that functions when we visually perceive patterns, including diagrams.

8.3.4 Diagrams as ways of tracking instances and alternatives

A diagram used in problem solving is often nothing more than a representation of a particular instance of the givens in a problem; a representation of some token situations, rather than of the entire class of situations mentioned in the problem statement. In some cases, diagrams can be useful even without the special properties of visual generalization, because they encode distinct cases and allow us to keep track of them.

For example, consider the following problem, discussed by Barwise and Etchemendy (1990). The problem is stated as follows: "You are to seat four people, A, B, C, and D, in a row of five chairs. A and C are to flank the empty chair. C must be closer to the center than D, who is to sit next to B. Who must be seated in the center chair and who is to be seated on either end?" Here is a straightforward way to solve this problem. First set out the five chair positions like this: – – – – –. Next consider the constraints. Since A and C are to flank the empty chair, there are six cases (where □ indicates the empty chair and – indicates a free or unallocated chair):

Case 1: A □ C – –   Case 1a: – – C □ A
Case 2: – A □ C –   Case 2a: – C □ A –
Case 3: – – A □ C   Case 3a: C □ A – –

Where cases 1a, 2a, and 3a are the mirror images of case 1, 2, and 3. Since none of the constraints refers to left or right, the problem can be solved without considering those cases separately, so we ignore the cases 1a, 1b, and 1c. Since C must be closer to the center than D we can eliminate case 3, which places C further from the center than D. Since D must be next to B we rule out case 2 because it does not have two adjoining unassigned seats. This leaves case 1, with B and D assigned as follows:

A □ C B D
A □ C D B

In these remaining cases (or their mirror images), all the stated constraints are satisfied. So the answer to the question is: C must occupy the middle seat and A must occupy one end seat, while either B or D can occupy the other end seat.

Although Barwise and Etchemendy present this as a problem that is easily solved with the aid of vision, in fact the diagram makes little use of vision's specific properties. The diagram primarily serves the function of setting out the distinct cases and keeping track of the names that occupy the five seat locations. Other than recognizing the letters and their relative location in a row, very little use is made of the capacity of the visual system in this example. Of course, a visual pattern is an excellent way to encode which position has which letter, and it does make it easy to "read off" the contents of the five locations. But no property of the pattern other than name and ordinal position is relevant. Any way of encoding name information and any way of representing ordinal position would do (e.g., this information could have been represented in the tactile modality or as a melody in the auditory/temporal modality).

I do not wish to make too much of the modality in which the figure is presented (vision is most likely the easiest if it is available), but it is important for our purpose to see exactly what function the "diagram" serves. It allows us to construct the distinct cases, to apply the problem constraints to each of them, and to access their contents readily. Because the constraints are stated in terms of the location in a row, a linear array is well suited to the problem. And because the visual form makes the array easiest to reaccess, it may offer an advantage over audition. The fact that only ordinal information together with the identity of individuals (as given in the problem statement) is relevant also means that the problem could easily be solved by a computer using a list representation.

Here is another way of characterizing what is special about such a use of a diagram: it is a constructed instance. In what I will call a pure qual-

itative construction such as in this example (one without symbolic annotations) there are no explicit magnitudes, no quantifiers (like "some," or
"all," or numerical quantifiers such as "some number greater than 2"),
there is no negation (the constructed instance cannot represent that something *may not* be the case), and no explicit disjunctions (they cannot represent that either one case or another holds except by the convention
of listing the entire disjunction of alternatives separately, as I did in the
above example, where disjunction is implied. The list format could
not directly represent the constraint that the item at the end had to be "A
or D"). Pure constructions contain individuals, not classes of individuals,
and properties or relations are ascribed to existing individuals. This
appears to be the essence of constructions such as those in this example.

To be sure, diagrams have other properties as well (e.g., they can represent metrical properties and other visual-appearance properties, such
as color, shape, orientation, and spatial frequency). I will put these aside
for now because I want to consider the function that can be played by
mental diagrams, where metrical properties present special problems
(contrary to claims often made about mental imagery). I will therefore
concentrate on the question of how pure constructions might be used in
reasoning if we abstracted from their metrical properties.

8.3.5   Diagrams as external memory of spatial patterns
There is little doubt of the importance of spatial constructs in
organizing our thoughts, including at the highly abstract levels. Spatial
metaphors abound when we are communicating complex ideas and
working through problems (Talmy, 2000). Yet it is far from clear how
the mind uses spatial concepts and spatial organization. This much seems
clear: we are able to exploit certain properties of vision in order to reason
in some nonvisual domains. For example, we can exploit such capacities
as the ability to individuate elements, to parse the world into figure and
ground, to rapidly recognize spatial patterns, to map a 2D display onto
a 3D shape, to perceive motion from successive displays, to complete
partially occluded patterns, and so on. Deductive reasoning can exploit
a figure's stability and accessibility in various ways, such as using logical
diagrams (such as Venn diagrams) or simply allowing expressions to be
written down and transformed while being visually examined.

As a concrete example of the use of what I call a pure qualitative
construction consider the following problem that involves the use of

qualitative spatial relations (based on an example of Mani and Johnson-Laird, 1982). A subject is read sentences such as (1) through (4) and then asked to recall them or to draw conclusions about the relative location of specified objects:

(1)   The spoon is to the left of the knife.

(2)   The plate is to the right of the knife.

(3)   The fork is in front of the spoon.

(4)   The cup is in front of the knife.

This description is satisfied by the layout of objects shown in (5):

(5)   spoon knife plate
       fork   cup

But a change to one word in sentence (2), making it "The plate is to the right of the spoon," results in the description being satisfied by two layouts, shown in (6):

(6)   spoon knife plate   *or*   spoon plate knife
       fork   cup   fork   cup

As might be expected, the second set of the sentences, with revised (2), results in subjects' having poorer recognition memory as well as taking longer to draw conclusions concerning such questions as where the fork is in relation to the plate. From examples such as these, Johnson-Laird (1989, 2001) conclude that (a) propositional reasoning is carried out by constructing models and (b) having to deal with a single model results in better performance than having to deal with several such models. This appears quite plausible (at least for reasoning about spatial arrangements) when subjects are allowed to sketch the layouts. We can see from the example that with physical diagrams (e.g., sketched on paper), the properties being exploited include the ones discussed earlier: the visual recognition of relations like "above" and "to the right of," the visual capacity to detect relations between disparate objects while ignoring their intrinsic properties (perhaps by using visual indexes), and the capacity of the visual system to generalize by ignoring properties that are accidental or secondary (like the exact alignment of the names or their length). With a physical diagram, the reasoning proceeds more easily because the diagram provides a rapidly accessible memory that simultaneously contains the given relations between the specified objects while ensuring that certain relations remain fixed as the objects are examined. The use of the model in this example also involves many inferences that are made tacitly and unconsciously and that are aided by seeing the figure. Having the diagram in front of you not only lessens the burden on memory, but also encourages certain assumptions and ways of thinking about the problem. For example, when we are given the new version of (2) above, telling us that the plate is to the right of the spoon, we see that there are two ways of arranging this, depending on whether or not we allow the knife to be interspersed between spoon and plate as shown in (6). The fact that placing the knife between spoon and plate does not alter the relations between spoon and plate or between plate and cup is attributable to our knowledge that the relation "to the right of" survives interpolation by another object and to our knowledge that the "in front of" relations had been previously specified, so it must not be altered by the move (which means that columns must be moved as a unit). The pairwise cohesiveness of plate and cup is aided by seeing them as forming a column in the figure and thus making it natural to move the entire column rather than the knife alone. Such properties do not hold when the figure is imagined rather than perceived. In a mental image the question of what remains fixed when some things are changed raises a deep problem that we have already encountered under the name "frame problem" (pp. 435–436). Because objects in a mental image do not literally have spatial locations on a rigid surface, there is nothing to ensure that certain relations will remain fixed when others are changed. Also a mental model does not have the advantage conferred by the use of early vision to create cohesive clusters such as columns. Only knowledge and inference confers special status to some relations over others. So the question naturally arises how we can get any advantage in reasoning through the use of mental models without a visual counterpart. I will return to this question presently.

8.3.6 Diagrams drawn from memory can allow you to make explicit what you knew implicitly

Closely related to the use of diagrams to construct qualitative models of spatial relations (as in the earlier example) is the use of spatial displays, together with the operations provided by vision, to carry out inferences concerning spatial properties that depend on quantitative relations. Consider the following example. Suppose you have seen a map that contains five objects (including, e.g., a beach, a windmill, and a church) located as in figure 6.4 (a portion of which is reproduced as figure 8.7).

Looking at the map, we can see many spatial relations that hold between the elements and their locations. If I asked you which elements are collinear you could easily provide the answer just by looking. Similarly for questions like, which elements are halfway between two others? Or which elements are at approximately the same latitude? Or which are furthest south (or east or west) or furthest inland? We have excellent spatial relation detectors in our visual system (I have already discussed the sorts of easily detectable n-place predicates that rely on what we call "visual routines"). But we have seen that if you are asked to detect such properties in your mental image you will not do very well on those that rely on real vision. Your exquisite visual facility does not apply to your mental image.

Now suppose you memorize this map so that you are able to reproduce the locations of the five distinct features. You may have remembered the locations of these features in any of a large number of ways: you might, for example, have noticed the cluster of four features at the top right, or you might have remembered the places in terms of units of measurement in relation to the width of the island, or you might have recognized a similarity of shape of the island to the African continent and remembered the map features by associating them with some African countries, and so on. Whatever the mnemonic you use, it must of necessity fail to encode an indefinite number of additional relationships that hold between these five places, since it is possible to reproduce the location of the five objects accurately without having encoded all the binary or triple relations between subsets of the objects.[5] Thus, even though you

5. Even if you had a so-called photographic memory (eidetic memory) your memory representation would be incomplete in many ways. Few psychologists believe that quantitatively accurate long-term photographic memory exists, and in any case, information-theoretic considerations suggest that it would have to be an approximation. Evidence from studies of visual memory show that it tends to be vague in qualitative ways (see pp. 30–36), rather then just fuzzy or low-grade the way a poor TV picture would be approximate. There are a number of studies of eidetikers, and few of the claims of detailed photographic memory have stood up to repeated tests. The principal study by Stromeyer and Psotka (1970) has not been replicated. The search for true eidetic imagery remains elusive (Haber, 1979).

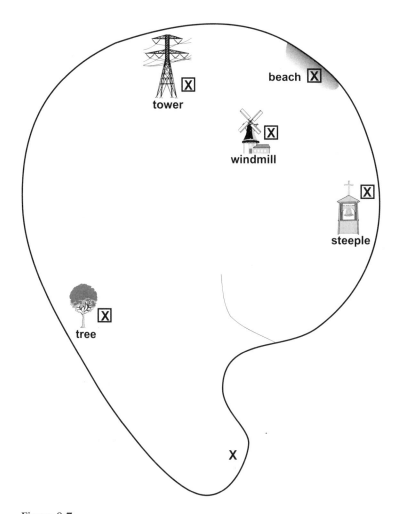

Figure 8.7
This is a portion of the map discussed in chapter 6, and shown in figure 6.4, as it might be recalled from memory. If we can recall the approximate locations of these five landmarks, regardless of how we encoded their locations, we can then draw this part of the map. Having drawn the map we can then notice geometrical relations (like collinearity, or relative location among new groupings of landmarks) that might not have been noticed and encoded initially.

memorized the map accurately, you might not have noticed that the tower is at about the same latitude as the beach, or that <tower, windmill, steeple> or <beach, windmill, tree> are collinear, or that <tower, beech, steeple>, <tower, beech, windmill>, and <tower, steeple, tree> form isosceles triangles, and so on. Since there are a large number of such relationships, you are bound to have failed to explicitly encode many of them. Yet despite your failing to encode such relationships explicitly, if the representation allows an accurate diagram to be drawn, it would be possible to notice these and indefinitely many other such relationships by drawing the map from the information you did encode and then *looking at the resulting drawing*. The missing relationships are implicit in the accurate location of the five features.

This, in a nutshell, is the advantage of drawing a diagram from what you know: it enables you in principle to *see* the relationships that are entailed by what you recalled, however sparse the set of explicitly encoded (i.e., "noticed") relationships might be. Even if such additional relationships might in principle be inferable from what you recalled, making them explicit without drawing the map might be extremely difficult. One might say that in most cases spatial relations are best represented spatially in a diagram in order to exploit the extraordinary capacity that vision has for extracting spatial relationships. But what about the proposal that something similar occurs even when the figure is not externalized on paper, but is internalized as a mental image or "mental model"? It is to this question that I now turn.

8.4   Thinking with Mental Diagrams

8.4.1   Using mental images

Given the advantages of visual displays in aiding certain kinds of reasoning, it is tempting to think that mental diagrams can do the same, especially since it feels like you are looking at a diagram when you imagine one. Indeed, many of the scholars who have studied the role of diagrams in reasoning have taken it for granted that their analysis applies to mental diagrams as well, so that visual thinking has come to mean thinking with the aid of visualized (mental) diagrams (e.g., Jamnek, 2001).

There is no denying that in some ways mental images may help reasoning; the problem is to say in what ways they might help reasoning despite the fact that many of the features of visually augmented reasoning discussed in the previous section do not apply to mental images. For example, as I argued in the last chapter, you cannot visually perceive new patterns in images (except for simple ones that you arguably "figure out" rather than visually perceive); you do not have a special facility to detect such mental image properties as region inclusion or intersection (as in figures 8.3 and 8.5); you cannot "see" properties in an image you did not independently know were there, or detect the similarity of figures constructed as a result of drawing new lines (as in figure 8.4); you cannot rely on being able to access several items at once to detect relational properties (such as collinearity and enclosure); and you cannot construct a set of distinct cases (such as those on pp. 451 and 454) and use them as an extended memory (since the "internal" memory of your mental image is not literally spatial and is also severely limited).

We saw (in chapter 1, and in various places in the last 3 chapters) that there is a great deal of evidence that both visual percepts and imagined pictures are very different from physical drawings. When we imagine carrying out certain operations on mental images (e.g., scanning them, or drawing a line on them) what we "see" happening in our mind's eye is just what we believe would happen if we were looking at a scene and carrying out the real operation—nothing more or less than that. As a result, we cannot rely on discovering something by observing what actually happens in our mental image, as we might if we were drawing on a piece of paper. Our mental image also does not have the benefit of being a rigid surface, so it does not have the stability and invariance of properties that a physical picture has when various operations are applied to it. For example, unlike a physical diagram, a mental image does not automatically retain its rigid shape when we transform it say, by rotating it, moving its parts around, folding it over, or adding new elements to it. This is because there is no inner drawing surface to give a mental image its rigidity and enduring shape and because there is no credible evidence for visually "noticing" new patterns or new construals in an image (see chapter 7).

To recall the ephemeral quality of image properties, try to imagine a diagram in which you do not know in advance where the elements will fall. For example, imagine an arbitrary triangle and draw lines from each vertex to the midpoint of the opposite side. Do the three lines you draw this way cross at a single common point, or do they form a small triangle inside the original triangle (and does this remain true for any triangle whatsoever)? Imagine a triangle drawn between a pair of parallel horizontal lines (with its base on the bottom parallel and its remaining vertex on the top parallel). Now transform the triangle by sliding the top vertex along the line it is on until the triangle becomes highly skewed. (What happens to its area?) Now draw a vertical line from the top vertex to the bottom parallel and two other vertical lines from the bottom vertices of the triangle to the top parallel. How many triangles are there now, and are any of them identical? Imagine a string wrapped around two partially embedded nails and held taut by a pencil (so that the string makes a triangle). Now move the pencil around wherever it can go while keeping the string taut and let it draw a figure on the table: what does this figure look like? Or, to repeat an example I cited earlier, imagine a pair of identical parallelograms, one above the other, with corresponding vertices of the two parallelograms joined by vertical lines. Think about it carefully and note what it looks like. Now draw it and look at the drawing (and do the same with the other examples: draw them and see how they look compared with how they looked in your imagination).

Geoff Hinton (1987) provides another example of how mental images lack many of the properties that one naturally attributes to them. His example focuses on the role of horizontal and vertical axes in determining how one represents a solid shape. Imagine a cube (about one foot on each edge). Place a finger on one of the vertices and place the diagonally opposite vertex on a table, so that the two vertices are directly above one another (and the cube is now being held with its diagonal vertical). Without first thinking about it, examine your image and count the remaining vertices of the figure as they appear in your image, pointing to them with your free hand as you count. Before reading on you should try this on yourself. Most people get the answer surprisingly wrong: they find themselves saying that there are four remaining vertices that lie in a plane, which of course results in the cube having only six vertices whereas we know it has eight. Hinton argues that in rotating the imagined cube we must alter a description of it to conclude what it would look like in the new orientation, and in doing so we are deceived by thinking of the solid not as a cube but as an octahedron that is symmetrical about the new vertical axis.

We saw in chapter 7 that mental figures are not *visually* reinterpreted after we make changes or combine several figures, except in cases where the figures are sufficiently simple that we can figure out (by reasoning) what familiar shape they would look like. If we were to try to prove the Pythagorean Theorem by constructing the squares in our mind (as in figure 8.4), we would not be able to use our power of recognition to notice that there were four identical triangles, one in each corner—a recognition that is critical to determining how to proceed with the proof. Some people explain such differences between pictures and mental images by saying that mental images are limited in their capacities (e.g., Posner and Raichle, 1994). But although the capacities of mental imagery clearly are limited, the limitation is one we specify not in terms of how many lines can be drawn, but in terms of how many conceptual units there are (as we saw in the examples on pp. 28–36). Moreover, such limitations are not compatible with the claims often made about what we are able to do with more complex images in reasoning, including operations like scanning and rotation.

The point here is the one that occupied the last 3 chapters of this book: it is a mistake to think that when we are visualizing, there is something in our head that is being seen or is being *visually* interpreted. Yet one might still ask, if mental diagrams are so different from real diagrams, why then is it easier to do a problem such as the one I discussed earlier, illustrated in figure 8.5, by imagining that figure in one's "mind's eye"? There is no doubt that it would be very difficult to do this extremely simple problem if one were barred from using a mental image, regardless of what formal properties underly the experienced image.[6] Why should this be so if the mental image does not have essentially pictorial properties?

6. Notice that even here one needs a broader understanding of a "mental image" than the picture theory provides, since blind people can solve such problems without the experience of "seeing." Presumably other sensory modalities or even unconscious spatial constructions of some sort could also be involved and therefore ought to be accommodated in our understanding of what it means to "imagine."

8.4.2   What happens during visualization?

If images (and mental models) have such serious, inherent problems, why then do they appear to help—at least in some circumstances—in reasoning? Perhaps the reason does not lie in any of the intrinsic properties of images or models that are tacitly assumed. Perhaps it is because of the content of the image or model, and not its alleged spatial form or the architecture of the imagery or visual system.

It is a general property of mental life that we tend to think different thoughts (thoughts with different contents) when we are presented with a problem in different ways (as Hayes and Simon, 1976, showed clearly). In fact, a major step in problem solving is formulating or representing the problem in an appropriate way. (Herb Simon, 1969, goes so far as to claim, "Solving a problem simply means representing it so as to make the solution transparent.") It appears that we think about different things (or at least we highlight different properties) when we *visualize* a situation than when we do not; and so perhaps the thoughts that arise under these conditions are helpful in solving certain kinds of problems, especially problems that concern spatial patterns.

So part of the answer to the question of why imagining a figure is sometimes helpful may simply be that when we think in terms of spatial layouts we tend to think about different things and represent the problem in different ways than when we think in terms of abstract properties. Such thinking is rightly viewed as more concrete, but that's because its contents concern spatiotemporal and visual properties rather than abstract properties, not because its form is any more "concrete" than the form of abstract thoughts. Concrete thoughts, according to this view, are thoughts about perceptual properties of individuals, including relations between them. When we think of a rectangle in the abstract we cannot readily understand the instruction to draw lines from the two bottom vertices to a point on the opposite side because we may not have individuated those vertices: you can think "rectangle" without also thinking of each of the four vertices, but when you visualize a rectangle you generally do think of each of its four vertices.

My experience in using the example of figure 8.5 in class is that the hardest part of solving the problem, without using the blackboard, is communicating the problem's specifications. Invariably, I am forced to ask students to imagine a rectangle whose vertices are labeled, starting from the bottom left corner and going clockwise, as A, B, C, and D, and then drawing a line from A to any point on CD and from D to any point on AB. By conveying the problem in this way I ensure that the individual vertices will be distinct parts of their representation of the figure, and I also provide a way to refer to these parts individually. This makes the task easier precisely because this way of describing the problem sets up thoughts about a particular rectangle and about particular, individuated and labeled vertices and sides. But even then one usually cannot select the side labeled CD without going through the vertex labels in order. Thus it may be that imaging certain figures is helpful in solving problems because this way of thinking about the problem focuses attention on individual elements and their relational properties. Viewing the role of imagined figures in this way is neutral on the question of the form of the representation of mental images, and indeed it may help to reduce the temptation to reify an inner diagram with its implication that the visual system's involvement in the visualization process is that of inspecting the mental image.

But why should imagery lead us to entertain certain kinds of representational contents, such as those just alluded to? In chapter 7 (pp. 423–426), I discussed ways in which representations underlying mental images might differ from other sorts of cognitive representations. The main points were that images are a more restricted form of representation because they are confined to representing individual instances rather than the more general situations that can be described using quantified statements: they do not represent the belief that all crows are black but only that crow #1 is black, crow #2 is black, crow #3 is black, and so on. They individuate elements of a situation and may represent parts of a scene by distinct parts of the representation. They also tend to attribute properties to particular elements (e.g., "crow #1 is black"). They do not contain quantifiers or negation, except by the addition of annotations that have to be interpreted by mechanisms outside the imagery system (by the sorts of mechanisms that interpret symbolic expressions).

Thus, such representations are more like a relational database or a restricted representational language, like Levesque's "vivid representation" (Levesque, 1986). Beyond such properties, which images do share with pictures (but also with relational databases), there are few pictorial properties whose attribution to mental images can withstand careful scrutiny, including the widely believed spatial nature of images. Finally, there is a way in which mental images or mental models can be spatial by taking advantage of our spatial sense. As I suggested earlier (section 7.3), once several discrete objects have been individuated in one's imagination, one can associate each of them with perceived objects in the environment and thereby gain some of the advantage of a real spatial layout. By thinking in terms of individuals rather than abstractions we are in a position to deploy the mechanism of FINST visual indexes (or nonvisual Anchors) to make it possible for us to entertain thoughts such as "line 1 goes from <index-1> to <index-2>" and "line 2 goes from <index-3> to <index-4>." Since these imagined lines have actual spatial locations in the world, to which their endpoints are bound, one can scan along these imagined lines and see, at least roughly, whether and where the lines intersect. In cases involving "mental models" where only qualitative spatial relations between a small number of objects are relevant, it is easy to see how binding these model objects to scene locations might allow us to construct and use these models to solve problems. So long as we do not exceed the indexing capacity of the indexing mechanism, we can set out distinct cases and capitalize on the indexes to keep track of the spatial configuration among imagined objects. One could then reason just the way that was postulated by Johnson-Laird. The important point is that none of this requires a mental picture or a reified space inside the head in which to locate the objects of the model.

8.5   Imagery and Imagination

One of the most interesting questions one might ask about mental imagery is how it serves as a vehicle for creative imagination, for there is no doubt that creativity often starts with imagining things that do not exist (or, in some cases, that *cannot* exist). Before considering this question, I want to point out a systematic ambiguity in discussions about imagination.

There are two senses in which we can imagine something. One is the sense in which a person might imagine *seeing* something (often referred to as "imaging" or as "visualizing"). The other is the sense in which a person simply considers a (counterfactual) situation in which something might be true. This is the difference between "imagining X" and "imagining *that X is the case*," or between imagining seeing X and considering the implications of X being the case (as in "what if X were true?"). Clearly, the latter is essential not only for creative invention but also for mundane planning. To make a plan one needs to consider nonactual (or counterfactual or fictitious) situations; one must be able to think "If I did this then it would result in such-and-such," which entails considering (and therefore representing) some nonactual state of affairs. There is much that can be said about this subjunctive or "imagining-that" form of reasoning (see, e.g., Harper, Stalnaker, and Pearce, 1981), but it clearly does not require generating a mental image. The other sense of imagining does require entertaining such a mental image, since it in effect means "imagine what it would look like if you were to see" some particular situation. What is less clear is whether the second sense of imagining (the one that does involve mental images) has a special place in creativity.

Libraries are full of books about the creativity of visual thinking. The history of science abounds in examples of important discoveries made when a scientist thinks about a problem without apparently using any logical reasoning (this idea is discussed widely; see Shepard, 1978a, for a good summary of this point with extensive biographical citations). How do these reports square with what I have been saying about the nature of imagery and especially about the nonpictorial nature of thinking and reasoning? Are these reports simply misled or romanticized? The simple answer is that these reports of experiences do not constitute a theory of what goes on in the mind that is causally responsible for episodes of creative thinking. Such reports are thus neutral on the question of whether thinking using mental images consists of examining pictorial entities in one's head. Moreover, such reports are usually about the "intuitive" (i.e., free of conscious experience) nature of creative thoughts, so they are very much in agreement with what I have been saying about thought in general (i.e., that the real work of reasoning is never experienced).

Take, for example, the widely cited case of Albert Einstein (discussed on pp. 428–429). What Einstein claimed was that (a) his thoughts were not expressed in words, at least not initially; (b) his discoveries were not made in a strictly logical manner; and (c) many of his ideas were developed in the course of carrying out "thought experiments," in which, for example, he imagined himself traveling at the front of a beam of light. Interpreting this to mean that a "visual" mode of reasoning leads to creative ideas more readily than other modes requires acceptance of a naive version of the dual code idea (i.e., that what is not logical is not verbal and what is not verbal is pictorial). It also requires conflating the two senses of "imagine" that I mentioned at the beginning of this section. Evidence that scientists do not "think in words" or that they do not discover new theories by following (deductive) logic tells us nothing about the process they do go through—nobody thinks in "words" (although they may think *about* words), nor do they use deductive logic in forming hypothesis. But to say that they do it "by intuition" is not to say that it involves pictorial mental images; it is just another way of saying that we have no idea how it happens.

While admitting our current state of ignorance about such things as the source of creative ideas, it is worthwhile to keep in mind where the real mystery lies. It lies not in questions about the nature or format of mental images, but in questions about the nature of creative thought, and in particular in the question of where new ideas come from. Whatever their underlying form, both imagery and language are at most a vehicle for expressing ideas. They cannot explain the origins of the ideas, much as it may be tempting to think that we simply "notice" something new or are "inspired" to have novel thoughts by observing our images unfold. The fact that a new idea may arrive accompanied by a particular image (e.g., Kekulé's dream of the snake swallowing its tail, which suggested the shape of the benzene molecule) is not the central fact; what is central is the idea that caused this image in the first place, and we have not the lightest notion where that came from. The act of creating, or calling to mind, is equally mysterious whether it is accompanied by the experience of a mental image or the experience of inner dialogue (especially since neither form is capable of fully expressing our thoughts). Having a new idea is, as Kant (1998) put it, "an art, hidden in the depths of the human soul, whose true modes of action we shall only with difficulty discover and unveil." But that is no reason to substitute one mystery (the role of imagery in creative insights) for another (where new thoughts come from).

Most writing about the role of imagery in creative problem solving, as well as in psychotherapy, typically does not make assumptions about the medium or the format of images, nor need it even take a position on whether thoughts experienced as images are different in any way from thoughts experienced as dialogue, *except for what they are about.* Clearly, when we imagine or visualize a scene we attend to different properties than we would if we were to, say, formulate a written description of it. The question of whether when we have the experience of "seeing in our mind's eye" we are thinking about different things, whether the subject or the meaning of our thoughts is different, is not in contention. It is obvious that when I think about a painting I am thinking of different things than when I think about mathematics. The difference between the contents in the two cases may be sufficient to explain why different experimental results are observed when subjects have imagery-thoughts than when they have nonimagery-thoughts.

For example, I can think about my office with or without visualizing it. But when I visualize it, the subject matter of my thought includes the appearance of the room and the appearance of some of the individual things in it. When I think about my office without visualizing it I have selected certain aspects of the room to be the subject of my thoughts. Although I can think some thoughts about specific visual features, such as where a chair is located, without visualizing the room, the subject matter is still different. The thought may not contain explicit references to colors or sizes or shapes. But this difference is still a difference in content and not in form. The same is true of other uses of mental imagery, say, in problem solving, as we saw in the previous section. The difference between thinking about geometrical theorems with and without visualizing is largely that in the former case I am thinking of the details of a *particular token* figure (a particular triangle or diagram). The interesting question of whether this entails a different form of representation is not addressed by the fact that in one case I visualize something and in another I do not.

One of the reasons why imagery is widely thought to contain the secret of creative imagination lies in its apparent autonomy and freedom from conscious ratiocination; it often seems to us that we "see" new meanings in images or that new ideas are "suggested" to us in a quasi-visual mode, and that this process follows a different logic, or perhaps no logic at all but some other intuitive principles.[7] The terminology of "seeing" is frequently used to indicate a new way of conceptualizing a problem or idea (as in "Now I see what you mean"). It has even been suggested that the process of *seeing as* hides the secret of the role of imagery in creative imagination. But as I argued in chapter 2, seeing as is the clearest example of an aspect of visual perception that is not unique to vision but involves inferences. Unlike the processes of early vision, seeing as occurs in the stage of visual perception that is shared with cognition generally. Seeing as involves not only seeing, but also reasoning, recalling, and recognizing. It is the part of the visual process where belief-fixation occurs, as opposed to the part of the process in which the appearance of a scene as a set of three-dimensional surfaces is computed. Consequently, seeing as is where vision crosses over to memory, recognition, inference, decision making, and problem solving.

Logical and quasi-logical reasoning occurs with every mental act we perform, including seeing something as a member of some particular category. But it is not the case, as many writers have assumed, that the sorts of semantically coherent processes that operate over beliefs and lead to new beliefs consist only of rigorous logical reasoning (for a critique of the use of logic to model intelligence, see McDermott, 1989). Although the processes I refer to as "reasoning" do respect the meaning of representations, and therefore, the content of thoughts has some connection to the content of those thoughts that trigger them, these processes need not be confined to logical or rational processes; semantic coherence is also true of creative innovation. The difference is that although we know something about logical reasoning (thanks to work over the past century on the foundations of logic), we know next to nothing about non-demonstrative, abductive, or commonsense reasoning and even less about creative reasoning. Nevertheless, this ignorance is not aided by talk of the role of the mind's eye in creativity since that just substitutes one mystery for another.

7. The notion that ideas interact according to special mental principles is close to the British empiricist notion of "mental chemistry," according to which the formation of concepts and the flow of thought is governed by principles such as temporal and spatial contiguity, repetition, similarity, and vividness, which were believed to favor the formation of associations.

8.5.1 How does creativity connect with imagery?

One idea that plays a role in virtually every theory of creative thinking is the notion that at some stage thinking makes a nonlogical leap; reasoning happens, as has sometimes been said, "outside the box." Of course, not everything outside the box is creative reasoning; most of it is just nonsense. The creative step must not be a total *non sequitur*: it must be related somehow to the topic at hand. So anything that can encourage a nondeductive yet content-related progression of thoughts could conceivably serve as a stage of or a catalyst for creative thinking. Indeed, several theories explicitly posit stages in which representations are altered in random ways, and many methods that teach creative thinking using imagery encourage people to come up with nondeductive connections, to create associations based on similarities, and to follow leads based on ideas suggested by images. Random perturbations by themselves serve no function (as they say in the computer field, "garbage in, garbage out"). But some randomness in conjunction with selectivity can, at least in principle, lead to creative leaps (this is the idea of a mental "dithering device"—see note 8 and the discussion of aids to creativity in the next section).

Yet even selective randomness is not enough. The proverbial thousand monkeys at typewriters will never produce Shakespearian prose, even if the probability is finite. What is needed for genuine creativity (other than skill) is content-restricted thought transitions that are nondeductive, in the sense that they are not like valid proofs, but are more like the heuristic process of formulating conjectures that occurs in abductive reasoning (the process of going from a set of facts to a hypothesis that explains them). People have looked to imagery as a mechanism that would allow transitions that are nonlogical (or perhaps *alogical*). For example, it has been suggested that when we examine a drawing or sketch we have made based on ideas that are relevant to the problem at hand, we might "notice" consequences that we would be unlikely to infer explicitly, or we might be reminded of something by virtue of its similarity in appearance to the object depicted in the drawing, or we might use the drawing as a metaphor for some abstract concept with which we are struggling, and so on. This kind of visual aid provided by one's own sketches is unproblematic, as we saw on pages 455–458, and it happens often (some people carry around a sketchpad for just this purpose). But this is not what happens in mental imagery.

Despite the caveats I have offered concerning the significant differences between drawings and mental images, it could still be the case that the mere fact that one is visualizing (whatever that means in terms of information processes) brings to the fore certain properties of the object of our thoughts, for example, properties that are related to shape and appearance. Whatever else happens when we visualize, it is a matter of definition that we consider the appearance of the objects we visualize. So even though there need be no difference in the form of the information in thought and vision, the difference in content and in the salience of difference properties of what we are thinking about could mean that when we visualize different principles come into play in determining what we think of next. For example, thinking about the shape of particular figures may remind you of other figures that have a similar shape, so it may be that the "remindings" run along a shape-similarity dimension rather than some other dimension (e.g., similarity of function or meaning) that might be more salient when thought is focused on more abstract aspects.

Roger Shepard (1978a) has given a great deal of thought to the question of why images should be effective in creative thought and invention. He lists four general properties of imagery that he claims make them especially suitable for creative thought. These are (p. 156) "their private and therefore not socially, conventionally, or institutionally controlled nature; their richly concrete and isomorphic structure; their engagement of highly developed, innate mechanisms of spatial intuition; and their direct emotional impact." These are perfectly reasonable speculations, though they vary in degree of plausibility. The first general property (imagery is more private) rests on the dual code assumption, since there is no reason why a pictorial form of representation is any more immune from external control than the form that I have discussed in this book (i.e., a conceptual system or "language of thought"). The second property (isomorphic structure) relies on an insufficiently constraining theory of image structure. As we saw on pages 314–316, the sort of isomorphism Shepard has in mind (which he calls "second-order isomorphism") leaves open the crucial question of whether the isomorphism arises from intrinsic properties of the representation or from inferences based on tacit knowledge. Consequently, although the idea that images have a concrete and isomorphic structure is not unreasonable, it does not favor one theory of image representation over another.

The third property Shepard mentions (images engage mechanisms of spatial intuition) is also reasonable and very much in accord with proposals I made earlier in section 7.3, where I discuss reasons why mental images appear to have "spatial" properties. There is no doubt that our spatial sense is central in how we cognize the world and may be particularly relevant when we think about shape-related properties, for example, when we think about the operation of mechanical devices. But, according to the analysis presented in chapter 7, what we do in imagining a scene is think of individual things as located in a space that we are currently perceiving, either visually or proprioceptively. We may use the real physical space that we perceive with one or another sense to provide the framework onto which we can project spatial patterns that we are thinking about, and in this way make use of the "highly developed, innate mechanisms of spatial intuition" that Shepard speaks of. In fact, we can even use this spatial sense to individuate and keep track of abstract ideas, as is done in American Sign Language.

The last property Shepard proposes as a basis for the superiority of mental images over words in promoting creative thought is their "direct emotional impact." Once again, this is a reasonable proposal that nevertheless does not favor one theory of the nature of mental images over another. It is true that if I think the sentence "I am about to be hit by a falling brick" I am not nearly as moved to action, or to emotion, as I am if I visualize a brick is falling down on me. There has not been a great deal of emphasis placed on this aspect of mental imagery, but it is surely important.

The power of images to create states of fear, anxiety, arousal, or sudden flinching or recoil (as when one imagines oneself at the edge of a precipice) is a property that in the past (e.g., as I was writing my first critique of mental imagery, Pylyshyn, 1973) made it most difficult for me to fully accept the symbolic view of mental imagery. Dealing with this power of imagery requires continually reminding oneself that the crucial parallel between seeing and emotional states, on the one hand, and imagery and emotional states on the other, very likely arises from common properties of the two types of mental representations, neither of which has anything to do with their having a pictorial format. Although they clearly both possess a vividness that may be absent in more deliberate forms of ratiocination, this vividness does not argue for one format of representation over another. The vividness may have more to do with the fact that images and visual representations both focus on the particular—on particular objects and individual episodes. Mental representations are powerful forces in our lives and representations of *particular* things, and events are more powerful to us as individuals than are representations of general principles.

8.5.2   Enhancing creative thinking

Creativity is much prized in our culture. It is also much misunderstood (for example, it is associated with being a misfit, with nearness to insanity, and so on). Measures of intelligence and of creativity, despite their many shortcomings, have generally shown the two to be highly related. This is not surprising since it is hard to be creative in finding a solution if you don't understand the problem or are unable to reason about it well.

Because creativity is especially prized in certain fields (e.g., science and art), people have tried to find specific factors that are associated with high creativity, including personality traits, styles of problem solving, and the use of strategies that enhance creative expression. Some of the studies have led to interesting findings and have connected creativity to nonstandard values. For example, Getzels and Jackson (1962) found that creative students had a more playful attitude toward problems and placed a higher value on finding and formulating problems for its own sake (they also valued humor more highly than other equally intelligent students).

Discovering what we consider to be creative solutions to a problem often requires that the problem solver generate a space of options that goes beyond the expected or the obvious. For this reason many creativity-enhancing techniques encourage free association, exploration of unusual similarities and relationships between elements of the problem, and other tricks to help bring to the fore aspects that might not readily come to mind in connection with the problem at hand—all in the interest of temporarily subverting habitual modes of thought and reasoning. An example of the use of mental imagery to generate associations and to trigger alternative ideas in this way is the game developed by Finke (1990) in his study of the role of mental imagery in creativity. This game asks people to make a sketch of what they think of when they think about a certain problem (or just to sketch some object involved in that problem) and then to modify it in certain ways or just think of what it reminds them of. The game relies on the fact that the manipulation of shapes and the recognition of similarity of shapes can remind one of things that are not connected to the problem in a logical, goal-directed way, and thereby may influence the sequence of thoughts one goes through in coming up with an idea. There are many examples of the use of such techniques to enhance creativity. In fact, the World Wide Web is filled with "creativity resources" consisting of everything from computer programs to actual physical devices, all designed to inhibit one's normal problem-solving habits.

Much of the advice for enhancing creative problem solving is focused specifically on encouraging nonstandard ways of thinking about a problem by emphasizing the association of ideas over more logical ways of working on a problem, such as deduction and means-ends analysis. In fact, some of the tools that have been claimed to enhance creativity are just tools for inhibiting the usual habits of problem solving. Gardner (1982, p. 27) describes what he calls "whimsical" devices for breaking away from "vertical thinking" into "lateral thinking." For example, there is a device called the "Think Tank," which has a rotating drum containing 13,000 tiny plastic chips, each with a word printed on it. When the drum is rotated, different words come into view and the user is invited to free-associate with each word or phrase. Related tools are being sold today that run on computers and produce graphic pictures that allow you to connect ideas (e.g., the "Mind Mapper"). Some years ago there was even a special room, called the *Imaginarium* (McKim, 1978), for training people to think creatively by leading them through a sequence from relaxation, through imagining the superposition and transformation of images (done with the help of slides and sounds), through a series of fantasies involving metaphors, to Zen-like attention to the here-and-now, coupled with physical exercises. What all these ideas and methods have in common is this: they tend to encourage you to do things differently than you normally do (and perhaps even to feel different about what you are doing).

Of course, not every way that is different from how you usually go about solving a problem is a good way, and inhibiting the usual ways need not lead to more creative solutions. But when you are stuck, it may well be a useful starting heuristic.[8] And so it is with many uses of imagery. Free-associating with images may be different from free-associating with words, but does free association necessarily enhance creativity? After looking at a wide range of claims about how imagery enhances creativity, I find it to be a mixed bag: it includes everything from advice on the use of graphics and other tools to the equivalent of giving a thousand monkeys graphics software instead of typewriters. It is safe to say that in the present state of our understanding of both creativity and mental imagery, this heterogeneous collection of talismans tells us little about the nature of creativity; and even if imagery techniques do enhance one's creativity, finding this out would be no more informative than the discovery of the power of placebos to alter one's somatic complaints. They may work, but they tell us nothing about the underlying mechanisms.

8. There is a technique used in servomechanisms (which can also be seen in some thermostats) that allows for more precise control by inhibiting static friction, which is always higher than dynamic friction (it takes more force to get something static to move than to keep it moving). The technique is to introduce some random perturbation into the control loop, using what is sometimes called a "dithering device." In a thermostat one can sometimes here a buzz that keeps the contact points from sticking, and in military applications involving the control of heavy arms, dithering can be introduced as noise in the position controller. Without some random noise search processes that seek to maximize some quantity using a method such as "steepest ascent" can become locked in a local maximum and thereby miss the optimum global maximum. It has been suggested that problem solving and thinking could use a dithering device to keep people from getting stuck in a "local maximum." Perhaps the sorts of creativity-enhancing ideas discussed above are just varieties of dithering devices.

References

Abernethy, B. (1991). Visual search strategies and decision-making in sport. Special issue: Information processing and decision making in sport. *International Journal of Sport Psychology*, 22(3–4), 189–210.

Abernethy, B., Neil, R. J., and Koning, P. (1994). Visual-perceptual and cognitive differences between expert, intermediate, and novice snooker players. *Applied Cognitive Psychology*, 8(3), 185–211.

Acton, B. (1993). *A Network Model of Visual Indexing and Attention*. Unpublished ms., University of Western Ontario, London, Ontario.

Aglioti, S., DeSouza, J. F. X., and Goodale, M. A. (1995). Size-contrast illusions deceive the eye but not the hand. *Current Biology*, 5(6), 679–685.

Allwein, G., and Barwise, J. (eds.). (1996). *Logical Reasoning with Diagrams*. New York: Oxford University Press.

Anderson, B., and Johnson, W. (1966). Two kinds of set in problem solving. *Psychological Reports*, 19(3), 851–858.

Anderson, J. R. (1978). Argument concerning representations for mental imagery. *Psychological Review*, 85, 249–277.

Anderson, R. A., Snyder, L. H., Bradley, D. C., and Xing, J. (1997). Multimodal representation of space in the posterior parietal cortex and its use in planning movements. *Annual Review of Neuroscience*, 29, 303–330.

Annan, V., and Pylyshyn, Z. W. (2002). Can indexes be voluntarily assigned in multiple object tracking? [Abstract] *Journal of Vision*, 2(7), 243a.

Ashby, F. G., Prinzmetal, W., Ivry, R., and Maddox, W. T. (1996). A formal theory of feature binding in object perception. *Psychological Review*, 103(1), 165–192.

Attneave, F. (1954). Some informational aspects of visual perception. *Psychological Review*, 61, 183–193.

Attneave, F., and Farrar, P. (1977). The visual world behind the head. *American Journal of Psychology*, 90(4), 549–563.

Attneave, F., and Pierce, C. R. (1978). Accuracy of extrapolating a pointer into perceived and imagined space. *American Journal of Psychology*, 91(3), 371–387.

Avant, L. L. (1965). Vision in the ganzfeld. *Psychological Bulletin*, 64, 246–258.

Bachmann, T. (1989). Microgenesis as traced by the transient paired-forms paradigm. *Acta Psychologica*, *70*, 3–17.

Backus, J. (1978). Can programming be liberated from the von neumann style? A functional style and its algebra of programs. *Communications of the Association for Computing Machinery*, *21*, 613–641.

Ballard, D. H., Hayhoe, M. M., Pook, P. K., and Rao, R. P. N. (1997). Deictic codes for the embodiment of cognition. *Behavioral and Brain Sciences*, *20*(4), 723–767.

Banks, W. P. (1981). Assessing relations between imagery and perception. *Journal of Experimental Psychology: Human Perception and Performance*, *7*, 844–847.

Barolo, E., Masini, R., and Antonietti, A. (1990). Mental rotation of solid objects and problem-solving in sighted and blind subjects. *Journal of Mental Imagery*, *14*(3–4), 65–74.

Baron-Cohen, S., Harrison, J., Goldstein, L. H., and Wyke, M. (1993). Coloured speech perception: Is synaesthesia what happens when modularity breaks down? *Perception*, *22*(4), 419–426.

Baron-Cohen, S., and Harrison, J. E. (eds.). (1997). *Synaesthesia: Classic and Contemporary Readings*. Cambridge, Mass.: Blackwell.

Barsalou, L. (1999). Perceptual symbol systems. *Behavioral and Brain Sciences*, *22*(4), 577–660.

Bartolomeo, P. (2002). The relationship between visual perception and visual mental imagery: A reappraisal of the neuropsychological evidence. *Cortex*, *38*(3), 357–378.

Bartolomeo, P., Bachoud-levi, A. C., and Denes, G. (1997). Preserved imagery for colours in a patient with cerebral achromatopsia. *Cortex*, *33*(2), 369–378.

Bartolomeo, P., and Chokron, S. (2002). Orienting of attention in left unilateral neglect. *Neuroscience and Biobehavioral Reviews*, *26*(2), 217–234.

Barwise, J., and Etchemendy, J. (1990). Information, infons, and inference. In R. Cooper, K. Mukai, and J. Perry (eds.), *Situation Theory and Its Applications, I*. Chicago: University of Chicago Press.

Baylis, G. C. (1994). Visual attention and objects: Two-object cost with equal convexity. *Journal of Experimental Psychology: Human Perception and Performance*, *20*, 208–212.

Baylis, G. C., and Driver, J. (1993). Visual attention and objects: Evidence for hierarchical coding of location. *Journal of Experimental Psychology: Human Perception and Performance*, *19*, 451–470.

Behrmann, M. (2000). The mind's eye mapped onto the brain's matter. *Current Directions in Psychological Science*, *9*(2), 50–54.

Behrmann, M., Moscovitch, M., and Winocur, G. (1994). Intact visual imagery and impaired visual perception in a patient with visual agnosia. *Journal of Experimental Psychology: Human Perception and Performance*, *20*(5), 1068–1087.

Behrmann, M., and Tipper, S. (1994). Object-based visual attention: Evidence from unilateral neglect. In C. Umiltà and M. Moscovitch (eds.), *Attention and Performance 15: Conscious and Unconscious Processing and Cognitive Functioning* (vol. 19, pp. 351–375). Cambridge, Mass.: MIT Press.

Behrmann, M., and Tipper, S. P. (1999). Attention accesses multiple reference frames: Evidence from visual neglect. *Journal of Experimental Psychology: Human Perception and Performance, 25*(1), 83–101.

Behrmann, M., Winocur, G., and Moscovitch, M. (1992). Dissociation between mental imagery and object recognition in a brain-damaged patient. *Nature, 359*(6396), 636–637.

Bennett, B., Hoffman, D., and Prakash, K. (1989). *Observer Mechanics: A Formal Theory of Perception.* New York: Academic Press.

Berger, G. H., and Gaunitz, S. C. (1977). Self-rated imagery and vividness of task pictures in relation to visual memory. *British Journal of Psychology, 68*(3), 283–288.

Bernbaum, K., and Chung, C. S. (1981). Müller-Lyer illusion induced by imagination. *Journal of Mental Imagery, 5*(1), 125–128.

Beschin, N., Basso, A., and Sala, S. D. (2000). Perceiving left and imagining right: Dissociation in neglect. *Cortex, 36*(3), 401–414.

Beschin, N., Cocchini, G., Della Sala, S., and Logie, R. H. (1997). What the eyes perceive, the brain ignores: A case of pure unilateral representational neglect. *Cortex, 33*(1), 3–26.

Biederman, I. (1987). Recognition-by-components: A theory of human image interpretation. *Psychological Review, 94,* 115–148.

Biederman, I. (1995). Visual object recognition. In S. M. Kosslyn and D. N. Osherson (eds.), *Visual Cognition* (second ed.). Cambridge, Mass.: MIT Press.

Biederman, I., and Bar, M. (1999). One-shot viewpoint invariance in matching novel objects. *Vision Research, 39*(17), 2885–2899.

Biederman, I., and Cooper, E. E. (1992). Size invariance in visual object priming. *Journal of Experimental Psychology: Human Perception Performance, 18,* 121–133.

Biederman, I., and Gerhardstein, P. C. (1993). Recognizing depth-rotated objects: Evidence and conditions for three-dimensional viewpoint invariance. *Journal of Experimental Psychology: Human Perception and Performance, 19*(6), 1162–1182.

Biederman, I., and Shiffrar, M. S. (1987). Sexing day-old chicks: A case study and expert systems analysis of a difficult perceptual-learning task. *Journal of Experimental Psychology: Learning, Memory, and Cognition, 13*(4), 640–645.

Binford, T. O. (1971). Visual perception by computer. Paper presented at the IEEE Systems Science and Cybernetics Conference, December 1971, Miami, Florida.

Bisiach, E., and Luzzatti, C. (1978). Unilateral neglect of representational space. *Cortex, 14*(1), 129–133.

Bisiach, E., Ricci, R., Lualdi, M., and Colombo, M. R. (1998). Perceptual and response bias in unilateral neglect: Two modified versions of the Milner Landmark task. *Brain and Cognition, 37*(3), 369–386.

Blackmore, S. J., Brelstaff, G., Nelson, K., and Troscianko, T. (1995). Is the richness of the visual world an illusion? Transsaccadic memory for complex scenes. *Perception, 24*(9), 1075–1081.

Blanchard, R. (1975). The effect of S- on observing behavior. *Learning and Motivation, 6*(1), 1–10.

Blaser, E., Pylyshyn, Z. W., and Holcombe, A. (2000a). With two objects at one location, attention is "object-based" (abstract). Presented at the 2000 meeting of the Association for Research in Vision and Ophthalmology, Ft. Lauterdale, Florida.

Blaser, E., Pylyshyn, Z. W., and Holcombe, A. O. (2000b). Tracking an object through feature-space. *Nature, 408* (Nov. 9), 196–199.

Block, N. (1981). Introduction: What is the issue? In N. Block (ed.), *Imagery* (pp. 1–16). Cambridge, Mass.: MIT Press.

Block, N. (1995). On a confusion about a function of consciousness. *Behavioral and Brain Sciences, 18*, 227–247.

Block, N. (2001). Is the content of experience the same as the content of thought? In E. Dupoux (ed.), *Language, Brain, and Cognitive Development: Essays in Honor of Jacques Mehler.* Cambridge, Mass.: MIT Press/Bradford Books.

Block, N., Flanagan, O., and Güzeldere, G. (eds.). (1997). *The Nature of Consciousness: Philosophical Debates.* Cambridge, Mass.: MIT Press.

Bolles, R. C. (1969). The role of eye movements in the Müller-Lyer illusion. *Perception and Psychophysics, 6*(3), 175–176.

Bower, G. H., and Glass, A. L. (1976). Structural units and the reintegrative power of picture fragments. *Journal of Experimental Psychology: Human Learning and Memory, 2*, 456–466.

Brawn, P. T., and Snowden, R. J. (2000). Attention to overlapping objects: Detection and discrimination of luminance changes. *Journal of Experimental Psychology: Human Perception and Performance, 26*(1), 342–358.

Bregman, A. (1990). *Auditory Scene Analysis: The Perceptual Organization of Sound.* Cambridge, Mass.: MIT Press.

Bridgeman, B. (1992). Conscious vs. unconscious processes: The case of vision. *Theoretical Psychology, 2*, 73–88.

Bridgeman, B. (1995). Dissociation between visual processing modes. In M. A. Arbib (ed.), *The Handbook of Brain Theory and Neural Networks.* Cambridge, Mass.: MIT Press.

Brigell, M., Uhlarik, J., and Goldhorn, P. (1977). Contextual influence on judgments of linear extent. *Journal of Experimental Psychology: Human Perception and Performance, 3*(1), 105–118.

Broadbent, D. E. (1958). *Perception and Communication.* London: Pergamon Press.

Broerse, J., and Crassini, B. (1981). Misinterpretations of imagery-induced McCollough effects: A reply to Finke. *Perception and Psychophysics*, *30*, 96–98.

Broerse, J., and Crassini, B. (1984). Investigations of perception and imagery using CAEs: The role of experimental design and psychophysical method. *Perception and Psychophysics*, *35*(2), 155–164.

Brooks, L. R. (1968). Spatial and verbal components of the act of recall. *Canadian Journal of Psychology*, *22*(5), 349–368.

Brooks, R. A. (1991). Intelligence without representation. *Artificial Intelligence*, *47*, 139–159.

Brown, C. M. (1984). Computer vision and natural constraints. *Science*, *224*(4655), 1299–1305.

Bruner, J., and Postman, L. (1949). On the perception of incongruity: A paradigm. *Journal of Personality*, *18*, 206–223.

Bruner, J. S. (1957). On perceptual readiness. *Psychological Review*, *64*, 123–152.

Bruner, J. S., and Minturn, A. L. (1955). Perceptual identification and perceptual organization. *Journal of General Psychology*, *53*, 21–28.

Bruner, J. S., and Potter, M. C. (1964). Interference in visual recognition. *Science*, *144*, 424–425.

Burkell, J., and Pylyshyn, Z. W. (1997). Searching through subsets: A test of the visual indexing hypothesis. *Spatial Vision*, *11*(2), 225–258.

Cai, R. H., and Cavanagh, P. (2002). Motion interpolation of a unique feature into gaps and blind spots. *Journal of Vision*, *2*(7), 30a.

Calis, G. J., Sterenborg, J., and Maarse, F. (1984). Initial microgenetic steps in single-glance face recognition. *Acta Psychologica*, *55*(3), 215–230.

Canon, L. K. (1970). Intermodality inconsistency of input and directed attention as determinants of the nature of adaptation. *Journal of Experimental Psychology*, *84*(1), 141–147.

Canon, L. K. (1971). Directed attention and maladaptive "adaptation" to displacement of the visual field. *Journal of Experimental Psychology*, *88*(3), 403–408.

Carraher, R. G., and Thurston, J. B. (1966). *Optical Illusions and the Visual Arts*. New York: Reinholt.

Carey, S., and Xu, F. (2001). Infants' knowledge of objects: Beyond object files and object tracking. *Cognition*, *80*(1/2), 179–213.

Carlson-Radvansky, L. A. (1999). Memory for relational information across eye movements. *Perception and Psychophysics*, *61*(5), 919–934.

Carpenter, P. A., and Eisenberg, P. (1978). Mental rotation and the frame of reference in blind and sighted individuals. *Perception and Psychophysics*, *23*(2), 117–124.

Casey, E. (1976). *Imagining: A Phenomenological Study*. Bloomington, Ind.: Indiana University Press.

Castiello, U., and Umiltà, C. (1992). Orienting attention in volleyball players. *International Journal of Sport Psychology*, 23(4), 301–310.

Cavanagh, P. (1988). Pathways in early vision. In Z. W. Pylyshyn (ed.), *Computational Processes in Human Vision: An Interdisciplinary Perspective* (pp. 239–262). Norwood, N.J.: Ablex.

Cavanagh, P. (1999). Attention: Exporting vision to the mind. In C. Taddei-Ferretti and C. Musio (eds.), *Neuronal Basis and Psychological Aspects of Consciousness* (pp. 129–143). Singapore: World Scientific.

Chakravarty, I. (1979). A generalized line and junction labeling scheme with applications to scene analysis. *IEEE Transactions, PAMI*, 202–205.

Chalmers, D. J. (1996). *The Conscious Mind: In Search of a Fundamental Theory*. New York: Oxford University Press.

Chambers, D., and Reisberg, D. (1985). Can mental images be ambiguous? *Journal of Experimental Psychology*, 11, 317–328.

Chara, P. J., and Hamm, D. A. (1989). An inquiry into the construct validity of the vividness of visual imagery questionnaire. *Perceptual and Motor Skills*, 69(1), 127–136.

Charlot, V., Tzourio, N., Zilbovicius, M., Mazoyer, B., and Denis, M. (1992). Different mental imagery abilities result in different regional cerebral blood flow activation patterns during cognitive tasks. *Neuropsychologia*, 30(6), 565–580.

Chase, W. G., and Simon, H. A. (1973). Perception in chess. *Cognitive Psychology*, 5, 55–81.

Chastain, G. (1995). Location coding with letters versus unfamiliar, familiar, and labeled letter-like forms. *Canadian Journal of Experimental Psychology*, 49(1), 95–112.

Chatterjee, A., and Southwood, M. H. (1995). Cortical blindness and visual imagery. *Neurology*, 45(12), 2189–2195.

Cheng, K. (1986). A purely geometric module in the rat's spatial representation. *Cognition*, 23, 149–178.

Cherry, C. (1957). *On Human Communication* (second ed.). Cambridge, Mass.: MIT Press.

Chiang, W.-C., and Wynn, K. (2000). Infants' tracking of objects and collections. *Cognition*, 75, 1–27.

Chomsky, N. (1957). Review of B. F. Skinner's verbal behavior. In J. A. Fodor and J. J. Katz (eds.), *The Structure of Language*. Englewood Cliffs: Prentice-Hall.

Chomsky, N. (1976). *Reflections on Language*. New York: Fontana.

Churchland, P. M. (1988). Perceptual plasticity and theoretical neutrality: A reply to Jerry Fodor. *Philosophy of Science*, 55, 167–187.

Clark, E. V. (1973). Nonlinguistic strategies and the acquisition of word meanings. *Cognition*, 2, 161–182.

Clark, H. H. (1969). Linguistic processes in deductive reasoning. *Psychological Review*, 76(4), 387–404.

Clowes, M. B. (1971). On seeing things. *Artificial Intelligence*, 2, 79–116.

Cocude, M., Mellet, E., and Denis, M. (1999). Visual and mental exploration of visuospatial configurations: Behavioral and neuroimaging approaches. *Psychology Research*, 62(2–3), 93–106.

Cohen, M. S., Kosslyn, S. M., Breiter, H. C., DiGirolamo, G. J., Thompson, W. L., Anderson, A. K., et al. (1996). Changes in cortical activity during mental rotation: A mapping study using functional MRI. *Brain*, 119, 89–100.

Cordes, S., Gelman, R., Gallistel, C. R., and Whalen, J. (2001). Variability signatures distinguish verbal from nonverbal counting for both large and small numbers. *Psychonomic Bulletin and Review*, 8(4), 698–707.

Coren, S. (1986). An efferent component in the visual perception of direction and extent. *Psychological Review*, 93(4), 391–410.

Coren, S., and Porac, C. (1983). The creation and reversal of the Mueller-Lyer illusion through attentional manipulation. *Perception*, 12(1), 49–54.

Cornoldi, C., Bertuccelli, B., Rocchi, P., and Sbrana, B. (1993). Processing capacity limitations in pictorial and spatial representations in the totally congenitally blind. *Cortex*, 29(4), 675–689.

Cornoldi, C., Calore, D., and Pra-Baldi, A. (1979). Imagery ratings and recall in congenitally blind subjects. *Perceptual and Motor Skills*, 48(2), 627–639.

Coslett, H. B. (1997). Neglect in vision and visual imagery: A double dissociation. *Brain*, 120, 1163–1171.

Coslett, H. B., and Saffran, E. (1991). Simultanagnosia: To see but not two see. *Brain*, 113(1523–1545).

Craig, E. M. (1973). Role of mental imagery in free recall of deaf, blind, and normal subjects. *Journal of Experimental Psychology*, 97(2), 249–253.

Crick, F., and Koch, C. (1995). Are we aware of neural activity in primary visual cortex? *Nature*, 375(11), 121–123.

Currie, C. B., McConkie, G. W., and Carlson-Radvansky, L. A. (2000). The role of the saccade target object in the perception of a visually stable world. *Perception and Psychophysics*, 62, 673–683.

Currie, G. (1995). Visual imagery as the simulation of vision. *Mind and Language*, 10(1–2), 25–44.

Cytowic, R. E. (1989). *Synaesthesia: A Union of the Senses*. New York: Springer Verlag.

Cytowic, R. E. (1993). *The Man Who Tasted Shapes*. New York: Putnam.

Cytowic, R. E. (1997). Synaesthesia: Phenomenology and neuropsychology. In S. Baron-Cohen and J. E. Harrison (eds.), *Synaesthesia: Classic and Contemporary Readings* (pp. 17–42). Cambridge, Mass.: Blackwell.

Dai, H., Scharf, B., and Buss, S. (1991). Effective attenuation of signals in noise under focused attention. *Journal of the Acoustical Society of America*, 89(6), 2837–2842.

Dalla Barba, G., Rosenthal, V., and Visetti, Y.-V. (2002). The nature of mental imagery: How "null" is the null hypothesis? *Behavioral and Brain Sciences*, 25(2), 187–188.

Dalman, J. E., Verhagen, W. I. M., and Huygen, P. L. M. (1997). Cortical blindness. *Clinical Neurology and Neurosurgery* (Dec.), 282–286.

Dauterman, W. L. (1973). A study of imagery in the sighted and the blind. *American Foundation for the Blind, Research Bulletin*, 95–167.

Davies, T. N., and Spencer, J. (1977). An explanation for the Mueller-Lyer illusion. *Perceptual and Motor Skills*, 45(1), 219–224.

Davis, G., Driver, J., Pavani, F., and Shepherd, A. (2000). Reappraising the apparent costs of attending to two separate visual objects. *Vision Research*, 40(10–12), 1323–1332.

Dawson, M., and Pylyshyn, Z. W. (1988). Natural constraints in apparent motion. In Z. W. Pylyshyn (ed.), *Computational Processes in Human Vision: An Interdisciplinary Perspective* (pp. 99–120). Stamford, Conn.: Ablex.

De Soto, C. B., London, M., and Handel, S. (1965). Social reasoning and spatial paralogic. *Journal of Personality and Social Psychology*, 2(4), 513–521.

De Vreese, L. P. (1991). Two systems for colour-naming defects: Verbal disconnection vs. colour imagery disorder. *Neuropsychologia*, 29(1), 1–18.

Dehaene, S. (1995). Electrophysiological evidence for category-specific word processing in the normal human brain. *Neuroreport: An International Journal for the Rapid Communication of Research in Neuroscience*, 6(16), 2153–2157.

Dehaene, S., and Naccache, L. (2001). Towards a cognitive neuroscience of consciousness: Basic evidence and a workspace framework. *Cognition*, 79(1–2), 1–37.

DeLucia, P. R., and Liddell, G. W. (1998). Cognitive motion extrapolation and cognitive clocking in prediction motion tasks. *Journal of Experimental Psychology: Human Perception and Performance*, 24(3), 901–914.

Démonet, J.-F., Wise, R., and Frackowiak, R. S. J. (1993). Language functions explored in normal subjects by positron emission tomography: A critical review. *Human Brain Mapping*, 1, 39–47.

Denis, M., and Kosslyn, S. M. (1999). Scanning visual mental images: A window on the mind. *Cahiers de Psychologie Cognitive / Current Psychology of Cognition*, 18(4), 409–465.

Dennett, D. C. (1978). *Brainstorms*. Cambridge, Mass.: MIT Press / Bradford Books.

Dennett, D. C. (1991). *Consciousness Explained*. Boston: Little, Brown.

Dennett, D. C., and Kinsbourne, M. (1992). Time and the observer: The where and when of consciousness in the brain. *Behavioral and Brain Sciences*, 15(2), 183–247.

DeSchepper, B., and Treisman, A. (1996). Visual memory for novel shapes: Implicit coding without attention. *Journal of Experimental Psychology: Learning, Memory, and Cognition*, 22(1), 27–47.

Desimone, R. (1996). Neural mechanisms for visual memory and their role in attention. *Proceedings of the National Academy of Science, USA, 93*(24), 13494–13497.

D'Esposito, M., Detre, J. A., Aguirre, G. K., Stallcup, M., Alsop, D. C., Tippet, L. J., et al. (1997). A functional MRI study of mental image generation. *Neuropsychologia, 35*(5), 725–730.

Dodds, A. G. (1983). Mental rotation and visual imagery. *Journal of Visual Impairment and Blindness, 77*(1), 16–18.

Driver, J. (1998). The neuropsychology of spatial attention. In H. Pashler (ed.), *Attention* (pp. 297–340). New York: Psychological Press.

Driver, J., Baylis, G., Goodrich, S., and Rafal, R. D. (1994). Axis-based neglect of visual shapes. *Neuropsychologia, 32*, 1353–1365.

Driver, J., and Halligan, P. (1991). Can visual neglect operate in object-centered coordinates? An affirmative single case study. *Cognitive Neuropsychology, 8*, 475–494.

Driver, J., and Vuilleumier, P. (2001). Perceptual awareness and its loss in unilateral neglect and extinction. *Cognition, 79*(1–2), 39–88.

Duncan, J. (1984). Selective attention and the organization of visual information. *Journal of Experimental Psychology: General, 113*(4), 501–517.

Duncan, J. (1993). Coordination of what and where in visual attention. *Perception, 22*(11), 1261–1270.

Dunham, W. (1994). *The Mathematical Universe.* New York: Wiley.

Easterbrook, J. A. (1959). The effect of emotion on cue utilization and the organization of behavior. *Psychological Review, 66*, 183–201.

Easton, R. D., and Bentzen, B. L. (1987). Memory for verbally presented routes: A comparison of strategies used by blind and sighted people. *Journal of Visual Impairment and Blindness, 81*(3), 100–105.

Egeth, H. E., Virzi, R. A., and Garbart, H. (1984). Searching for conjunctively defined targets. *Journal of Experimental Psychology, 10*(1), 32–39.

Egly, R., Driver, J., and Rafal, R. D. (1994). Shifting visual attention between objects and locations: Evidence from normal and parietal lesion subjects. *Journal of Experimental Psychology: General, 123*(2), 161–177.

Epstein, W. (1982). Percept-percept couplings. *Perception, 11*, 75–83.

Eriksen, C. W., and Schultz, D. W. (1977). Retinal locus and acuity in visual information processing. *Bulletin of the Psychonomic Society, 9*, 81–84.

Eriksen, C. W., and St. James, J. D. (1986). Visual attention within and around the field of focal attention: A zoom lens model. *Perception and Psychophysics, 40*, 225–240.

Escher, M. C. (1960). *The Graphic Work of M. C. Escher.* New York: Hawthorn Books.

Farah, M. J. (1988). Is visual imagery really visual? Overlooked evidence from neuropsychology. *Psychological Review, 95*(3), 307–317.

Farah, M. J. (1989). Mechanisms of imagery-perception interaction. *Journal of Experimental Psychology: Human Perception and Performance, 15*, 203–211.

Farah, M. J. (1990). *Visual Agnosia: Disorders of Object Recognition and What They Tell Us about Normal Vision.* Cambridge, Mass.: MIT Press.

Farah, M. J. (1994). Beyond "pet" methodologies to converging evidence. *Trends in Neurosciences, 17*(12), 514–515.

Farah, M. J. (1995). The neural bases of mental imagery. In M. S. Gazzaniga (ed.), *The Cognitive Neurosciences* (pp. 963–975). Cambridge, Mass.: MIT Press.

Farah, M. J., Hammond, K. M., Levine, D. N., and Calvanio, R. (1988). Visual and spatial mental imagery: Dissociable systems of representation. *Cognitive Psychology, 20*(4), 439–462.

Farah, M. J., Soso, M. J., and Dasheiff, R. M. (1992). Visual angle of the mind's eye before and after unilateral occipital lobectomy. *Journal of Experimental Psychology: Human Perception Performance, 18*(1), 241–246.

Farrell, M. J., and Robertson, I. H. (1998). Mental rotation and the automatic updating of body-centered spatial relationships. *Journal of Experimental Psychology: Learning, Memory, and Cognition, 21*, 483–500.

Felleman, D. J., and Van Essen, D. C. (1991). Distributed hierarchical processing in the primate cerebral cortex. *Cerebral Cortex, 1*(1), 1–47.

Festinger, L., White, C. W., and Allyn, M. R. (1968). Eye Movements and decrement in the Müller-Lyer Illusion. *Perception and Psychophysics, 3*(5-B), 376–382.

Feyerabend, P. (1962). Explanation, reduction, and empiricism. In H. Feigl and G. Maxwell (eds.), *Minnesota Studies in Philosophy of Science* (volume 3). Minneapolis, Minn.: University of Minnesota Press.

Fidelman, U. (1994). A misleading implication of the metabolism scans of the brain. *International Journal of Neuroscience, 74*(1–4), 105–108.

Finke, R. A. (1979). The functional equivalence of mental images and errors of movement. *Cognitive Psychology, 11*, 235–264.

Finke, R. A. (1980). Levels of equivalence in imagery and perception. *Psychological Review, 87*, 113–132.

Finke, R. A. (1989). *Principles of Mental Imagery.* Cambridge, Mass.: MIT Press.

Finke, R. A. (1990). *Creative Imagery: Discoveries and Inventions in Visualization.* Hillsdale, N.J.: Erlbaum.

Finke, R. A., and Freyd, J. J. (1989). Mental extrapolation and cognitive penetrability: Reply to Ranney and proposals for evaluative criteria. *Journal of Experimental Psychology: General, 118*(4), 403–408.

Finke, R. A., and Kosslyn, S. M. (1980). Mental imagery acuity in the peripheral visual field. *Journal of Experimental Psychology: Human Perception and Performance, 6*(1), 126–139.

Finke, R. A., and Kurtzman, H. S. (1981a). Mapping the visual field in mental imagery. *Journal of Experimental Psychology: General, 110*(4), 501–517.

Finke, R. A., and Kurtzman, H. S. (1981b). Methodological considerations in experiments on imagery acuity. *Journal of Experimental Psychology: Human Perception and Performance, 7*(4), 848–855.

Finke, R. A., and Pinker, S. (1982). Spontaneous imagery scanning in mental extrapolation. *Journal of Experimental Psychology: Learning, Memory, and Cognition, 8*(2), 142–147.

Finke, R. A., Pinker, S., and Farah, M. J. (1989). Reinterpreting visual patterns in mental imagery. *Cognitive Science, 13*(1), 51–78.

Finke, R. A., and Schmidt, M. J. (1977). Orientation-specific color aftereffects following imagination. *Journal of Experimental Psychology: Human Perception and Performance, 3*(4), 599–606.

Fisher, G. H. (1976). Measuring ambiguity. *American Journal of Psychology, 80,* 541–557.

Fletcher, P. C., Shallice, T., Frith, C. D., Frackowiak, R. S. J., and Dolan, R. J. (1996). Brain activity during memory retrieval: The influence of imagery and semantic cueing. *Brain, 119*(5), 1587–1596.

Fodor, J. A. (1968). The appeal to tacit knowledge in psychological explanation. *Journal of Philosophy, 65,* 627–640.

Fodor, J. A. (1975). *The Language of Thought.* New York: Crowell.

Fodor, J. A. (1981). Imagistic representation. In N. Block (ed.), *Imagery.* Cambridge, Mass.: MIT Press.

Fodor, J. A. (1983). *The Modularity of Mind: An Essay on Faculty Psychology.* Cambridge, Mass.: MIT Press Bradford Books.

Fodor, J. A. (1998). *Concepts: Where Cognitive Science Went Wrong.* Oxford: Oxford University Press.

Fodor, J. A. (2001). Language, thought, and compositionality. *Mind and Language, 16*(1), 1–15.

Fodor, J. A., and Pylyshyn, Z. W. (1981). How direct is visual perception? Some reflections on Gibson's "ecological approach." *Cognition, 9,* 139–196.

Fodor, J. A., and Pylyshyn, Z. W. (1988). Connectionism and cognitive architecture: A critical analysis. *Cognition, 28,* 3–71.

Ford, K., and Pylyshyn, Z. W. (eds.), (1996). *The Robot's Dilemma Revisited.* Stamford, Conn.: Ablex.

Fox, E. (1995). Negative priming from ignored distractors in visual selection: A review. *Psychonomic Bulletin and Review, 2*(2), 145–173.

Fox, P. T., Mintun, M. A., Raichle, M. E., Miezin, F. M., Allman, J. M., and Van Essen, D. C. (1986). Mapping human visual cortex with positron emission tomography. *Nature, 323*(6091), 806–809.

Fraisse, P. (1963). *The Psychology of Time.* New York: Harper and Row.

Freuder, E. C. (1986). Knowledge-mediated perception. In H. C. Nusbaum and Schwab, E. C. (ed.), *Pattern Recognition by Humans and Machines: Visual Perception* (vol. 2). Orlando: Academic Press.

Freyd, J. J., and Finke, R. A. (1984). Representational momentum. *Journal of Experimental Psychology: Learning, Memory, and Cognition*, *10*(1), 126–132.

Friedman, A. (1978). Memorial comparisons without the "mind's eye." *Journal of Verbal Learning and Verbal Behavior*, *17*(4), 427–444.

Friedman-Hill, S., and Wolfe, J. M. (1995). Second-order parallel processing: Visual search for odd items in a subset. *Journal of Experimental Psychology: Human Perception and Performance*, *21*(3), 531–551.

Frisby, J. P., and Clatworthy, J. L. (1975). Learning to see complex random-dot stereograms. *Perception*, *4*(2), 173–178.

Galilei, G. (1610/1983). The starry messenger. In S. Drake (ed.), *Telescopes, Tides, and Tactics*. Chicago: University of Chicago Press.

Gallistel, C. R. (1990). *The Organization of Learning*. Cambridge, Mass.: MIT Press / Bradford Books.

Gallistel, C. R. (1994). Foraging for brain stimulation: Toward a neurobiology of computation. *Cognition*, *50*, 151–170.

Gallistel, C. R., and Cramer, A. E. (1996). Computations on metric maps in mammals: Getting oriented and choosing a multi-destination route. *Journal of Experimental Biology*, *199*(1), 211–217.

Gardner, M. (1982). *Logic Machines and Diagrams* (second ed.). Chicago: University of Chicago Press.

Gazzaniga, M. S. (2000). Cerebral specialization and interhemispheric communication: Does the corpus callosum enable the human condition? *Brain*, *123*(7), 1293–1326.

Georgeff, M. P. (1987). Planning. In J. F. Traub, B. J. Grosz, B. W. Lampson, and N. J. Nilsson (eds.), *Annual Review of Computer Science* (vol. 2). Palo Alto: Annual Reviews.

Getzels, J. W., and Jackson, P. W. (1962). *Creativity and Intelligence: Explorations with Gifted Students*. New York: Wiley.

Gibson, B. (1994). Visual attention and objects: One versus two or convex versus concave? *Journal of Experimental Psychology: Human Perception and Performance*, *20*, 203–207.

Gibson, E. J. (1991). *An Odyssey in Learning and Perception*. Cambridge, Mass.: MIT Press.

Gibson, J. J. (1966). *The Senses Considered as Perceptual Systems*. Boston: Houghton Mifflin.

Gibson, J. J. (1979). *An Ecological Approach to Visual Perception*. Boston: Houghton Mifflin.

Gilchrist, A. (1977). Perceived lightness depends on perceived spatial arrangement. *Science*, *195*, 185–187.

Gilden, D., Blake, R., and Hurst, G. (1995). Neural adaptation of imaginary visual motion. *Cognitive Psychology*, *28*(1), 1–16.

Gillam, B., and Chambers, D. (1985). Size and position are incongruous: Measurements on the Mueller-Lyer figure. *Perception and Psychophysics*, 37(6), 549–556.

Girgus, J. J., Rock, I., and Egatz, R. (1977). The effect of knowledge of reversibility on the reversibility of ambiguous figures. *Perception and Psychophysics*, 22(6), 550–556.

Gnadt, J. W., Bracewell, R. M., and Anderson, R. A. (1991). Sensorimotor transformation during eye movements to remembered visual targets. *Vision Research*, 31, 693–715.

Gogel, W. C. (1997/1973). The organization of perceived space. In I. Rock (ed.), *Indirect Perception* (pp. 361–386). Cambridge, Mass.: MIT Press.

Goldenberg, G. (1992). Loss of visual imagery and loss of visual knowledge: A case study. *Neuropsychologia*, 30(12), 1081–1099.

Goldenberg, G., and Artner, C. (1991). Visual imagery and knowledge about the visual appearance of objects in patients with posterior cerebral artery lesions. *Brain and Cognition*, 15(2), 160–186.

Goldenberg, G., Mullbacher, W., and Nowak, A. (1995). Imagery without perception: A case study of anosognosia for cortical blindness. *Neuropsychologia*, 33(11), 1373–1382.

Goldstone, R. L. (1994). Influences of categorization on perceptual discrimination. *Journal of Experimental Psychology: General*, 123(2), 178–200.

Goldstone, R. L. (1995). The effect of categorization on color perception. *Psychological Science*, 6(5), 298–304.

Gollin, E. S. (1960). Developmental studies of visual recognition of incomplete objects. *Perceptual and Motor Skills*, 11, 289–298.

Goodale, M. A. (1983). Vision as a sensorimotor system. In T. E. Robinson (ed.), *Behavioral Approaches to Brain Research* (pp. 41–61). New York: Oxford University Press.

Goodale, M. A. (1988). Modularity in visuomotor control: From input to output. In Z. W. Pylyshyn (ed.), *Computational Processes in Human Vision: An Interdisciplinary Perspective* (pp. 262–285). Norwood, N.J.: Ablex.

Goodale, M. A., Jacobson, J. S., and Keillor, J. M. (1994). Differences in the visual control of pantomimed and natural grasping movements. *Neuropsychologia*, 32(10), 1159–1178.

Goodale, M. A., and Milner, A. D. (1982). Fractionating orientation behavior in rodents. In D. J. Ingle, M. A. Goodale, and R. J. W. Mansfield (eds.), *Analysis of Visual Behavior*. Cambridge, Mass.: MIT Press.

Goodale, M. A., Pelisson, D., and Prablanc, C. (1986). Large adjustments in visually guided reaching do not depend on vision of the hand or perception of target displacement. *Nature*, 320, 748–750.

Goodman, N. (1968). *Languages of Art*. Indianapolis: Bobbs-Merrill.

Gordon, R. D., and Irwin, D. E. (1996). What's in an object file? Evidence from priming studies. *Perception and Psychophysics*, 58(8), 1260–1277.

Goryo, K., Robinson, J. O., and Wilson, J. A. (1984). Selective looking and the Mueller-Lyer illusion: The effect of changes in the focus of attention on the Mueller-Lyer illusion. *Perception*, 13(6), 647–654.

Green, B. F., and Anderson, L. K. (1956). Color coding in a visual search task. *Journal of Experimental Psychology*, 51, 19–24.

Greenfield, P. M., deWinstanley, P., Kilpatrick, H., and Kaye, D. (1994). Action video games and informal education: Effects on strategies for dividing visual attention. Special issue: Effects of interactive entertainment technologies on development. *Journal of Applied Developmental Psychology*, 15(1), 105–123.

Gregory, R. L. (1968). Visual illusions. *Scientific American*, 219(5), 66–76.

Gregory, R. L. (1970). *The Intelligent Eye*. New York: McGraw-Hill.

Grice, H. P. (1975). Logic and conversation. *Syntax and Semantics*, 3, 41–58.

Grimes, J. (1996). Failure to detect changes in scenes across saccades. In K. Akins (ed.), *Perception*. New York: Oxford University Press.

Grimson, W. E. L. (1990). The combinatorics of object recognition in cluttered environments using constrained search. *Artificial Intelligence*, 44(1–2), 121–166.

Guariglia, C., Padovani, A., Pantano, P., and Pizzamiglio, L. (1993). Unilateral neglect restricted to visual imagery. *Nature*, 364(6434), 235–237.

Gumperz, J., and Levinson, S. (eds.). (1996). *Rethinking Linguistic Relativity: Studies in the Social and Cultural Foundations of Language*. Cambridge: Cambridge University Press.

Haber, R. N. (1966). Nature of the effect of set on perception. *Psychological Review*, 73, 335–351.

Haber, R. N. (1968). Perceptual reports vs. recognition responses: A reply to Parks. *Perception and Psychophysics*, 4(6), 374.

Haber, R. N. (1979). Twenty years of haunting eidetic imagery: Where's the ghost? *Behavioral and Brain Sciences*, 2(4), 583–629.

Haber, R. N., and Nathanson, L. S. (1968). Post-retinal storage? Some further observations on Park's Camel as seen through the eye of a needle. *Perception and Psychophysics*, 3, 349–355.

Haenny, P., and Schiller, P. (1988). State dependent activity in money visual cortex I. Single cell activity in V1 and V4 on visual tasks. *Experimental Brain Research*, 69, 225–244.

Hagenzieker, M. P., van der Heijden, A. H. C., and Hagenaar, R. (1990). Time course in visual-information processing: Some empirical evidence for inhibition. *Psychological Research*, 52, 13–21.

Haier, R. J., Siegel, B. V., Neuchterlein, K. H., Hazlett, E., Wu, J. C., Paek, J., et al. (1988). Cortical glucose metabolic rate correlates of abstract reasoning and attention studied with positron emission tomography. *Intelligence*, 12, 199–217.

Hampson, P. J., and Duffy, C. (1984). Verbal and spatial interference effects in congenitally blind and sighted subjects. *Canadian Journal of Psychology, 38*(3), 411–420.

Hans, M. A. (1974). Imagery and modality in paired-associate learning in the blind. *Bulletin of the Psychonomic Society, 4*(1), 22–24.

Hanson, N. R. (1958). *Patterns of Discovery*. Cambridge: Cambridge University Press.

Harper, W. L., Stalnaker, R., and Pearce, G. (eds.). (1981). *Ifs: Conditionals, Belief, Decision, Chance, and Time*. Boston, Mass.: D. Reidel.

Harris, J. P. (1982). The VVIQ imagery-induced McCollough effects: An alternative analysis. *Percept Psychophys, 32*(3), 290–292.

Harrison, J. E., and Baron-Cohen, S. (1997). Synaesthesia: A review of psychological theories. In S. Baron-Cohen and J. E. Harrison (eds.), *Synaesthesia: Classic and Contemporary Readings* (pp. 109–122). Cambridge, Mass.: Blackwell.

Hayes, J. R. (1973). On the function of visual imagery in elementary mathematics. In W. G. Chase (ed.), *Visual Information Processing*. New York: Academic Press.

Hayes, J. R., and Simon, H. A. (1976). The understanding process: Problem isomorphs. *Cognitive Psychology, 8*, 165–180.

Hayhoe, M. M., Bensinger, D. G., and Ballard, D. H. (1998). Task constraints in visual working memory. *Vision Research, 38*(1), 125–137.

He, S., Cavanagh, P., and Intriligator, J. (1997). Attentional resolution. *Trends in Cognitive Sciences, 1*(3), 115–121.

He, Z. J., and Nakayama, K. (1994). Perceiving textures: Beyond filtering. *Vision Research, 34*, 151–162.

Hebb, D. O. (1949). *Organization of Behavior*. New York: Wiley.

Heller, M. A., and Kennedy, J. M. (1990). Perspective taking, pictures, and the blind. *Perception and Psychophysics, 48*(5), 459–466.

Henderson, J. M. (1991). Stimulus discrimination following covert attentional orienting to an exogenous cue. *Journal of Experimental Psychology: Human Perception and Performance, 11*, 409–430.

Henderson, J. M., and Hollingworth, A. (1999). The role of fixation position in detecting scene changes across saccades. *Psychological Science, 10*(5), 438–443.

Hernandez-Péon, R., Scherrer, R. H., and Jouvet, M. (1956). Modification of electrical activity in the cochlear nucleus during "attention" in unanesthetized cats. *Science, 123*, 331–332.

Heywood, C. A., and Zihl, J. (1999). Motion blindness. In G. W. Humphreys (ed.), *Case Studies in the Neuropsychology of Vision* (pp. 1–16). Sussex: Psychology Press/Taylor and Francis.

Hikosaka, O., Miyauchi, S., and Shimojo, S. (1993). Voluntary and stimulus-induced attention detected as motion sensation. *Perception, 22*, 517–526.

Hinton, G. E. (1987). The horizontal-vertical delusion. *Perception, 16*(5), 677–680.

Hirsch, E. (1982). *The Concept of Identity*. Oxford University Press: Oxford.

Hochberg, J. (1968). In the mind's eye. In R. N. Haber (ed.), *Contemporary Theory and Research in Visual Perception* (pp. 309–331). New York: Holt, Rinehart, and Winston.

Hochberg, J., and Gellman, L. (1977). The effect of landmark features on mental rotation times. *Memory and Cognition*, *5*(1), 23–26.

Hoenig, P. (1972). The effects of eye movements, fixation and figure size on decrement in the Muller-Lyer illusion. *Dissertation Abstracts International*, *33*(6-B), 2835.

Hoffman, D. D. (1998). *Visual Intelligence: How We Create What We See*. New York: W. W. Norton.

Hollingworth, A., and Henderson, J. M. (1999). Vision and cognition: Drawing the line. *Behavioral and Brain Sciences*, *22*(3), 380–381.

Hollingworth, A., and Henderson, J. M. (1998). Does consistent scene context facilitate object perception? *Journal of Experimental Psychology: General*, *127*(4), 398–415.

Holmes, G. (1918). Disturbances in visual orientation. *British Journal of Ophthalmology*, *2*, 449–506.

Holmes, G., and Horax, G. (1919). Disturbances of spatial orientation and visual attention, with loss of stereoscopic vision. *Archives of Neurology and Psychiatry*, *1*, 385–407.

Howard, I. P. (1982). *Human Visual Orientation*. New York: Wiley.

Howard, R. J., ffytche, D. H., Barnes, J., McKeefry, D., Ha, Y., Woodruff, P. W., et al. (1998). The functional anatomy of imagining and perceiving colour. *Neuroreport*, *9*(6), 1019–1023.

Hubel, D. H., and Wiesel, T. N. (1962). Receptive fields, binocular interaction, and functional architecture in the cat's visual cortex. *Journal of Physiology*, *160*, 106–154.

Humphrey, G. (1951). *Thinking: An Introduction to Its Experimental Psychology*. London: Methuen.

Humphreys, G. W., and Riddoch, M. J. (1987). *To See but Not to See: A Case Study of Visual Agnosia*. Hillsdale, N.J.: Erlbaum.

Humphreys, G. W., and Riddoch, M. J. (1993). Interactions between object and space systems revealed through neuropsychology. In D. Meyer and S. Kornblum (eds.), *Attention and Performance XIV* (pp. 183–218). Cambridge, Mass.: MIT Press.

Humphreys, G. W., and Riddoch, M. J. (1994). Visual object processing in normality and pathology: Implications for rehabilitation. In Jane, Riddoch, and G. W. Humphreys (eds.), *Cognitive Neuropsychology and Cognitive Rehabilitation* (pp. 39–76). Hillsdale, N.J.: Erlbaum.

Humphreys, G. W., and Riddoch, M. J. (1995). Separate coding of space within and between perceptual objects: Evidence from unilateral visual neglect. *Cognitive Neuropsychology*, *12*, 283–311.

Huntley-Fenner, G., Carey, S., and Salimando, A. (2002). Objects are individuals but stuff doesn't count: Perceived rigidity and cohesiveness influence infants' representation of small number of discrete entities. *Cognition*, 85(3), 203–221.

Huttenlocher, J. (1968). Constructing spatial images: A strategy in reasoning. *Psychological Review*, 75(6), 550–560.

Ingle, D. J. (1973). Two visual systems in the frog. *Science*, 181, 1053–1055.

Ingle, D. J. (2002). Problems with a "cortical screen" for visual imagery. *Behavioral and Brain Sciences*, 29(2), 195–196.

Ingle, D. J., Goodale, M. A., and Mansfield, R. J. W. (eds.). (1982). *Analysis of Visual Behavior*. Cambridge, Mass.: MIT Press.

Intons-Peterson, M. J. (1983). Imagery paradigms: How vulnerable are they to experimenters' expectations? *Journal of Experimental Psychology: Human Perception and Performance*, 9(3), 394–412.

Intons-Peterson, M. J., and White, A. R. (1981). Experimenter naivete and imaginal judgments. *Journal of Experimental Psychology: Human Perception and Performance*, 7(4), 833–843.

Intriligator, J., and Cavanagh, P. (1992). Object-specific spatial attention facilitation that does not travel to adjacent spatial locations. *Investigative Ophthalmology and Visual Science*, 33, 2849 (abstract).

Intriligator, J. M. (1997). The spatial resolution of attention. Unpublished dissertation. Harvard, Cambridge, Mass.

Irwin, D. E. (1991). Information integration across saccadic eye movements. *Cognitive Psychology*, 23, 420–456.

Irwin, D. E. (1993). Perceiving an integrated visual world. In D. E. Meyer and S. Kornblum (eds.), *Attention and Performance XIV*. Cambridge, Mass.: MIT Press.

Irwin, D. E. (1996). Integrating information across saccadic eye movements. *Current Directions in Psychological Science*, 5(3), 94–100.

Irwin, D. E., McConkie, G. W., Carlson-Radvansky, L. A., and Currie, C. (1994). A localist evaluation solution for visual stability across saccades. *Behavioral and Brain Sciences*, 17, 265–266.

Ishai, A., and Sagi, D. (1995). Common mechanisms of visual imagery and perception. *Science*, 268(5218), 1772–1774.

Ittelson, W. H., and Ames, A. J. (1968). *The Ames Demonstrations in Perception*. New York: Hafner.

Jamnek, M. (2001). *Mathematical Reasoning with Diagrams: From Intuition to Automation*. Chicago, Ill.: University of Illinois Press.

Jankowiak, J., Kinsbourne, M., Shalev, R. S., and Bachman, D. L. (1992). Preserved visual imagery and categorization in a case of associative visual agnosia. *Journal of Cognitive Neuroscience*, 4(2), 119–131.

Jastrow, J. (1900). *Fact and Fable in Psychology*. New York: Houghton Mifflin.

Jensen, E., Reese, E., and Reese, T. (1950). The subitizing and counting of visually presented fields of dots. *Journal of Psychology*, *30*, 363–392.

Johansson, G. (1950). *Configurations in Event Perception*. Boston: Houghton Mifflin.

Johnson, M. H., and Gilmore, R. O. (1998). Object-centered attention in 8-month-old infants. *Developmental Science*, *1*(2), 221–225.

Johnson, R. A. (1980). Sensory images in the absence of sight: Blind versus sighted adolescents. *Perceptual and Motor Skills*, *51*(1), 177–178.

Johnson-Laird, P. N. (1989). Mental models. In M. I. Posner (ed.), *Foundations of Cognitive Science* (pp. 469–499). Cambridge, Mass.: MIT Press.

Johnson-Laird, P. N. (2001). Mental models and deduction. *Trends in Cognitive Sciences*, *5*(10), 434–442.

Jolicoeur, P., Ullman, S., and MacKay, M. F. (1986). Curve Tracing: A possible basic operation in the perception of spatial relations. *Memory and Cognition*, *14*(2), 129–140.

Jonides, J., Kahn, R., and Rozin, P. (1975). Imagery instructions improve memory in blind subjects. *Bulletin of the Psychonomic Society*, *5*(5), 424–426.

Julesz, B. (1971). *Foundations of Cyclopean Perception*. Chicago: University of Chicago Press.

Julesz, B. (1990). Early vision is bottom up, except for focal attention. *Cold Spring Harbor Symposium on Quantitative Biology*, *55*, 973–978.

Julesz, B., and Papathomas, T. V. (1984). On spatial-frequency channels and attention. *Perception and Psychophysics*, *36*(4), 398–399.

Just, M. A., and Carpenter, P. A. (1976). Eye fixations and cognitive processes. *Cognitive Psychology*, *8*(4), 441–480.

Kabanza, F., Barbeau, M., and St-Denis, R. (1997). Planning control rules for reactive agents. *Artificial Intelligence*, *95*, 67–113.

Kahneman, D., and Treisman, A. (1984). Changing views of attention and automaticity. In R. Parasuraman and D. R. Davies (eds.), *Varieties of Attention* (pp. 29–62). New York: Academic Press.

Kahneman, D., Treisman, A., and Gibbs, B. J. (1992). The reviewing of object files: Object-specific integration of information. *Cognitive Psychology*, *24*(2), 175–219.

Kanizsa, G. (1969). Perception, past experience, and the impossible experiment. *Acta Psychologica*, *31*, 66–96.

Kanizsa, G. (1976). Subjective contours. *Scientific American*, *234*, 48–52.

Kanizsa, G. (1985). Seeing and thinking. *Acta Psychologica*, *59*, 23–33.

Kanizsa, G., and Gerbino, W. (1982). Amodal completion: Seeing or thinking? In B. Beck (ed.), *Organization and Representation in Perception* (pp. 167–190). Hillsdale, N.J.: Erlbaum.

Kant, E. (1998). *The Critique of Pure Reason (Kritik der reinen Vernunft. English)* (P. Guyer and A. Wood, trans.). Cambridge: Cambridge University Press.

Kanwisher, N. (2001). Neural events and perceptual awareness. *Cognition, 79,* 89–113.

Karni, A., and Sagi, D. (1995). A memory system in the adult visual cortex. In B. Julesz and I. Kovacs (eds.), *Maturational Windows and Adult Cortical Plasticity* (pp. 95–109). Reading, Mass.: Addison-Wesley.

Kaufman, E., Lord, M., Reese, T., and Volkman, J. (1949). The discrimination of visual number. *American Journal of Psychology, 62,* 498–525.

Kawabata, N. (1986). Attention and depth perception. *Perception, 15(5),* 563–572.

Keele, S. W. (1973). *Attention and Human Performance.* Pacific Palisades, Calif.: Goodyear Publishing.

Kelly, M. D. (1971). Edge detection by computer using planning. In B. Meltzer and D. Michie (eds.), *Machine Intelligence 6.* Edinburgh: University of Edinburgh Press.

Kelso, J. A. S., Cook, E., Olson, M. E., and Epstein, W. (1975). Allocation of attention and the locus of adaptation to displaced vision. *Journal of Experimental Psychology: Human Perception and Performance, 1,* 237–245.

Kerr, N. H. (1983). The role of vision in "visual imagery" experiments: Evidence from the congenitally blind. *Journal of Experimental Psychology: General, 112(2),* 265–277.

Klein, G., and Crandall, B. W. (1995). The role of mental simulation in problem solving and decision making. In P. Hancock (ed.), *Local applications of the ecological approach to human-machine systems, Volume 2: Resources for ecological psychology* (pp. 324–358). Mahwah, N.J.: Erlbaum.

Klein, R. (2000). Inhibition of return. *Trends in Cognitive Sciences, 4(4),* 138–147.

Koch, C., and Ullman, S. (1985). Shifts in selective visual attention: Towards the underlying neural circuitry. *Human Neurobiology, 4,* 219–227.

Koenderink, J. J. (1990). *Solid Shape.* Cambridge, Mass.: MIT Press.

Kosslyn, S. M. (1973). Scanning visual images: Some structural implications. *Perception and Psychophysics, 14,* 90–94.

Kosslyn, S. M. (1978). Measuring the visual angle of the mind's eye. *Cognitive Psychology, 10,* 356–389.

Kosslyn, S. M. (1980). *Image and Mind.* Cambridge, Mass.: Harvard University Press.

Kosslyn, S. M. (1981). The medium and the message in mental imagery: A theory. *Psychological Review, 88,* 46–66.

Kosslyn, S. M. (1983). *Ghosts in the Mind's Machine.* New York: Norton.

Kosslyn, S. M. (1994). *Image and Brain: The Resolution of the Imagery Debate.* Cambridge, Mass.: MIT Press.

Kosslyn, S. M., Ball, T. M., and Reiser, B. J. (1978). Visual images preserve metric spatial information: Evidence from studies of image scanning. *Journal of Experimental Psychology: Human Perception and Performance, 4,* 46–60.

Kosslyn, S. M., Pascual-Leone, A., Felican, O., Camposano, S., Keenan, J. P., Thompson, W. L., et al. (1999). The role of area 17 in visual imagery: Convergent evidence from PET and rTMS. *Science, 284* (April 2), 167–170.

Kosslyn, S. M., Pinker, S., Smith, G., and Shwartz, S. P. (1979). On the demystification of mental imagery. *Behavioral and Brain Science, 2,* 535–581.

Kosslyn, S. M., Sukel, K. E., and Bly, B. M. (1999). Squinting with the mind's eye: Effects of stimulus resolution on imaginal and perceptual comparisons. *Memory and Cognition, 27*(2), 276–287.

Kosslyn, S. M., and Sussman, A. L. (1995). Roles of imagery in perception: Or, there is no such thing as immaculate perception. In M. S. Gazzaniga (ed.), *The Cognitive Neurosciences* (pp. 1035–1042). Cambridge, Mass.: MIT Press.

Kosslyn, S. M., Thompson, W. L., Kim, I. J., and Alpert, N. M. (1995). Topographical representations of mental images in primary visual cortex. *Nature, 378* (Nov. 30), 496–498.

Kosslyn, S. M., Thomson, W. L., and Ganis, G. (2002). Mental imagery doesn't work like that. *Behavioral and Brain Sciences, 25*(2), 198–200.

Kotovsky, K., Hayes, J. R., and Simon, H. A. (1985). Why are some problems hard? Evidence from Tower of Hanoi. *Cognitive Psychology, 17*(2), 248–294.

Kowler, E. (1989). Cognitive expectations, not habits, control anticipatory smooth oculomotor pursuit. *Vision Research, 29,* 1049–1057.

Kowler, E. (1990). The role of visual and cognitive processes in the control of eye movement. In E. Kowler (ed.), *Eye Movements and Their Role in Visual and Cognitive Processes* (pp. 1–70). Amsterdam: Elsevier Science.

Kowler, E., Anderson, E., Dosher, B., and Blaser, E. (1995). The role of attention in the programming of saccades. *Vision Research, 35*(13), 1897–1916.

Kowler, E., and Steinman, R. M. (1977). The role of small saccades in counting. *Vision Research, 17*(1), 141–146.

Krekelberg, B. (2001). The persistence of position. *Vision Research, 41*(4), 529–539.

Kubovy, M., and Van Valkenburg, D. (2001). Auditory and visual objects. *Cognition, 80*(1/2), 97–126.

Kuhn, T. (1972). *The Structure of Scientific Revolutions.* Chicago: University of Chicago Press.

Kunen, S., and May, J. G. (1980). Spatial frequency content of visual imagery. *Perception and Psychophysics, 28*(6), 555–559.

Kunen, S., and May, J. G. (1981). Imagery-induced McCollough effects: Real or imagined? *Perception and Psychophysics, 30*(1), 99–100.

Lackner, J. R., and Garrett, M. F. (1972). Resolving ambiguity: Effects of biasing context in the unattended ear. *Cognition*, *1*, 359–372.

Landis, T. (2000). Disruption of space perception due to cortical lesions. *Spatial Vision*, *13*(2–3), 179–191.

Lee, D. N., and Lishman, J. R. (1975). Visual proprioceptive control of stance. *Journal of Human Movement Studies*, *1*, 87–95.

Lee, E. K. B., and Simon, H. (1993). Parallel implementation of the extended square-root covariance filter for tracking applications. *IEEE Transactions on Parallel and Distributed Systems*, *4*, 446–457.

Leslie, A. M., Xu, F., Tremoulet, P. D., and Scholl, B. J. (1998). Indexing and the object concept: Developing "what" and "where" systems. *Trends in Cognitive Sciences*, *2*(1), 10–18.

Lespérance, Y., and Levesque, H. J. (1995). Indexical knowledge and robot action: A logical account. *Artificial Intelligence*, *73*, 69–115.

Levesque, H. (1986). Making believers out of computers. *Artificial Intelligence*, *30*, 81–108.

Leyton, M. (1992). *Symmetry, Causality, Mind*. Cambridge, Mass.: MIT Press.

Li, P., and Gleitman, L. (2002). Turning the tables: Language and spatial reasoning. *Cognition*, *83*, 265–294.

Lindberg, D. C. (1976). *Theories of Vision from al-Kindi to Kepler*. Chicago: University of Chicago Press.

Lindsay, P. H., and Norman, D. A. (1977). *Human Information Processing: An Introduction to Psychology* (second edition). New York: Academic Press.

Livingstone, M. S., and Hubel, D. H. (1987). Psychophysical evidence for separate channels for the perception of form, color, movement, and depth. *Journal of Neuroscience*, *7*(11), 3416–3468.

Loftus, E. F. (1975). Leading questions and the eyewitness report. *Cognitive Psychology*, *7*, 560–572.

Lowe, D. G. (1987). Three-dimensional object recognition from single two-dimensional images. *Artificial Intelligence*, *31*, 355–395.

Luce, R. D., D'Zmura, M., Hoffman, D. D., Iverson, G. J., and Romney, A. K. (eds.). (1995). *Geometric Representations of Perceptual Phenomena: Papers in Honor of Tarow Indow on His 70th Birthday* (vol. 356). Mahwah, N.J.: Erlbaum.

Luchins, A. S. (1942). Mechanization in problem solving. *Psychological Monographs*, *54*(6), 248.

Luck, S., and Vogel, E. (1997). The capacity of visual working memory for features and conjunctions. *Nature*, *390*, 279–281.

Luria, A. R. (1959). Disorders of "simultaneous perception" in a case of bilateral occipito-parietal brain injury. *Brain*, *83*, 437–449.

Lynch, J. C. (1980). The functional organization of posterior parietal cortex. *Behavioral and Brain Sciences*, *3*, 485–534.

Mack, A., Heuer, F., Villardi, K., and Chambers, D. (1985). The dissociation of position and extent in Mueller-Lyer figures. *Perception and Psychophysics*, *37*(4), 335–344.

Mack, A., and Rock, I. (1998a). *Inattentional Blindness*. Cambridge, Mass.: MIT Press.

Mack, A., and Rock, I. (1998b). Inattentional blindness: Perception without attention. In R. D. Wright (ed.), *Visual Attention*. New York: Oxford University Press.

Mackworth, A. K. (1973). Interpreting pictures of polyhedral scenes. *Artificial Intelligence*, *4*, 121–137.

Maloney, L. T., and Wandell, B. A. (1990). Color constancy: A method for recovering surface spectral reflectance. In S. Ullman and W. Richards (eds.), *Image Understanding 1989* (vol. 3). Norwood, N.J.: Ablex.

Mandler, G., and Shebo, B. (1982). Subitizing: An analysis of its component processes. *Journal of Experimental Psychology: General*, *111*, 1–22.

Mani, K., and Johnson-Laird, P. N. (1982). The mental representation of spatial descriptions. *Memory and Cognition*, *10*(2), 181–187.

Marmor, G. S., and Zaback, L. A. (1976). Mental rotation by the blind: Does mental rotation depend on visual imagery? *Journal of Experimental Psychology: Human Perception and Performance*, *2*(4), 515–521.

Marr, D. (1982). *Vision: A Computational Investigation into the Human Representation and Processing of Visual Information*. San Francisco: W. H. Freeman.

Marr, D., and Nishihara, H. K. (1976). *Representation and Recognition of Spatial Organization of Three-dimensional Shapes*. (MIT A. I. Memo 377).

Marr, D., and Nishihara, H. K. (1978). Representation and recognition of spatial organization of three-dimensional shapes. *Proceedings of the Royal Society of London, B, 200,* 269–294.

Marr, D., and Poggio, T. (1979). A theory of human stereo vision. *Proceedings of the Royal Society of London, 204*(1156), 301–328.

Marshall, J. C. (2001). Auditory neglect and right parietal cortex. *Brain*, *124*(4), 645–646.

Mather, J. A., and Lackner, J. R. (1977). Adaptation to visual rearrangement: Role of sensory discordance. *Quarterly Journal of Experimental Psychology*, *29*(2), 237–244.

Mather, J. A., and Lackner, J. R. (1980). Visual tracking of active and passive movements of the hand. *Quarterly Journal of Experimental Psychology*, *32*(2), 307–315.

Mather, J. A., and Lackner, J. R. (1981). Adaptation to visual displacement: Contribution of proprioceptive, visual, and attentional factors. *Perception*, *10*(4), 367–374.

McBeath, M. K., Shaffer, D. M., and Kaiser, M. K. (1995). How baseball outfielders determine where to run to catch fly balls. *Science*, *278* (April 28), 569–573.

McConkie, G. M., and Currie, C. B. (1996). Visual stability across saccades while viewing complex pictures. *Journal of Experimental Psychology: Human Perception and Performance, 22*(3), 563–581.

McCormick, P. A., and Klein, R. (1990). The spatial distribution of attention during covert visual orienting. *Acta Psychologica, 75*, 225–242.

McDermott, D. (1989). A critique of pure reason. *Computational Intelligence, 3*, 151–160.

McGinn, C. (1999). *The Mysterious Flame: Conscious Minds in a Material World*. New York: Basic Books.

McGlinchey-Berroth, R., Milberg, W. P., Verfaellie, M., and Grande, L. (1996). Semantic processing and orthographic specificity in hemispatial neglect. *Journal of Cognitive Neuroscience, 8*(3), 291–304.

McKeever, P. (1991). Nontarget numerosity and identity maintenance with FINSTs: A two component account of multiple-target tracking. Unpublished master's thesis, University of Western Ontario, London, Ontario.

McKelvie, S. J. (1994). The vividness of visual imagery questionnaire as a predictor of facial recognition memory performance. *British Journal of Psychology, 85*(Pt 1), 93–104.

McKim, R. H. (1978). The Imaginarium: An environment and program for opening the mind's eye. In B. S. Randhawa and W. E. Coffman (eds.), *Visual Learning, Thinking, and Communication* (pp. 61–91). New York: Academic Press.

McLeod, P., Driver, J., Dienes, Z., and Crisp, J. (1991). Filtering by movement in visual search. *Journal of Experimental Psychology: Human Perception and Performance, 17*(1), 55–64.

Mellet, E., Petit, L., Mazoyer, B., Denis, M., and Tzourio, N. (1998). Reopening the mental imagery debate: Lessons from functional anatomy. *Neuroimage, 8*(2), 129–139.

Mellet, E., Tzourio, N., Crivello, F., Joliot, M., Denis, M., and Mazoyer, B. (1996). Functional anatomy of spatial mental imagery generated from verbal instructions. *Journal of Neuroscience, 16*(20), 6504–6512.

Merikle, P. M., Smilek, D., and Eastwood, J. D. (2001). Perception without awareness: Perspectives from cognitive psychology. *Cognition, 79*, 115–134.

Michie, D. (1986). *On Machine Intelligence*. New York: Halstead Press.

Miller, G. A. (1956). The magical number seven, plus or minus two: Some limits on our capacity for processing information. *Psychological Review, 63*, 81–97.

Miller, G. A. (1962). Decision units in the perception of speech. *Institute of Radio Engineers: Transactions on Information Theory, 8*, 81–83.

Miller, G. A. (1984). Informavores. In F. Machlup and U. Mansfield (eds.), *The Study of Information: Interdisciplinary Messages*. New York: Wiley.

Miller, G. A., Bruner, J. S., and Postman, L. (1954). Familiarity of letter sequences and tachistoscopic identification. *Journal of General Psychology, 50*, 129–139.

Miller, J., and Festinger, L. (1977). Impact of oculomotor retraining on the visual perception of curvature. *Journal of Experimental Psychology: Human Perception and Performance*, 3(2), 187–200.

Miller, N. (2001). A diagrammatic formal system for Euclidean geometry. Unpublished doctoral dissertation, Cornell University, Ithica, New York.

Milner, A. D., and Goodale, M. A. (1995). *The Visual Brain in Action*. New York: Oxford University Press.

Mitchell, D. B., and Richman, C. L. (1980). Confirmed reservations: Mental travel. *Journal of Experimental Psychology: Human Perception and Performance*, 6, 58–66.

Moffatt, H. K. (2000). Euler's disk and its finite-time singularity. *Nature*, 404(6780), 833–834.

Moore, C., Yantis, S., and Vaughan, B. (1998). Object-based visual selection: Evidence from perceptual completion. *Psychological Science*, 9, 104–110.

Moran, J., and Desimone, R. (1985). Selective attention gates visual processing in the extrastriate cortex. *Science*, 229(4715), 782–784.

Morton, J., Hammersley, R. H., and Bekerian, D. A. (1985). Headed records: A model for memory and its failures. *Cognition*, 20(1), 1–23.

Mountcastle, V., Motter, B., Steinmetz, M., and Sestokas, A. (1987). Common and differential effects of attentive fixation on the excitability of parietal and pre-striate (V4) cortical visual neurons in the macaque monkey. *Journal of Neuroscience*, 7(7), 2239–2255.

Mueller, H. J., and Findlay, J. M. (1988). The effect of visual attention on peripheral discrimination thresholds in single and multiple element displays. *Acta Psychologica*, 69(2), 129–155.

Mueller, H. J., and Rabbitt, P. M. (1989). Reflexive and voluntary orienting of visual attention: Time course of activation and resistance to interruption. *Journal of Experimental Psychology: Human Perception and Performance*, 15(2), 315–330.

Nakayama, K., He, Z. J., and Shimojo, S. (1995). Visual surface representation: A critical link between lower-level and higher-level vision. In S. M. Kosslyn and D. N. Osherson (eds.), *Visual Cognition* (second edition, pp. 1–70). Cambridge, Mass.: MIT Press.

Nakayama, K., and Mackeben, M. (1989). Sustained and transient components of focal visual attention. *Vision Research*, 29, 1631–1647.

Nakayama, K., and Silverman, G. H. (1986). Serial and parallel processing of visual feature conjunctions. *Nature*, 320(6059), 264–265.

Nazir, T. A., and O'Regan, J. K. (1990). Some results on translation invariance in the human visual system. *Spatial Vision*, 5(2), 81–100.

Neisser, U., and Becklen, R. (1975). Selective looking: Attending to visually specified events. *Cognitive Psychology*, 7, 480–494.

Newell, A. (1972). A theoretical exploration of mechanisms for coding the stimulus. In A. W. Melton and E. Martin (eds.), *Coding Processes in Human Memory*. Edinburgh: Edinburgh University Press.

Newell, A. (1980a). HARPY, production systems, and human cognition. In R. A. Cole (ed.), *Perception and Production of Fluent Speech*. Hillsdale, N.J.: Erlbaum.

Newell, A. (1980b). Physical symbol systems. *Cognitive Science*, 4(2), 135–183.

Newell, A. (1990). *Unified Theories of Cognition*. Cambridge, Mass.: Harvard University Press.

Newell, A., and Simon, H. A. (1972). *Human Problem Solving*. Englewood Cliffs, N.J.: Prentice-Hall.

Nichols, S., Stich, S., Leslie, A., and Klein, D. (1996). Varieties of on-line simulation. In P. Carruthers and P. Smith (eds.), *Theories of Theories of Mind* (pp. 39–74). Cambridge: Cambridge University Press.

Nicod, J. (1970). *Geometry and Induction*. Berkeley: University of California Press.

Nijhawan, R. (1991). Three-dimensional Müller-Lyer Illusion. *Perception and Psychophysics*, 49(9), 333–341.

Nijhawan, R. (1994). Motion extrapolation in catching. *Nature*, 370(6487), 256–257.

Nissen, M. J. (1985). Accessing features and objects: Is location special? In M. I. Posner and O. S. Marin (eds.), *Attention and Performance XI* (pp. 205–219). Hillsdale, N.J.: Erlbaum.

Norman, D. A. (1969). *Memory and Attention*. New York: Wiley.

Norman, D. A. (1988). *The Psychology of Everyday Things*. New York: Basic Books.

Norman, D. A. (1991). Cognitive artifacts. In J. M. Carroll (ed.), *Designing Interaction: Psychology at the Human-Computer Interface* (pp. 17–38). New York: Cambridge University Press.

Nougier, V., Ripoll, H., and Stein, J.-F. (1989). Orienting of attention with highly skilled athletes. *International Journal of Sport Psychology*, 20(3), 205–223.

Ogawa, H., and Yagi, A. (2002). The processing of untracked objects during multiple object tracking [abstract]. *Journal of Vision*, 2(7), 242a.

Ohkuma, Y. (1986). A comparison of image-induced and perceived Mueller-Lyer illusion. *Journal of Mental Imagery*, 10(4), 31–38.

O'Kane, B. L., Biederman, I., Cooper, E. E., and Nystrom, B. (1997). An account of object identification confusions. *Journal of Experimental Psychology: Applied*, 3(1), 21–41.

Olivers, C. N. J., Watson, D. G., and Humphreys, G. W. (1999). Visual marking of locations and feature maps: Evidence from within-dimension defined conjunctions. *Quarterly Journal of Experimental Psychology A*, 52A(3), 679–715.

O'Regan, J. K. (1992). Solving the "real" mysteries of visual perception: The world as an outside memory. *Canadian Journal of Psychology*, 46, 461–488.

O'Regan, J. K., Deubel, H., Clark, J. J., and Rensink, R. A. (2000). Picture changes during blinks: Looking without seeing and seeing without looking. *Visual Cognition*, 7, 191–212.

O'Regan, J. K., and Lévy-Schoen, A. (1983). Integrating visual information from successive fixations: Does trans-saccadic fusion exist? *Vision Research*, 23(8), 765–768.

O'Regan, J. K., and Noë, A. (2002). A sensorimotor account of vision and visual consciousness. *Behavioral and Brain Sciences*, 24(5), 939–1031.

Paivio, A. (1971). *Imagery and Verbal Processes*. New York: Holt, Rinehart, and Winston.

Paivio, A. (1986). *Mental Representations*. New York: Oxford University Press.

Paivio, A., and te Linde, J. (1980). Symbolic comparisons of objects on color attributes. *Journal of Experimental Psychology: Human Perception and Performance*, 6(4), 652–661.

Palmer, S. E. (1977). Hierarchical structure in perceptual representation. *Cognitive Psychology*, 9, 441–474.

Palmer, S. E. (1978). Structural aspects of visual similarity. *Memory and Cognition*, 6, 91–97.

Parks, T. E. (1965). Post-retinal visual storage. *American Journal of Psychology*, 78, 145–147.

Parks, T. E. (1968). Further comments on the evidence for post-retinal storage. *Perception and Psychophysics*, 4(6), 373.

Parks, T. E. (1994). On the microgenesis of illusory figures: A failure to replicate. *Perception*, 23, 857–862.

Parks, T. E. (1995). The microgenesis of illusory figures: Evidence for visual hypothesis testing. *Perception*, 24, 681–684.

Pashler, H. (1995). Attention and visual perception: analyzing divided attention. In S. M. Kosslyn and D. N. Osherson (eds.), *Visual Cognition* (second edition, pp. 71–100). Cambridge, Mass.: MIT Press.

Pashler, H. E. (1998). *The Psychology of Attention*. Cambridge, Mass.: MIT Press/Bradford Books.

Patterson, J., and Deffenbacher, K. (1972). Haptic perception of the Mueller-Lyer illusion by the blind. *Perceptual and Motor Skills*, 35(3), 819–824.

Pavani, F., Ladavas, E., and Driver, J. (2002). Selective deficit of auditory localisation in patients with visuospatial neglect. *Neuropsychologia*, 40(3), 291–301.

Pentland, A. P. (1986). Perceptual organization and the representation of natural form. *Artificial Intelligence*, 28, 293–331.

Perky, C. W. (1910). An experimental study of imagination. *American Journal of Psychology*, 21(3), 422–452.

Perrett, D. I., Harries, M. H., Benson, P. J., Chitty, A. J., and Mistlin, A. J. (1990). Retrieval of structure from rigid and biological motion: An analysis of the visual responses of neurons in the Macaque temporal cortex. In A. Blake and T. Troscianko (eds.), *AI and the Eye* (pp. 181–200). Chichester: Wiley.

Perrett, D. I., Mistlin, A. J., and Chitty, A. J. (1987). Visual neurons responsive to faces. *Trends in Neuroscience, 10,* 358–364.

Perry, J. (1979). The problem of the essential indexical. *Noûs, 13,* 3–21.

Pessoa, L., Thompson, E., and Noë, A. (1998). Finding out about filling in: A guide to perceptual completion for visual science and the philosophy of perception. *Behavioral and Brain Sciences, 21*(6), 723–802.

Peterson, M. A. (1993). The ambiguity of mental images: insights regarding the structure of shape memory and its function in creativity. In H. Roskos-Ewoldson, M. J. Intons-Peterson, and R. E. Anderson (eds.), *Imagery, Creativity, and Discovery: A Cognitive Perspective.* Advances in psychology, vol. 98. Amsterdam: North Holland/Elsevier Science.

Peterson, M. A., and Gibson, B. S. (1991). Directing spatial attention within an object: Altering the functional equivalence of shape description. *Journal of Experimental Psychology: Human Perception and Performance, 17*(1), 170–182.

Peterson, M. A., and Hochberg, J. (1983). Opposed-set measurement procedure: A quantitative analysis of the role of local cues and intention in form perception. *Journal of Experimental Psychology: Human Perception and Performance, 9,* 183–193.

Peterson, M. A., Kihlstrom, J. F., Rose, P. M., and Glisky, M. A. (1992). Mental images can be ambiguous: Recontruals and reference-frame reversals. *Memory and Cognition, 20*(2), 107–123.

Piaget, J., and Inhelder, B. (1957). *The Child's Conception of Space.* New York: Humanities Press.

Pike, K. L. (1967). *Language in Relation to a Unified Theory of the Structure of Human Behavior.* The Hague: Mouton.

Pinker, S. (1980). Mental imagery and the third dimension. *Journal of Experimental Psychology: General, 109*(3), 354–371.

Pinker, S. (1994). *The Language Instinct: How the Mind Creates Language.* New York: W. Morrow.

Pinker, S. (1997). *How the Mind Works.* New York: Norton.

Pinker, S., Choate, P. A., and Finke, R. A. (1984). Mental extrapolation in patterns constructed from memory. *Memory and Cognition, 12*(3), 207–218.

Pinker, S., and Finke, R. A. (1980). Emergent two-dimensional patterns in images rotated in depth. *Journal of Experimental Psychology: Human Perception and Performance, 6*(2), 244–264.

Planck, M. (1933). *Where Is Science Going?* (J. Murphy, trans.). London: Allen and Unwin.

Podgorny, P., and Shepard, R. N. (1978). Functional representations common to visual perception and imagination. *Journal of Experimental Psychology: Human Perception and Performance*, 4(1), 21–35.

Poggio, T., Torre, V., and Koch, C. (1990). Computational vision and regularization theory. In S. Ullman and W. Richards (eds.), *Image Understanding 1989* (vol. 3, pp. 1–18). Norwood, N.J.: Ablex.

Poincaré, H. (1963). Why space has three dimensions. In *Mathematics and Science: Last Essays*. New York: Dover.

Posner, M. I. (1978). *Chronometric Explorations of Mind.* Hillsdale, N.J.: Erlbaum.

Posner, M. I. (1980). Orienting of attention. *Quarterly Journal of Experimental Psychology*, 32, 3–25.

Posner, M. I., Nissen, M. J., and Ogden, W. C. (1978). Attended and unattended processing modes: The role of set for spatial location. In H. L. Pick and I. J. Saltzman (eds.), *Modes of Perceiving and Processing Information.* Hillsdale, N.J.: Erlbaum.

Posner, M. I., and Raichle, M. E. (1994). *Images of Mind.* New York: Freeman.

Potter, M. C. (1975). Meaning in visual search. *Science*, 187(4180), 965–966.

Predebon, J., and Wenderoth, P. (1985). Imagined stimuli: Imaginary effects? *Bulletin of the Psychonomic Society*, 23(3), 215–216.

Prinz, J. J. (2002). *Furnishing the Mind: Concepts and Their Perceptual Basis.* Cambridge, Mass.: MIT Press.

Proteau, L. (1992). On the specificity of learning and the role of visual information for movement control. In L. Proteau and D. Elliot (eds.), *Vision and Motor Control. Advances in Psychology No. 85* (pp. 67–103). Amsterdam: North-Holland.

Pylyshyn, Z. W. (1973). What the mind's eye tells the mind's brain: A critique of mental imagery. *Psychological Bulletin*, 80, 1–24.

Pylyshyn, Z. W. (1978). Imagery and artificial intelligence. In C. W. Savage (ed.), *Perception and Cognition: Issues in the Foundations of Psychology* (vol. 9). Minneapolis: University of Minnesota Press.

Pylyshyn, Z. W. (1979a). Do mental events have durations? *Behavioral and Brain Sciences*, 2(2), 277–278.

Pylyshyn, Z. W. (1979b). The rate of "mental rotation" of images: A test of a holistic analogue hypothesis. *Memory and Cognition*, 7, 19–28.

Pylyshyn, Z. W. (1979c). Validating computational models: A critique of Anderson's indeterminacy of representation claim. *Psychological Review*, 86(4), 383–394.

Pylyshyn, Z. W. (1980). Cognitive representation and the process-architecture distinction. *Behavioral and Brain Sciences*, 3(1), 154–169.

Pylyshyn, Z. W. (1981a). Complexity and the study of human and machine intelligence. In J. Haugeland (ed.), *Mind Design*. Cambridge, Mass.: MIT Press/ Bradford Books.

Pylyshyn, Z. W. (1981b). The imagery debate: Analogue media versus tacit knowledge. *Psychological Review, 88*, 16–45.

Pylyshyn, Z. W. (1984a). *Computation and Cognition: Toward a Foundation for Cognitive Science*. Cambridge, Mass.: MIT Press.

Pylyshyn, Z. W. (1984b). Plasticity and invariance in cognitive development. In J. Mehler and R. Fox (eds.), *Neonate Cognition: Beyond the Blooming, Buzzing Confusion*. Hillsdale, N.J.: Erlbaum.

Pylyshyn, Z. W. (1989). The role of location indexes in spatial perception: A sketch of the FINST spatial-index model. *Cognition, 32*, 65–97.

Pylyshyn, Z. W. (1991a). The role of cognitive architectures in theories of cognition. In K. VanLehn (ed.), *Architectures for Intelligence*. Hillsdale, N.J.: Erlbaum.

Pylyshyn, Z. W. (1991b). Rules and representation: Chomsky and representational realism. In A. Kashir (ed.), *The Chomskian Turn*. Oxford: Blackwell.

Pylyshyn, Z. W. (1996). The study of cognitive architecture. In D. Steier and T. Mitchell (eds.), *Mind Matters: Contributions to Cognitive Science in honor of Allen Newell*. Hillsdale, N.J.: Erlbaum.

Pylyshyn, Z. W. (1998). Visual indexes in spatial vision and imagery. In R. D. Wright (ed.), *Visual Attention* (pp. 215–231). New York: Oxford University Press.

Pylyshyn, Z. W. (1999). Is vision continuous with cognition? The case for cognitive impenetrability of visual perception. *Behavioral and Brain Sciences, 22*(3), 341–423.

Pylyshyn, Z. W. (2000). Situating vision in the world. *Trends in Cognitive Sciences, 4*(5), 197–207.

Pylyshyn, Z. W. (2001a). Connecting vision and the world: Tracking the missing link. In J. Branquinho (ed.), *The Foundations of Cognitive Science* (pp. 183–195). Oxford: Clarendon Press.

Pylyshyn, Z. W. (2001b). Visual indexes, preconceptual objects, and situated vision. *Cognition, 80*(1/2), 127–158.

Pylyshyn, Z. W. (2002). Mental imagery: In search of a theory. *Behavioral and Brain Sciences, 25*(2), 157–237.

Pylyshyn, Z. W. (ed.). (1987). *The Robot's Dilemma: The Frame Problem in Artificial Intelligence*. Norwood, N.J.: Ablex.

Pylyshyn, Z. W., Burkell, J., Fisher, B., Sears, C., Schmidt, W., and Trick, L. (1994). Multiple parallel access in visual attention. *Canadian Journal of Experimental Psychology, 48*(2), 260–283.

Pylyshyn, Z. W., and Cohen, J. (1999). Imagined extrapolation of uniform motion is not continuous. Paper presented at the Annual Conference of the

Association for Research in Vision and Ophthalmology, May 1999, Ft. Lauderdale, Florida.

Pylyshyn, Z. W., and Eagleson, R. A. (1994). Developing a network model of multiple visual indexing (abstract). *Investigative Ophthalmology and Visual Science*, 35(4), 2007.

Pylyshyn, Z. W., Elcock, E. W., Marmor, M., and Sander, P. (1978). Explorations in visual-motor spaces. Paper presented at the Proceedings of the Second International Conference of the Canadian Society for Computational Studies of Intelligence, University of Toronto.

Pylyshyn, Z. W., and Storm, R. W. (1988). Tracking multiple independent targets: Evidence for a parallel tracking mechanism. *Spatial Vision*, 3(3), 1–19.

Radeau, M. (1994). Auditory-visual spatial interaction and modularity. *Cahiers de Psychologie Cognitive / Current Psychology of Cognition*, 13(1), 3–51.

Rafal, R. D. (1997). Balint syndrome. In T. Feinberg and M. Farah (eds.), *Behavioral Neurology and Neuropsychology* (pp. 337–356). New York: McGraw-Hill.

Rafal, R. D. (1998). Neglect. In R. Parasuraman (ed.), *The Attentive Brain* (pp. 489–525). Cambridge, Mass.: MIT Press.

Ramachandran, V. S. (1976). Learning-like phenomena in stereopsis. *Nature*, 262(5567), 382–384.

Ramachandran, V. S. (1988). Perception of shape from shading. *Nature*, 331, 163–166.

Ramachandran, V. S., and Braddick, O. (1973). Orientation specific learning in stereopsis. *Perception*, 2, 371–376.

Ranney, M. (1989). Internally represented forces may be cognitively penetrable: Comment on Freyd, Pantzer, and Cheng (1988). *Journal of Experimental Psychology: General*, 118(4), 399–402.

Reddy, D. R. (ed.). (1975). *Speech Recognition*. New York: Academic Press.

Reed, S. K., Hock, H. S., and Lockhead, G. R. (1983). Tacit knowledge and the effect of pattern configuration on mental scanning. *Memory and Cognition*, 11, 137–143.

Reisberg, D., and Chambers, D. (1991). Neither pictures nor propositions: What can we learn from a mental image? *Canadian Journal of Psychology*, 45(3), 336–352.

Reisberg, D., and Morris, A. (1985). Images contain what the imager put there: A nonreplication of illusions in imagery. *Bulletin of the Psychonomic Society*, 23(6), 493–496.

Rensink, R. A. (2000). The dynamic representation of scenes. *Visual Cognition*, 7, 17–42.

Rensink, R. A., O'Regan, J. K., and Clark, J. J. (1997). To see or not to see: The need for attention to perceive changes in scenes. *Psychological Science*, 8(5), 368–373.

Rensink, R. A., O'Regan, J. K., and Clark, J. J. (2000). On the failure to detect changes in scenes across brief interruptions. *Visual Cognition*, 7, 127–145.

Reynolds, R. (1981). Perception of an illusory contour as a function of processing time. *Perception, 10*, 107–115.

Reynolds, R. I. (1978). The microgenetic development of the Ponzo and Zollner illusions. *Perception and Psychophysics, 23*, 231–236.

Reynolds, R. I. (1985). The role of object-hypotheses in the organization of fragmented figures. *Perception, 14*, 49–52.

Richards, W. (ed.). (1988). *Natural Computation*. Cambridge, Mass.: MIT Press/Bradford Books.

Richman, C. L., Mitchell, D. B., and Reznick, J. S. (1979). Mental travel: Some reservations. *Journal of Experimental Psychology: Human Perception and Performance, 5*, 13–18.

Richter, W., Somorjai, R., Summers, R., Jarmasz, M., Menon, R. S., Gati, J. S., et al. (2000). Motor area activity during mental rotation studied by time-resolved single-trial fMRI. *Journal of Cognitive Neuroscience, 12*(2), 310–320.

Rieser, J. J. (1989). Access to knowledge of spatial structure at novel points of observation. *Journal of Experimental Psychology: Human Perception and Performance, 15*, 1157–1165.

Rieser, J. J., Guth, D. A., and Hill, E. W. (1986). Sensitivity to perspective structure while walking without vision. *Perception, 15*, 173–188.

Riseman, E. M., and Hanson, A. R. (1987). A methodology for the development of general knowledge-based vision systems. In M. A. Arbib and A. R. Hanson (eds.), *Vision, Brain, and Cooperative Computation*. Cambridge, Mass.: MIT Press/Bradford Books.

Roberts, L. G. (1965). Machine perception of three-dimensional solids. In J. P. Tippett (ed.), *Optical and Electro-optical Information Processing*. Cambridge, Mass.: MIT Press.

Rock, I. (1973). *Orientation and Form*. New York: Academic Press.

Rock, I. (1981). Anorthoscopic perception. *Scientific American, 224*(2), 145–153.

Rock, I. (1983). *The Logic of Perception*. Cambridge, Mass.: MIT Press/Bradford Books.

Rock, I. (ed.). (1997). *Indirect Perception*. Cambridge, Mass.: MIT Press.

Rock, I., and Anson, R. (1979). Illusory contours as the solution to a problem. *Perception, 8*, 655–681.

Rock, I., and Gutman, D. (1981). The effect of inattention on form perception. *Journal of Experimental Psychology: Human Perception and Performance, 7*, 275–285.

Rode, G., Rossetti, Y., and Biosson, D. (2001). Prism adaptation improves representational neglect. *Neuropsychologia, 39*(11), 1250–1254.

Roland, P. E., and Gulyas, B. (1994a). Beyond "pet" methodologies to converging evidence: Reply. *Trends in Neurosciences, 17*(12), 515–516.

Roland, P. E., and Gulyas, B. (1994b). Visual imagery and visual representation. *Trends in Neurosciences, 17*(7), 281–287.

Roland, P. E., and Gulyas, B. (1995). Visual memory, visual imagery, and visual recognition of large field patterns by the human brain: Functional anatomy by positron emission tomography. *Cerebral Cortex*, 5(1), 79–93.

Rosch, E. H., Mervis, C. B., Gray, W. D., Johnson, D. M., and Boyes-Braem, P. (1976). Basic objects in natural categories. *Cognitive Psychology*, 8, 382–439.

Rosenblatt, F. (1959). Two theorems of statistical separability in the perceptron. In *National Physical Laboratory, Symposium on Mechanization of Thought Processes*. London: HM Stationery Office.

Rosenfeld, A., Hummel, R. A., and Zucker, S. W. (1976). Scene labeling by relaxation operators. *IEEE Transactions on Systems, Man, and Cybernetics, SMC-6,* 420–433.

Russell, B. (1918/1985). The philosophy of logical atomism. In D. F. Pears (ed.), *The Philosophy of Logical Atomism* (pp. 35–155). Lasalle: Open Court.

Sagi, D., and Julesz, B. (1984). Detection versus discrimination of visual orientation. *Perception*, 13, 619–628.

Samson, D., Pillon, A., and De Wilde, V. (1998). Impaired knowledge of visual and non-visual attributes in a patient with a semantic impairment for living entities: A case of a true category-specific deficit. *Neurocase: Case Studies in Neuropsychology, Neuropsychiatry, and Behavioural Neurology*, 4(4–5), 273–290.

Samuel, A. G. (1981). Phonemic restoration: Insights from a new methodology. *Journal of Experimental Psychology: General*, 110(4), 474–494.

Sarter, M., Berntson, G. G., and Cacioppo, J. T. (1996). Brain imaging and cognitive neuroscience: Toward strong inference in attributing function to structure. *American Psychologist*, 51(1), 13–21.

Saye, A., and Frisby, J. P. (1975). The role of monocularly conspicuous features in facilitating stereopsis from random-dot stereograms. *Perception*, 4(2), 159–171.

Schlingensiepen, K. H., Campbell, F. W., Legge, G. E., and Walker, T. D. (1986). The importance of eye movements in the analysis of simple patterns. *Vision Research*, 26(7), 1111–1117.

Schmidt, W. C., Fisher, B. D., and Pylyshyn, Z. W. (1998). Multiple-location access in vision: Evidence from illusory line motion. *Journal of Experimental Psychology: Human Perception and Performance*, 24(2), 505–525.

Scholl, B. J., and Pylyshyn, Z. W. (1999). Tracking multiple items through occlusion: Clues to visual objecthood. *Cognitive Psychology*, 38(2), 259–290.

Scholl, B. J., Pylyshyn, Z. W., and Feldman, J. (2001). What is a visual object: Evidence from target-merging in multiple-object tracking. *Cognition*, 80, 159–177.

Schulz, T. (1991). A microgenetic study of the Mueller-Lyer illusion. *Perception*, 20(4), 501–512.

Schweinberger, S. R., and Stief, V. (2001). Implicit perception in patients with visual neglect: Lexical specificity in repetition priming. *Neuropsychologia*, 39(4), 420–429.

Schyns, P., Goldstone, R. L., and Thibaut, F. P. (1998). The development of features in object concepts. *Behavioral and Brain Sciences, 21*, 1–54.

Searle, J. R. (1990). Consciousness, explanatory inversion, and cognitive science. *Behavioral and Brain Sciences, 13*(4), 585–642.

Searle, J. R. (1995). The problem of consciousness. In J. King and K. H. Pribram (eds.), *Scale in Conscious Experience: Is the Brain too Important to Be Left to Specialists to Study?* (pp. 13–22). Mahwah, N.J.: Erlbaum.

Sears, C. (1996). Visual indexing and inhibition of return of visual attention. Unpublished doctoral dissertation, University of Western Ontario, London, Ontario.

Sears, C. R., and Pylyshyn, Z. W. (2000). Multiple object tracking and attentional processes. *Canadian Journal of Experimental Psychology, 54*(1), 1–14.

Segal, S. J., and Fusella, V. (1969). Effects of imaging on signal-to-noise ratio, with varying signal conditions. *British Journal of Psychology, 60*(4), 459–464.

Segal, S. J., and Fusella, V. (1970). Influence of imaged pictures and sounds on detection of visual and auditory signals. *Journal of Experimental Psychology, 83*(3), 458–464.

Sekuler, A. B., and Palmer, S. E. (1992). Visual completion of partly occluded objects: A microgenetic analysis. *Journal of Experimental Psychology: General, 121*, 95–111.

Sekuler, R., and Blake, R. (1994). *Perception* (second edition). New York: McGraw-Hill.

Selfridge, O. (1959). Pandemonium: A paradigm for learning. In *Symposium on Mechanization of Thought Processes: National Physical Laboratory Symposium.* London: HM Stationery Office.

Sergent, J. (1994). Brain-imaging studies of cognitive functions. *Trends in Neurosciences, 17*, 221–227.

Servos, P., and Goodale, M. A. (1995). Preserved visual imagery in visual form agnosia. *Neuropsychologia, 33*(11), 1383–1394.

Shapiro, K. L., and Raymond, J. E. (1989). Training of efficient oculomotor strategies enhances skill acquisition. *Acta Psychologica, 71*(1–3), 217–242.

Sheingold, K., and Tenney, Y. J. (1982). Memory for a salient childhood event. In U. Neisser (ed.), *Memory Observed* (pp. 201–212). San Francisco: W. H. Freeman.

Shepard, R. N. (1978a). Externalization of mental images and the act of creation. In B. S. Randhawa and W. E. Coffman (eds.), *Visual Learning, Thinking, and Communication* (pp. 133–189). New York: Academic Press.

Shepard, R. N. (1978b). The Mental Image. *American Psychologist, 33*, 125–137.

Shepard, R. N. (1981). Psychophysical complementarity. In M. Kubovy and J. R. Pomerantz (eds.), *Perceptual Organization* (pp. 279–342). Hillsdale, N.J.: Erlbaum.

Shepard, R. N., and Chipman, S. (1970). Second-order isomorphism of internal representations: Shapes of states. *Cognitive Psychology, 1,* 1–17.

Shepard, R. N., and Feng, C. (1972). A chronometric study of mental paper folding. *Cognitive Psychology, 3,* 228–243.

Shepard, R. N., and Metzler, J. (1971). Mental rotation of three-dimensional objects. *Science, 171,* 701–703.

Shepherd, M., and Mueller, H. J. (1989). Movement versus focusing of visual attention. *Perception and Psychophysics, 46*(2), 146–154.

Shiffrin, R. M., and Nosofsky, R. M. (1994). Seven plus or minus two: A commentary on capacity limitations. *Psychological Review, 101*(2), 357–361.

Shioiri, S., Cavanagh, P., Miyamoto, T., and Yaguchi, H. (2000). Tracking the aparent location of targets in interpolated motion. *Vision Research, 40,* 1365–1376.

Shirai, Y. (1975). Analyzing intensity arrays using knowledge about scenes. In P. H. Winston (ed.), *Psychology of Computer Vision.* Cambridge, Mass.: MIT Press.

Shulman, G. L., Remington, R. W., and McLean, J. P. (1979). Moving attention through visual space. *Journal of Experimental Psychology: Human Perception and Performance, 15,* 522–526.

Shulman, G. L., and Wilson, J. (1987). Spatial frequency and selective attention to local and global information. *Perception, 16*(1), 89–101.

Shuren, J. E., Brott, T. G., Schefft, B. K., and Houston, W. (1996). Preserved color imagery in an achromatopsic. *Neuropsychologia, 34*(6), 485–489.

Sigman, E., and Rock, I. (1974). Stroboscopic movement based on perceptual intelligence. *Perception, 3*(1), 9–28.

Silbersweig, D. A., and Stern, E. (1998). Towards a functional neuroanatomy of conscious perception and its modulation by volition: Implications of human auditory neuroimaging studies. *Philosophical Transactions of the Royal Society of London, B, Biological Sciences, 353*(1377), 1883–1888.

Sillito, A. M., Jones, H. E., Gerstein, G. L., and West, D. C. (1994). Feature-linked synchronization of thalamic relay cell firing induced by feedback from the visual cortex. *Nature, 369*(6480), 479–482.

Simon, H. A. (1969). *The Sciences of the Artificial.* Cambridge, Mass.: MIT Press.

Simon, H. A. (1975). The functional equivalence of problem solving skills. *Cognitive Psychology, 7,* 268–288.

Simon, T. J., Hespos, S. J., and Rochat, P. (1995). Do infants understand simple arithmetic? A replication of Wynn (1992). *Cognitive Development, 10*(2), 253–269.

Simon, T. J., and Vaishnavi, S. (1996). Subitizing and counting depend on different attentional mechanisms: Evidence from visual enumeration in afterimages. *Perception and Psychophysics, 58*(6), 915–926.

Simons, D. J. (1996). In sight, out of mind: When object representations fail. *Psychological Science*, 7(5), 301–305.

Simons, D. J., and Levin, D. T. (1997). Change blindness. *Trends in Cognitive Sciences*, 1, 261–267.

Slemmer, J. A., and Johson, S. P. (2002). Object tracking in ecologically valid occlusion events. Paper presented at the Vision Sciences 2002, Sarasota, Florida.

Slezak, P. (1991). Can images be rotated and inspected? A test of the pictorial medium theory. *Proceedings of the Thirteenth Annual Meeting of the Cognitive Science Society* (pp. 55–60). Hillsdale, N.J.: Lawrence Erlbaum.

Slezak, P. (1992). When can images be reinterpreted: Non-chronometric tests of pictorialism. *Proceedings of the Fourteenth Conference of the Cognitive Science Society* (pp. 124–129). Hillsdale, N.J.: Lawrence Erlbaum.

Slezak, P. (1995). The "philosophical" case against visual imagery. In P. Slezak, T. Caelli, and R. Clark (eds.), *Perspective on Cognitive Science: Theories, Experiments, and Foundations* (pp. 237–271). Stamford, Conn.: Ablex.

Slezak, P. (2002). The Tripartite model of Representation. *Philosophical Psychology*, 15(3), 239–270.

Sloman, A. (1971). Interactions between philosophy and artificial intelligence: The role of intuition and non-logical reasoning in intelligence. *Artificial Intelligence*, 2, 209–225.

Snodgrass, J. G., and Feenan, K. (1990). Priming effects in picture fragment completion: Support for the perceptual closure hypothesis. *Journal of Experimental Psychology: General*, 119(3), 276–296.

Soloman, R. L., and Postman, L. (1952). Frequency of usage as a determinant of recognition thresholds for words. *Journal of Experimental Psychology*, 43, 195–201.

Spelke, E., Gutheil, G., and Van de Walle, G. (1995). The development of object perception. In S. M. Kosslyn and D. N. Osherson (eds.), *Visual Cognition* (second edition, vol. 2, pp. 297–330). Cambridge, Mass.: MIT Press.

Spelke, E. S. (1990). Principles of object perception. *Cognitive Science*, 14, 29–56.

Sperber, D., and Wilson, D. (1998). The mapping between the mental and the public lexicon. In P. Carruthers and J. Boucher (eds.), *Thought and Language* (pp. 184–200). Cambridge: Cambridge University Press.

Sperling, G. (1960). The information available in brief visual presentations. *Psychological Monographs*, 74(11, whole No. 498), 29.

Sperling, G., and Melchner, M. J. (1978). The attention operating characteristic: Examples from visual search. *Science*, 202(4365), 315–318.

Sperling, G., and Weichselgarter, E. (1995). Episodic theory of the dynamics of spatial attention. *Psychological Review*, 102(3), 503–532.

Squire, L. R., and Slater, P. C. (1975). Forgetting in very long-term memory as assessed by an improved questionnaire technique. *Journal of Experimental Psychology: Human Perception and Performance*, 104, 50–54.

Starkes, J., Allard, F., Lindley, S., and O'Reilly, K. (1994). Abilities and skill in basketball. Special issue: Expert-novice differences in sport. *International Journal of Sport Psychology*, 25(3), 249–265.

Steinbach, M. J. (1976). Pursuing the perceptual rather than the retinal stimulus. *Vision Research*, 16, 1371–1376.

Sternberg, S. (1969). The discovery of processing stages: Extensions of Donders' method. *Acta Psychologica*, 30, 276–315.

Stevens, J. K., Emerson, R. C., Gerstein, G. L., Kallos, T., Neufield, G. R., Nichols, C. W., et al. (1976). Paralysis of the awake human: Visual perceptions. *Vision Research*, 16, 93–98.

Stich, S. (1978). Beliefs and subdoxastic states. *Philosophy of Science*, 45, 499–518.

Stoerig, P. (1996). Varieties of vision: From blind responses to conscious recognition. *Trends in Neurosciences*, 19(9), 401–406.

Street, R. F. (1931). *A Gestalt Completion Test: A Study of a Cross Section of Intellect.* New York: Bureau of Publications, Teachers College, Columbia University.

Stromeyer, C. F., and Psotka, J. (1970). The detailed texture of eidetic images. *Nature*, 225(230), 346–349.

Suchman, L. A. (1987). *Plans and Situated Actions: The Problem of Human-Machine Communication.* Cambridge: Cambridge University Press.

Suganuma, M., and Yokosawa, K. (2002). Is multiple object tracking affected by three-dimensional rigidity? Paper presented at the Vision Sciences Society, Sarasota, Florida.

Suppes, P. (1995). Some foundational problems in the theory of visual space. In R. D. Luce, M. D'Zmura, et al. (eds.), *Geometric Representations of Perceptual Phenomena: Papers in Honor of Tarow Indow on His 70th Birthday* (pp. 37–45). Mahwah, N.J.: Erlbaum.

Swinney, D. A. (1979). Lexical access during sentence comprehension: (Re)consideration of context effects. *Journal of Verbal Learning and Verbal Behavior*, 18(6), 645–659.

Talmy, L. (2000). *Toward a Cognitive Semantics, vol. 1: Concept Structuring Systems.* Cambridge, Mass.: MIT Press.

Tanner, W. P., and Swets, J. A. (1954). A decision-making theory of human detection. *Psychological Review*, 61, 401–409.

Theeuwes, J., Kramer, A. F., and Atchley, P. (1998). Visual marking of old objects. *Psychonomic Bulletin and Review*, 5(1), 130–134.

Thomas, N. J. T. (1999). Are theories of imagery theories of imagination? Active perception approach to conscious mental content. *Cognitive Science*, 23(2), 207–245.

Tipper, S., Driver, J., and Weaver, B. (1991). Object-centered inhibition of return of visual attention. *Quarterly Journal of Experimental Psychology*, 43A, 289–298.

Tipper, S. P., and Behrmann, M. (1996). Object-centered not scene-based visual neglect. *Journal of Experimental Psychology: Human Perception and Performance*, 22(5), 1261–1278.

Tipper, S. P., Weaver, B., Jerreat, L. M., and Burak, A. L. (1994). Object-based and environment-based inhibition of return of selective attention. *Journal of Experimental Psychology: Human Perception and Performance*, 20, 478–499.

Titchener, E. B. (1915). *A Beginner's Psychology*. New York: Macmillan.

Tlauka, M., and McKenna, F. P. (1998). Mental imagery yields stimulus-response compatibility. *Acta Psychologica*, 67–79.

Todd, J. T., Tittle, J. S., and Norman, J. F. (1995). Distortions of three-dimensional space in the perceptual analysis of motion and stereo. *Perception*, 24(1), 75–86.

Tootell, R. B., Silverman, M. S., Switkes, E., and de Valois, R. L. (1982). Deoxyglucose analysis of retinotopic organization in primate striate cortex. *Science*, 218(4575), 902–904.

Treisman, A., and DeSchepper, B. (1995). Object tokens, attention, and visual memory. In T. Inui and J. McClelland (eds.), *Attention and Performance XVI: Information Integration in Perception and Communication* (pp. 15–46). Cambridge, Mass.: MIT Press.

Treisman, A., and Gelade, G. (1980). A feature integration theory of attention. *Cognitive Psychology*, 12, 97–136.

Treisman, A., and Schmidt, H. (1982). Illusory conjunctions in the perception of objects. *Cognitive Psychology*, 14(1), 107–141.

Treisman, A. M. (1964). Verbal cues, language, and meaning in selective attention. *American Journal of Psychology*, 77, 206–219.

Treisman, A. M. (1969). Strategies and models of selective attention. *Psychological Review*, 76, 282–299.

Tremoulet, P. D., Leslie, A. M., and Hall, D. G. (2001). Infant individuation and identification of objects. *Cognitive Development*, 15(4), 499–522.

Trick, L., and Pylyshyn, Z. W. (1993). What enumeration studies tell us about spatial attention: Evidence for limited capacity preattentive processing. *Journal of Experimental Psychology: Human Perception and Performance*, 19(2), 331–351.

Trick, L. M., and Pylyshyn, Z. W. (1994a). Cuing and counting: Does the position of the attentional focus affect enumeration? *Visual Cognition*, 1(1), 67–100.

Trick, L. M., and Pylyshyn, Z. W. (1994b). Why are small and large numbers enumerated differently? A limited capacity preattentive stage in vision. *Psychological Review*, 101(1), 80–102.

Trojano, L., and Grossi, D. (1994). A critical review of mental imagery defects. *Brain and Cognition*, 24(2), 213–243.

Tsal, Y. (1983). Movements of attention across the visual field. *Journal of Experimental Psychology: Human Perception and Performance*, 9, 523–530.

Tsotsos, J. K. (1988). How does human vision beat the computational complexity of visual perception? In Z. W. Pylyshyn (ed.), *Computational Processes in Human Vision: An Interdisciplinary Perspective* (pp. 286–340). Norwood, N.J.: Ablex.

Tufte, E. R. (1990). *Envisioning Information.* Cheshire, Conn.: Graphics Press.

Tye, M. (1991). *The Imagery Debate.* Cambridge, Mass.: MIT Press.

Uhlarik, J. J. (1973). Role of cognitive factors on adaptation to prismatic displacement. *Journal of Experimental Psychology, 98,* 223–232.

Ullman, S. (1976). On visual detection of light sources. *Biological Cybernetics, 21,* 205–212.

Ullman, S. (1979). *The Interpretation of Visual Motion.* Cambridge, Mass.: MIT Press.

Ullman, S. (1984). Visual routines. *Cognition, 18,* 97–159.

Ullman, S., and Richards, W. (eds.). (1990). *Image Understanding* (vol. 4). Norwood, N.J.: Ablex.

Ungerleider, L. G., and Mishkin, M. (1982). Two cortical visual systems. In J. Ingle, M. A. Goodale, and R. J. W. Mansfield (eds.), *Analysis of Visual Behavior* (pp. 549–586). Cambridge, Mass.: MIT Press.

Uttal, W. (1967). Evoked brain potentials: Signs or codes? *Perspectives in Biology and Medicine, 10,* 627–639.

Uttley, A. M. (1959). Conditional probability computing in the nervous system. In *National Physical Laboratory, Symposium on Mechanization of Thought Processes* (vol. 1, pp. 119–149). London: HM Stationery Office.

Van der Heijden, A. H., Schreuder, R., and Wolters, G. (1985). Enhancing single-item recognition accuracy by cueing spatial locations in vision. *Quarterly Journal of Experimental Psychology: A, Human Experimental Psychology, 37A(3),* 427–434.

van Essen, D. C., and Anderson, C. H. (1990). Information processing strategies and pathways in the primate retina and visual cortex. In S. F. Zornetzer, J. L. Davis, and C. Lau (eds.), *Introduction to Neural and Electronic Networks.* New York: Academic Press.

VanLehn, K., and Ball, W. (1991). Goal reconstruction: How TETON blends situated action and planned action. In K. VanLehn (ed.), *Architectures for Intelligence* (pp. 147–188). Hillsdale, N.J.: Erlbaum.

Virsu, V. (1971). Tendencies to eye movement, and misperception of curvature, direction, and length. *Perception and Psychophysics, 9(1-B),* 65–72.

Viswanathan, L., and Mingolla, E. (2002). Dynamics of attention in depth: Evidence from multi-element tracking. *Perception, 31(12),* 1415–1437.

von Holst, E., and Mittelstaedt, H. (1971/1950). The principle of reafference: Interactions between the central nervous system and the peripheral organs. In P. C. Dodwell (ed.), *Perceptual Processing: Stimulus Equivalence and Pattern Recognition* (pp. 41–71). New York: Appleton.

Vuilleumier, P., and Rafal, R. (1999). "Both" means more than "two": Localizing and counting in patients with visuospatial neglect. *Nature Neuroscience*, 2(9), 783–784.

Wallace, B. (1984a). Apparent equivalence between perception and imagery in the production of various visual illusions. *Memory and Cognition*, 12(2), 156–162.

Wallace, B. (1984b). Creation of the horizontal-vertical illusion through imagery. *Bulletin of the Psychonomic Society*, 22(1), 9–11.

Wallace, B. (1991). Imaging ability and performance in a proofreading task. *Journal of Mental Imagery*, 15(3–4), 177–188.

Wallach, H. (1976). *On Perception*. New York: Quadrangle/New York Times Book.

Wallach, H., and O'Connell, D. N. (1953). The kinetic depth effect. *Journal of Experimental Psychology*, 45, 205–217.

Waltz, D. (1975). Understanding line drawings of scenes with shadows. In P. H. Winston (ed.), *The Psychology of Computer Vision* (pp. 19–91). New York: McGraw-Hill.

Ward, R., Goodrich, S., and Driver, J. (1994). Grouping reduces visual extinction: Neuropsychological evidence for weight-linkage in visual selection. *Visual Cognition*, 1, 101–129.

Watanabe, K., and Shimojo, S. (1998). Attentional modulation in perception of visual motion events. *Perception*, 27(9), 1041–1054.

Watson, D. G., and Humphreys, G. W. (1997). Visual marking: Prioritizing selection for new objects by top-down attentional inhibition of old objects. *Psychological Review*, 104(1), 90–122.

Watson, D. G., and Humphreys, G. W. (1998). Visual marking of moving objects: A role for top-down feature-based inhibition in selection. *Journal of Experimental Psychology: Human Perception and Performance*, 24(3), 946–962.

Weinstein, E. L. (1974). The influence of symbolic systems on perspective drawings: A developmental approach. Unpublished master's thesis, University of Toronto, Toronto, Ontario.

Weiskrantz, L. (1995). Blindsight: Not an island unto itself. *Current Directions in Psychological Science*, 4(5), 146–151.

Weiskrantz, L. (1997). *Consciousness Lost and Found: A Neuropsychological Exploration*. New York: Oxford University Press.

Weiskrantz, L., Warrington, E., Sanders, M. D., and Marshall, J. (1974). Visual capacity in the hemianopic field following restricted occipital ablation. *Brain*, 97, 709–729.

Wexler, M., Kosslyn, S. M., and Berthoz, A. (1998). Motor processes in mental rotation. *Cognition*, 68(1), 77–94.

Wiggins, D. (1979). *Sameness and Substance*. London: Blackwell.

Wilson, J. A., and Robinson, J. O. (1986). The impossibly twisted Pulfrich pendulum. *Perception, 15*(4), 503–504.

Winston, P. H. (1974). *New Progress in Artificial Intelligence* (MIT-AI-74-310). Cambridge, Mass.: MIT Artificial Intelligence Laboratory.

Winston, P. H. (1984). *Artificial Intelligence* (second edition). Reading, Mass.: Addison-Wesley.

Wittgenstein, L. (1953). *Philosophical Investigations [Philosophische Untersuchungen]*. Oxford: Blackwell.

Wittreich, W. J. (1959). Visual perception and personality. *Scientific American, 200* (April), 56–75.

Wolfe, J. M., Cave, K. R., and Franzel, S. L. (1989). Guided search: An alternative to the feature integration model for visual search. *Journal of Experimental Psychology: Human Perception and Performance, 15*(3), 419–433.

Wong, E., and Mack, A. (1981). Saccadic programming and perceived location. *Acta Psychologia, 48*, 123–131.

Woods, W. A. (1978). Theory formation and control in a speech understanding system with extrapolations towards vision. In A. R. Hanson and E. M. Riseman (eds.), *Computer Vision Systems: Papers from the Workshop on Computer Vision Systems*. New York: Academic Press.

Wright, R. D., and Richard, C. M. (1995). Subitizing abrupt-onset visual stimuli. Paper presented at the Annual Meeting of the Canadian Society for Brain, Behavior and Cognitive Science, Halifax, Nova Scotia.

Wright, R. D., and Richard, C. M. (1996). Inhibition-of-return at multiple locations in visual space. *Canadian Journal of Experimental Psychology, 50*(3), 324–327.

Wyatt, H. J., and Pola, J. (1979). The role of perceived motion in smooth pursuit eye movements. *Vision Research, 19*, 613–618.

Wynn, K. (1992). Addition and subtraction by human infants. *Nature, 358*, 749–750.

Wynn, K. (1998). Psychological foundations of number: Numerical understanding in human infants. *Trends in Cognitive Sciences, 2*, 296–303.

Wynn, K., Bloom, P., and Chiang, W.-C. (2002). Enumeration of collective entities by 5-month-old infants. *Cognition, 83*(3), B55–B62.

Xu, F. (1997). From Lot's wife to a pillar of salt: Evidence that *physical object* is a sortal concept. *Mind and Language, 12*, 365–392.

Xu, F., and Carey, S. (1996). Infants' metaphysics: The case of numerical identity. *Cognitive Psychology, 30*, 111–153.

Yantis, S. (1992). Multielement visual tracking: Attention and perceptual organization. *Cognitive Psychology, 24*, 295–340.

Yantis, S. (1995). Perceived continuity of occluded visual objects. *Psychological Science, 6*(3), 182–186.

Yantis, S. (1998). Objects, attention, and perceptual experience. In R. Wright (ed.), *Visual Attention* (pp. 187–214). Oxford: Oxford University Press.

Yantis, S., and Gibson, B. S. (1994). Object continuity in apparent motion and attention. *Canadian Journal of Experimental Psychology*, 48(2), 182–204.

Yantis, S., and Jones, E. (1991). Mechanisms of attentional selection: Temporally modulated priority tags. *Perception and Psychophysics*, 50(2), 166–178.

Zhou, H., and May, J. G. (1993). Effects of spatial filtering and lack of effects of visual imagery on pattern-contingent color aftereffects. *Perception and Psychophysics*, 53, 145–149.

Zimler, J., and Keenan, J. M. (1983). Imagery in the congenitally blind: How visual are visual images? *Journal of Experimental Psychology: Learning, Memory, and Cognition*, 9(2), 269–282.

Zucker, S. W., Rosenfeld, A., and David, L. S. (1975). General purpose models: Expectations about the unexpected. Paper presented at the Fourth International Joint Conference on Artificial Intelligence, Tbilisi, Georgia, U.S.S.R.

Name Index

Subject Index

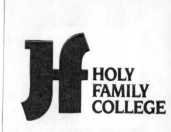

HOLY
FAMILY
COLLEGE